Healthcare-Associated Infections in Children

J. Chase McNeil • Judith R. Campbell
Jonathan D. Crews
Editors

Healthcare-Associated Infections in Children

A Guide to Prevention
and Management

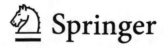 Springer

Editors
J. Chase McNeil
Department of Pediatrics
Section of Infectious Diseases
Baylor College of Medicine and Texas
Children's Hospital
Houston, TX
USA

Judith R. Campbell
Department of Pediatrics
Section of Infectious Diseases
Baylor College of Medicine and Texas
Children's Hospital
Houston, TX
USA

Jonathan D. Crews
Department of Pediatrics
Baylor College of Medicine and The
Children's Hospital of San Antonio
San Antonio, TX
USA

ISBN 978-3-319-98121-5   ISBN 978-3-319-98122-2   (eBook)
https://doi.org/10.1007/978-3-319-98122-2

Library of Congress Control Number: 2018957095

This Springer imprint is published by the registered company Springer Nature Switzerland AG
The registered company address is: Gewerbestrasse 11, 6330 Cham, Switzerland

To my wife, Carrie
To my sons, Noah and Sam
To my parents, Mark and Terri, and my sister,
Tanis

-J. Chase McNeil

To my wife, Lindsey
To my children, Will, Samuel, Sophie, and
Ellie
To my parents

-Jonathan D. Crews

To my husband, Reese, and our children,
Matthew, Emily, and Joseph

-Judith R. Campbell

Thank you for your love and support.

Preface

Continual advances in the field of medicine have allowed for countless patients to survive and have improved quality of life in the face of diseases that were once untreatable. These achievements include antibiotics, antineoplastic chemotherapeutic agents, medical devices, and improved surgical techniques to just name a few. Unfortunately, with these lifesaving interventions comes the potential for harm to the patient, principal among which is the risk for serious infection. Children in many ways are more challenging in this regard than their adult counterparts given their unique microbiology and epidemiology of infection, distinct pharmacology, and varied physiologic development. Furthermore, there is a relative paucity of data on the diagnosis, management, and prevention of these infections in children compared to adults.

In this text, *Healthcare-Associated Infections in Children: A Guide to Prevention and Management*, we have sought to provide an overview of the most common infections in children associated with the provision of medical care. This text includes contributions from authors with a wide array of expertise including pediatric infectious diseases, infection control and prevention, critical care medicine, hospital medicine, nephrology, oncology, and pediatric surgical subspecialties. It is our hope that this text will serve as a learning resource for students and medical trainees as well as a source of guidance to practicing clinicians caring for children in these often challenging situations. While we have strived to include the most up-to-date research and evidence-based practice guidelines, given the breadth and pace of advancements in medical knowledge, no single text can be truly comprehensive. Thus, while the information in this text may serve as a reference and starting place in patient management, sound clinical judgment must be exercised at all times.

This endeavor is the consequence of the work and influence of countless people, both directly and indirectly. We would like to acknowledge the many contributors to this text for their informative chapters. In addition, we extend our thanks to the editorial staff at Springer for their assistance with and interest in this project. We must also express thanks to our patients and their families for challenging us to be excellent clinicians who practice state-of-the-art care while minimizing risks to patients. Additionally we must recognize the tremendous impact of each of our numerous mentors, teachers, and colleagues who have shaped us as physicians and researchers. Finally, we wish to thank our respective institutions for providing environments supportive of academic pursuits.

Houston, TX, USA   J. Chase McNeil, MD
Houston, TX, USA   Judith R. Campbell, MD
San Antonio, TX, USA   Jonathan D. Crews, MD, MS

Contents

Contributors

Ayse Akcan-Arikan, MD Department of Pediatrics, Sections of Critical Care Medicine and Renal, Baylor College of Medicine, Houston, TX, USA

Amy S. Arrington, MD, PhD Pediatric Critical Care Medicine, Global Biologic Preparedness, Baylor College of Medicine/Texas Children's Hospital, Houston, TX, USA

Allison H. Bartlett, MD, MS Department of Pediatrics, Section of Infectious Diseases, The University of Chicago Medicine, Chicago, IL, USA

Judith R. Campbell, MD Department of Pediatrics, Section of Infectious Diseases, Baylor College of Medicine and Texas Children's Hospital, Houston, TX, USA

J. B. Cantey, MD Department of Pediatrics, University of Texas Health San Antonio, San Antonio, TX, USA

Luis A. Castagnini, MD, MPH Department of Pediatrics, Section of Infectious Diseases, Baylor College of Medicine and The Children's Hospital of San Antonio, San Antonio, TX, USA

Jonathan D. Crews, MD, MS Department of Pediatrics, Section of Infectious Diseases, Baylor College of Medicine, Houston, TX, USA

Pediatric Infectious Diseases, The Children's Hospital of San Antonio, San Antonio, TX, USA

John Darby, MD Department of Pediatrics, Wake Forest School of Medicine, Winston-Salem, NC, USA

Gail J. Demmler-Harrison, MD Department of Pediatrics, Baylor College of Medicine, Houston, TX, USA

Infectious Diseases Service, Texas Children's Hospital, Houston, TX, USA

Ankhi Dutta, MD, MPH Department of Pediatrics, Section of Pediatric Infectious Diseases, Texas Children's Hospital and Baylor College of Medicine, Houston, TX, USA

Carla Falco, MD Department of Pediatrics, Section of Hospital Medicine, Baylor College of Medicine, Houston, TX, USA

Ricardo Flores, MD Department of Pediatrics, Texas Children's Cancer and Hematology Centers and Baylor College of Medicine, The Woodlands, TX, USA

Catherine E. Foster, MD Department of Pediatrics, Section of Infectious Diseases, Baylor College of Medicine and Texas Children's Hospital, Houston, TX, USA

Johanna Goldfarb, MD Cleveland Clinic Lerner College of Medicine of Case Western Reserve University, Cleveland, OH, USA

Blanca E. Gonzalez, MD Cleveland Clinic Lerner College of Medicine of Case Western Reserve University, Cleveland Clinic Children's, Cleveland, OH, USA

Galit Holzmann-Pazgal, MD Department of Pediatrics, Section of Infectious Diseases, Baylor College of Medicine, Houston, TX, USA

Sarah Kubes, PharmD, BCPS Pharmacy, The Children's Hospital of San Antonio, San Antonio, TX, USA

Lucila Marquez, MD, MPH Pediatric Infectious Diseases, Baylor College of Medicine, Houston, TX, USA

J. Chase McNeil, MD Department of Pediatrics, Section of Infectious Diseases, Baylor College of Medicine and Texas Children's Hospital, Houston, TX, USA

Ann-Christine Nyquist, MD, MSPH Department of Pediatrics, Section of Infectious Diseases and Epidemiology, University of Colorado School of Medicine, Aurora, CO, USA

Infection Prevention and Control, Children's Hospital Colorado, Aurora, CO, USA

Scott Rosenfeld, MD Department of Orthopedic Surgery, Division of Pediatric Orthopedic Surgery, Baylor College of Medicine, Houston, TX, USA

Poyyapakkam R. Srivaths, MD Department of Pediatrics, Section of Renal, Baylor College of Medicine, Houston, TX, USA

Zachary Stinson, MD Department of Orthopedic Surgery, Division of Pediatric Orthopedic Surgery, Baylor College of Medicine, Houston, TX, USA

Sarah J. Swartz, MD Department of Pediatrics, Section of Renal, Baylor College of Medicine, Houston, TX, USA

Jesus G. Vallejo, MD Department of Pediatrics, Section of Infectious Diseases, Baylor College of Medicine, Houston, TX, USA

William Whitehead, MD, MPH Department of Neurosurgery, Division of Pediatric Neurosurgery, Baylor College of Medicine, Houston, TX, USA

Julie D. Wohrley, MD Department of Pediatrics, Section of Infectious Diseases, The University of Chicago Medicine, Chicago, IL, USA

Part I

Overview of Infection Control and Prevention

Basic Principles of Infection Control

Catherine E. Foster and Judith R. Campbell

Introduction

Healthcare-associated infections (HAIs) are defined as infections that patients acquire while receiving treatment for other conditions within a healthcare setting. These infections cause significant morbidity and mortality in children and adults worldwide. HAIs pose a major risk to patient safety and contribute substantially to healthcare costs and to increased hospital lengths of stay [1, 2]. In the United States, a HAI prevalence survey estimated that there were approximately 722,000 HAIs in US acute care hospitals in 2011 [3]. Nationally, institutions and organizations have prioritized programs and efforts to decrease rates of HAIs. Patrick and colleagues studied trends in HAIs specifically in the neonatal and pediatric populations in the United States and reported substantial reductions in the rates of central line-associated bloodstream infections (CLABSIs) and ventilator-associated pneumonias (VAPs) between 2007 and 2012 thought to be secondary to a national focus on quality and safety improvement efforts [4]. Hospital infection control and prevention programs are integral to quality healthcare and are designed to protect patients and healthcare workers (HCWs) from acquiring and transmitting infectious diseases.

Over the past three decades, HAIs have been increasingly recognized as a major patient safety concern. Infection control and prevention practitioners and hospital epidemiologists identify patients with HAIs and help identify and implement policies and practices to limit such events. Evidence-based guidelines from the Centers for Disease Control and Prevention (CDC), Society for Healthcare Epidemiology of America (SHEA), and the Association for Professionals in Infection Control and Epidemiology (APIC) are available to assist institutions in developing policies and

C. E. Foster · J. R. Campbell (✉)
Department of Pediatrics, Section of Infectious Diseases, Baylor College of Medicine and Texas Children's Hospital, Houston, TX, USA
e-mail: jrcampb1@texaschildrens.org

© Springer Nature Switzerland AG 2019
J. C. McNeil et al. (eds.), *Healthcare-Associated Infections in Children*,
https://doi.org/10.1007/978-3-319-98122-2_1

Table 1.1 Selected guidelines and resources for the prevention of healthcare-associated infections

Guidelines from the Centers for Disease Control and Prevention, the Healthcare Infection Control Practices Advisory Committee[a], and the Advisory Committee on Immunization Practices	
Hand hygiene	Guideline for Hand Hygiene in Healthcare Settings, 2002 https://www.cdc.gov/mmwr/PDF/rr/rr5116.pdf
Isolation precautions	Guideline for Isolation Precautions: Preventing Transmission of Infectious Agents in Healthcare Settings, 2007 https://www.cdc.gov/infectioncontrol/pdf/guidelines/isolation-guidelines.pdf
Device- or procedure-related infections	Guidelines for the Prevention of Intravascular Catheter-Related Infections, 2011 https://www.cdc.gov/infectioncontrol/pdf/guidelines/bsi-guidelines.pdf Guideline for Prevention of Catheter-Associated Urinary Tract Infections, 2009 https://www.cdc.gov/infectioncontrol/pdf/guidelines/cauti-guidelines.pdf Guideline for the Prevention of Surgical Site Infection, 2017 (Updated from 1999) https://jamanetwork.com/journals/jamasurgery/fullarticle/2623725
Antibiotic resistance	Management of Multi-Drug Resistant Organisms (MDROs) in Healthcare Settings, 2006 https://www.cdc.gov/infectioncontrol/pdf/guidelines/mdro-guidelines.pdf
Environment of care	Guidelines for Environmental Infection Control in Health-Care Facilities, 2003 https://www.cdc.gov/infectioncontrol/pdf/guidelines/environmental-guidelines.pdf Guideline for Disinfection and Sterilization in Healthcare Facilities, 2008 https://www.cdc.gov/infectioncontrol/pdf/guidelines/disinfection-guidelines.pdf
Immunization of healthcare workers	Immunization of Health-Care Personnel: Recommendations of the Advisory Committee on Immunization Practices (ACIP), 2011 (updated from 1997) https://www.cdc.gov/mmwr/preview/mmwrhtml/rr6007a1.htm.
Guidelines for infection prevention and control from additional professional organizations	
Infection control in nonhospital settings	Infection Prevention and Control in Pediatric Ambulatory Settings, 2017 (Updated from 2007) http://pediatrics.aappublications.org/content/140/5/e20172857 Infection Prevention and Control in Residential Facilities for Pediatric Patients and Their Families, 2013 (Updated from 2003) SHEA. Infect Control Hosp Epidemiol. 2013 Oct;34(10):1003–41.

Table 1.1   (continued)

Special populations	Infection Prevention and Control Guideline for Cystic Fibrosis, 2013 Update SHEA. Infect Control Hosp Epidemiol. 2014 Aug;35 Suppl 1:S1-S67. Guidelines for Preventing Infectious Complications among Hematopoietic Cell Transplantation Recipients: A Global Perspective, 2009 http://www.shea-online.org/images/guidelines/2009_HSCT_Guideline.pdf
For additional guidance	The Society for Healthcare Epidemiology of America (www.shea-online.org) Association for Professionals in Infection Control and Epidemiology (www.apic.org) Committee on Infectious Diseases, American Academy of Pediatrics (aap.org) Occupational Safety and Health Administration (www.osha.gov)

ªAdditional guidelines, including disease and organism-specific guidelines, are available through the Centers for Disease Control and Prevention/Healthcare Infection Control Practices Advisory Committee (HICPAC) website, https://www.cdc.gov/infectioncontrol/guidelines/index.html

practices on topics such as hand hygiene, isolation, device-associated infections, and surgical site infections (SSIs) (Table 1.1).

This chapter provides a brief overview of commonly encountered HAIs and the primary guiding principles of infection control and prevention. In addition, we briefly discuss general concepts and approaches to hospital outbreak investigation and implementation of infection control practices in outpatient settings.

Sources and Types of HAIs

Hospitalized infants and children are at risk for HAIs associated with treatment, procedures, and devices necessary to care for them. Bloodstream infections related to intravascular catheters, particularly central venous catheters, constitute a major proportion of pediatric HAIs. In the largest multinational prevalence study of HAIs in children performed to date, the European Center for Disease Prevention and Control found that bloodstream infections were the most common type of HAI and that the burden of HAIs in children is highest in the first year of life [5]. Risk factors for the development of a CLABSI include the catheter selection (multiple vs single lumen), catheter site, duration of catheterization, bacterial colonization at the exit site, and underlying condition and immune status of the patient [6]. Pathogens commonly causing CLABSIs in children are coagulase-negative staphylococci (CONS), *Staphylococcus aureus*, enterococci, and *Candida* spp. [7, 8]. Standardized practices of strict aseptic technique during catheter insertion and manipulation minimize risk of CLABSI [9].

Additional HAIs related to invasive devices and procedures include catheter-associated urinary tract infections (CAUTIs), ventilator-associated pneumonia

Table 1.2 Comparison between surveillance and clinical definitions of infection

Definition	Surveillance	Clinical
Goal	Identify incidence, prevalence, and trends in a specified population[a]	Diagnosis and treatment of an individual patient
Criteria	Limited to predefined data elements and timeframe	Consider all diagnostic information[b]
Interpretation	Should be standardized	Integrates clinical judgment

Adapted from the NHSN Patient Safety Component Protocol FAQs. March 2013. Available online at https://www.cdc.gov/nhsn/faqs/faq-psc.pdf
[a]The population of interest could be, for example, all patients with a central line
[b]This may include radiographic, microbiologic, epidemiologic, and clinical data

(VAP) or ventilator-associated events (VAEs), and surgical site infections (SSIs). For surveillance purposes, the National Healthcare Safety Network (NHSN) of CDC standardizes definitions for HAIs; however, clinicians need to understand that variables considered in epidemiologic surveillance definitions differ from that of clinical definitions (Table 1.2) [10, 11]. CDC's NHSN is the most widely used HAI tracking system, and it provides facilities with data needed to identify areas for improvement and to measure impact of prevention efforts.

Another consideration when evaluating a HAI is whether the source of the infection was the patient's skin or mucosal surfaces. Endogenous HAIs refer principally to infections caused by colonizing flora of the patient. Impairment of host defenses, from an underlying disease, immunosuppressive therapy, or invasive devices or procedures, may increase the risk of infection due to endogenous organisms. Endogenous pathogens can include microorganisms that colonize the skin such as *S. epidermidis* and other CONS or colonize the gastrointestinal tract such as gram-negative bacilli. Exogenous sources typically include organisms acquired through contact with the environment, visitors, and HCWs in the healthcare setting. Examples of exogenous organisms include multidrug-resistant (MDR) pathogens such as vancomycin-resistant *Enterococcus* transmitted from another patient or acute viral illnesses such as influenza acquired in a healthcare setting.

Children hospitalized with community acquired infections may serve as a source of transmission of viruses within the healthcare setting. Common healthcare-associated respiratory infections include respiratory syncytial virus (RSV) and influenza. RSV, influenza, and other viral infections can be acquired from patients, visitors, or HCWs. Premature infants, those with immunodeficiency, congenital heart disease, or chronic lung disease are at increased risk of severe disease. RSV can spread through direct contact with respiratory secretions or indirectly by contact with contaminated environmental surfaces harboring viruses such as RSV. Patients or HCWs then may inoculate their mucous membranes, thus transmitting the virus. Strict hand hygiene practices are integral to preventing the transmission of viral pathogens such as RSV [12, 13].

Similarly, children hospitalized with gastrointestinal infections are potential sources for transmission of gastrointestinal viruses within the hospital. Rotavirus and norovirus are two frequent causes of healthcare-associated gastrointestinal infections, though rotavirus is more common in the pediatric population [14, 15].

The risk of healthcare-associated rotavirus increases during periods of increased hospitalizations in seasonal community outbreaks. While rotavirus is still a significant cause of diarrhea in infants and young children in the United States, rotavirus vaccination has substantially decreased the burden of the disease and thus reduced the number of hospitalizations each year. Indirect fecal-oral contact, often via contaminated hands, is the predominant mode of transmission of gastrointestinal viruses such as rotavirus.

Transmission of Infectious Pathogens

An in-depth understanding of both the common causes of HAIs in children and the mode of transmission of these pathogens is critical to prevent the transmission of infections [16]. Transmission of pathogens occurs by four principle mechanisms: direct contact, indirect contact, droplet, and airborne. Contact is the dominant mode of transmission and can occur when there is direct contact of an infected person with a susceptible person or direct contact with an infected person's body fluids (including blood, urine, feces, draining purulent material, or respiratory tract secretions) to a susceptible person. Indirect transmission occurs when there is an intermediate contaminated person, object, or surface. Fomites (such as medical equipment) and environmental surfaces have been shown to be a contributing factor in the transmission of certain pathogens, including the following: RSV, norovirus, *Clostridium difficile*, *Acinetobacter* spp., and methicillin-resistant *S. aureus* (MRSA) [17, 18]. Environmental surfaces are also a possible source of transmission of emerging MDR pathogens such as *Candida auris*, carbapenemase-producing *Enterobacteriaceae*, and vancomycin-resistant enterococci, especially in outbreak situations [19, 20]. Droplet transmission involves the transfer of microorganisms by large respiratory droplets (e.g., via coughing and sneezing) to a susceptible person within 3–6 ft of the patient. A few examples of organisms transmitted by droplet include influenza virus, adenovirus, and *Bordetella pertussis*. Airborne transmission refers to spread of infection through droplet nuclei which are small particles, $\leq$ 5 μm, and can remain suspended in air for longer periods of time. Examples of pathogens transmitted by airborne route include varicella-zoster virus, *Mycobacterium tuberculosis*, and measles (rubeola) virus [16].

Hand Hygiene

Hand hygiene is the leading measure in protecting patients against HAIs and decreasing the transmission of pathogens, including MDR pathogens, from patient to patient and the surrounding healthcare environment [21, 22]. In the late 1840s, Dr. Ignaz Semmelweis observed that pregnant women attended by medical students and physicians in the First Clinic at the General Hospital of Vienna had a considerably higher post-delivery mortality (termed childbed fever) rate compared to those women delivered by midwives in the Second Clinic. This observation prompted him to consider several hypotheses including that the morality rate was higher in women delivered by medical students because they performed autopsies and had exposure to "cadaverous particles," while the midwives did not have contact with the corpses. As a result, he initiated a mandatory hand-cleansing procedure with a chlorinated lime solution for anyone attending autopsies prior to entering the maternity ward. Shortly thereafter, the mortality rate of the First Clinic fell to that of the Second Clinic which was staffed by the midwives [23, 24].

Even though Dr. Semmelweis attempted to convince his contemporaries of the value of handwashing, it wasn't until later with the acceptance of germ theory and the development of antiseptic techniques that his views were adopted [23]. He is now posthumously credited as the "father of infection control." While hand hygiene techniques and the formulations of various antiseptics have changed considerably over the past 150 years, the basic principle remains unchanged: hand hygiene prevents the transmission of infectious agents.

The introduction of alcohol-based hand rubs for hand hygiene eliminated many barriers to performing hand hygiene, such as access to sinks, soap, and water, and improved efficacy and efficiency of the hand hygiene process [22, 25]. In 2002, the CDC published a detailed Guideline for Hand Hygiene in Healthcare Settings (https://www.cdc.gov/handhygiene/providers/guideline.html) [21]. Hand hygiene should be performed before and after all patient contact and after exposure to blood, body fluids, secretions, excretions, or contaminated items and after glove removal. Gloves should not be considered a substitute for hand hygiene [26]. Alcohol-based hand rubs are preferred for use in most instances of patient care, except if hands are visibly soiled with dirt, blood, or bodily fluid or following care of patients with *Clostridium difficile* colonization or infection. Alcohol rubs do not kill the spores, and the movement of hand washing is more effective in removing spores [22]. Soap and water are also preferred in the setting of a norovirus outbreak [27].

A study at the University of Geneva Hospitals was one of the first to show sustained improvement in hand hygiene compliance coinciding with a simultaneous reduction of nosocomial infections and MRSA transmission [28]. The most successful approaches to improving and sustaining hand hygiene compliance are multifaceted programs that include reinforced education and monitored compliance paired with performance feedback [29]. Hand hygiene compliance rates are improved by identifying and removing potential barriers such as providing adequate supply of hand hygiene product that is easily accessible and convenient with HCW workflows. A culture of safety and peer accountability also have been shown to improve compliance with hand hygiene [30].

Unfortunately, adherence to recommended hand hygiene practices often remains below targeted thresholds. Understaffing and overcrowding present challenges to improving hand hygiene rates. Hand hygiene rates vary substantially among and within institutions. Additionally, there can be significant variability in compliance rates among HCWs. Physician hand hygiene compliance rates are often below that of nonphysician staff members [31]. Many factors, including the behavior of other HCWs, can positively or negatively impact hand hygiene rates. Lankford *et al.* found that HCWs in a room with a high-ranking medical staff member who did not wash hands were significantly less likely to wash their own hands [32], underscoring the importance of role modeling particularly in the teaching hospital setting.

Due to the complexity of hand hygiene behaviors, many educational and motivational programs geared toward improving hand hygiene have been developed. As part of the World Health Organization (WHO) First Global Patient Safety Challenge "Clean Care is Safer Care," the "My 5 Moments for Hand Hygiene" concept was developed. This strategy is a practical tool to help HCWs recognize when hand hygiene should be performed. The five key moments for when hand hygiene is required include before touching a patient, before a clean or aseptic procedure, after body fluid exposure, after touching a patient, and after contact with patient surroundings [33].

Hand hygiene compliance may be determined by direct observation (e.g., "secret shopper" method) or with newer innovative, electronic monitoring systems [34]. Ward and colleagues performed a systematic review of hand hygiene monitoring systems and identified 42 articles which employed various methods: electronically assisted or enhanced direct observation (5), video-monitored direct observation (4), electronic dispenser counter systems (15), and automated hand hygiene monitoring networks (18) [35]. Cost-effectiveness analyses of these tools are needed before recommendations can be made regarding their routine inclusion into hand hygiene programs.

Patients and parents should also participate in hand hygiene and should be encouraged to discuss hand hygiene with their HCWs. A review article identified 11 studies, mostly observational, that evaluated the role of parents in promoting hand hygiene and found that parents feel more comfortable about reminding HCWs to clean their hands if they had previously been invited to do so [36].

Isolation Practices

The intent of isolation precautions is to prevent transmission and acquisition of infections. In 2007, Healthcare Infection Control Practices Advisory Committee (HICPAC) updated guidelines for preventing the transmission of infectious agents in healthcare settings [16]. Isolation precautions include use of standard precautions for all patients, regardless of whether the patient has a suspected or confirmed infection. Standard precautions include hand hygiene before and after all patient contacts as described above. Additionally, gloves should be worn whenever touching blood, bodily fluids, secretions, or excretions or items contaminated with any of these fluids. In instances where these fluids may be sprayed or splashed, protective masks, face shields, and eye wear should be worn. Gowns are also used when needed to protect skin and clothing.

Additional transmission-based precautions may be needed if patients are infected with agents transmitted by contact, droplet, or airborne routes (Table 1.3). Contact

Table 1.3 Isolation precautions for hospitalized children [16, 26]

Precaution classification	Example	Hand hygiene	Gown and gloves	Mask	Recommended room type
Standard	HIV	Yes	No[a]	No[b]	No requirement
Contact	RSV	Yes	Yes	No[b]	Single-patient preferred[e]
Droplet	*B. Pertussis*	Yes	No[a]	Surgical mask[c]	Single-patient preferred[e]
Airborne	*M. Tuberculosis*	Yes	No[a]	Fitted respirator (N95 or N100)[d]	Single-patient, with negative airflow, 6–12 air exchanges per hour, HEPA filtration

[a]Gown and gloves are required when performing activities that involve exposure to blood, bodily fluids, secretions, or excretions
[b]Mask (and eye protection or face shield) is required when preforming activities that are likely to create splashes or sprays of blood, bodily fluids, or secretions
[c]Mask should be donned *upon* entry into the room
[d]Mask should be donned *before* entry into the room
[e]The potential for transmission of infectious agents should be considered when making patient placement decisions. Cohorting patients with like infections is acceptable if a single-patient room is not available. Ensure physical separation of the patients (>3 ft) and change protective attire and perform hand hygiene between all contacts with different patients in the room

precautions involve use of gown and gloves and should be used for patients with infections transmitted by contact or for those infected or colonized with resistant bacteria. A few examples of infectious agents transmitted by the contact route include enteroviruses, herpes simplex virus (HSV), RSV, and rotavirus. Contact precautions due to colonization or infection with MDR bacteria may be institution specific, depending on local, regional, or national recommendations. For example, contact precautions may be implemented in patients with MRSA. The CDC recommends contact precautions when the facility deems MRSA to be of special clinical and epidemiologic significance. Increasingly, MDR organisms have emerged as a serious threat, and there are evolving infection control and antimicrobial stewardship strategies to reduce the incidence of HAIs caused by MDR organisms; such organisms typically warrant contact precautions [37]. To interrupt horizontal transmission in the setting of an outbreak, contact precautions may be implemented even with susceptible organisms.

Droplet precautions involve use of masks in addition to standard precautions when entering a patient room. Patients with infections spread by droplets can include influenza, pertussis, rhinovirus, and adenovirus (pneumonia). Droplet precautions should be employed when within 3–6 ft of the patient. These patients should be placed in a single room or if needed may be cohorted with patients with the same infection. Given that adenovirus, influenza, and rhinovirus are common, some institutions implement combination droplet and contact precautions for infants and young children presenting with respiratory tract infections until the respiratory viral pathogen is identified [38].

Lastly, airborne precautions necessitate the use of N95 or N100 respirators that have been fitted to the healthcare provider. Measles (rubeola) virus, *M.*

tuberculosis, and varicella-zoster virus are all examples of infections that require airborne precautions. Patients with any of these pathogens need to be placed in a single room with a negative pressure airflow in which the air should enter from the surrounding corridor into the room and exit directly outside or through a high-efficiency particulate air (HEPA) filter. Special air handling and ventilation are required to prevent airborne transmission because of the small size of the droplet nuclei and their ability to remain suspended in the air for an extended period.

Prevention of Other Potential Sources of Transmission

As described above, some infectious agents may remain viable on environmental surfaces. Infection control practitioners work closely with environmental services and facilities departments to assure appropriate cleaning of the patient care environment and equipment. Given the complexity of the healthcare environment, detailed policies and procedures are needed for the process and persons responsible for adequately cleaning each item based on manufacturer's instructions.

Although no standardized approach exists, many pediatric hospitals and their specialized units, including neonatal intensive care units (NICUs), bone marrow transplant units, and oncology units, have visitor screening protocols. Screening protocols may be applied differently depending on the person (e.g., parent, sibling, or nonrelative) or on the time of year (e.g., during respiratory viral season) and may play an important role in limiting the transmission of viral HAIs [39, 40]. A nationwide UK survey revealed significant practice variation in visitor protocols across 143 neonatal units [41]. Washam and colleagues recently reported a 37% reduction in the incidence of suspected healthcare-associated respiratory viral infections after standardization of a visitation protocol at a pediatric quaternary care hospital [42].

Lastly, the WHO identified eight core components for the establishment of effective infection control and prevention programs and included avoiding overcrowding of facilities and optimizing the HCW to patient ratio as methods to reduce the risk of HAIs [43].

Challenges in Infection Prevention

MDR Pathogens

Antibiotic resistance among pathogens has risen significantly over the past three decades. According to the CDC report on "Antibiotic resistance threats in the United States, 2013," an estimated two million people acquire serious infections from organisms resistant to at least one or more antimicrobial agents resulting in at least 23,000 deaths each year in the United States [44]. Several studies have reported increasing trends of extended-spectrum β-lactamase-producing and carbapenem-resistant *Enterobacteriaceae* in children nationally in both inpatient and ambulatory settings [45, 46]. In 2006, HICPAC published guidelines on the management of MDR pathogens in healthcare settings (https://www.cdc.gov/infectioncontrol/pdf/guidelines/mdro-guidelines.pdf) [37]. In general, successful control of MDR pathogens involves a multifaceted approach including hand hygiene, environmental cleaning, education, active surveillance cultures, and isolation precautions for the target MDR organism [37]. Antimicrobial stewardship programs promoting judicious use of antimicrobials (including use of narrow-spectrum agents and appropriate duration of therapy) are also integral to the control of MDR pathogens [37, 47].

Reporting of HAIs

As infection control and prevention is within the realm of healthcare quality improvement, accountability to governmental agencies and quality networks is important. Public reporting of HAIs is one facet of how healthcare organizations are held accountable for outcomes. Furthermore in a value-based reimbursement system, HAI outcomes impact hospital reimbursement [48, 49]. Mandatory reporting of HAIs varies by state; thus, it is important to know the regulatory requirements and consequences for your practice location. In general, states require reporting HAI data to the NHSN. Reportable HAIs that are mandated by the state health authority include device-associated HAIs such as CLABSIs and CAUTIs in intensive care units (ICUs) and SSIs including ventricular shunt placement, spinal fusion/refusion, laminectomy, cardiac surgery, and cardiac transplant. SSIs associated with other procedures such as cholecystectomies and colorectal surgeries are required by the Centers for Medicare and Medicaid Services (CMS) but are not common in the pediatric population. Beyond mandatory reporting, participation in quality improvement networks such as the Children's Hospitals' Solutions for Patient Safety (SPS) (http://www.solutionsforpatientsafety.org/about-us/our-goals/) enables institutions to benchmark with similar pediatric hospitals and to collaborate to develop interventions that take into consideration the unique challenges in the care of pediatric patients.

Basic Principles of Outbreak Investigation

Outbreak investigations are often performed when clusters of HAIs due to the same pathogen (or other common factors) are identified or suspected. The key component of any outbreak investigation is identification of likely predisposing factors or conditions followed by interventions to decrease the incidence of additional cases. A successful outbreak investigation requires multidisciplinary teamwork with infection control and prevention, hospital epidemiologists, clinical teams, laboratory support, and hospital administration. Outbreaks due to unusual pathogens or that continue despite interventions may warrant consultation with local, regional, or national health authorities. A basic approach for an outbreak investigation is illustrated in Figs. 1.1 and 1.2. Online courses and modules for training in outbreak response are available through the CDC and SHEA.

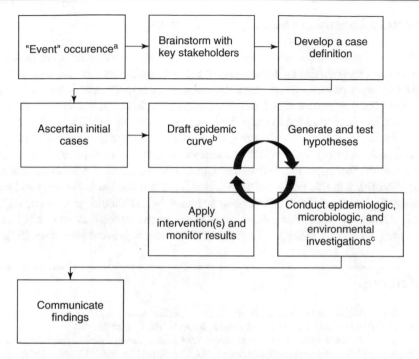

Fig. 1.1 Basic approach to hospital outbreak investigation. [a]An event or outbreak may be suspected due to increased incidence of an unusual pathogen or a typical pathogen considering seasonality, community epidemiology, or timing and location (e.g., several cases in closely located units). [b]An epidemic curve is a graph which depicts a measure of time on the horizontal x-axis and the number of cases on the vertical y-axis. [c]See Fig. 1.2 for further details

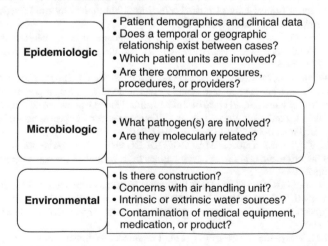

Fig. 1.2 Select epidemiologic, microbiologic, and environmental considerations during outbreak investigations

Infection Control in the Outpatient Setting

While most of the literature on infection control focuses on acute care facilities, infection control remains an integral part of patient care in outpatient clinics, offices, and ambulatory procedure and surgical centers. Most principles of infection control including hand hygiene and isolation precautions should be applied in the outpatient setting. Clinicians working in outpatient settings may find the CDC guideline and checklist helpful (https://www.cdc.gov/infectioncontrol/pdf/outpatient/guide.pdf) as well as the recently updated 2017 American Academy of Pediatrics (AAP) policy statement on Infection Prevention and Control in Pediatric Ambulatory Settings [50]. According to this policy statement, policies for infection prevention and control should be updated routinely at 2-year intervals and should be written, widely available, and enforced. The policy also emphasizes the importance of public health measures, such as vaccination of patients and HCWs, to prevent infections [50].

References

1. Graves N, Weinhold D, Tong E, et al. Effect of healthcare-acquired infection on length of hospital stay and cost. Infect Control Hosp Epidemiol. 2007;28(3):280–92.
2. Cosgrove SE. The relationship between antimicrobial resistance and patient outcomes: mortality, length of hospital stay, and health care costs. Clin Infect Dis. 2006;42(Suppl 2):S82–9.
3. Magill SS, Edwards JR, Bamberg W, et al. Multistate point-prevalence survey of health care–associated infections. N Engl J Med. 2014;370(13):1198–208.
4. Patrick SW, Kawai AT, Kleinman K, et al. Health care-associated infections among critically ill children in the US, 2007-2012. Pediatrics. 2014;134(4):705–12.
5. Zingg W, Hopkins S, Gayet-Ageron A, et al. Health-care-associated infections in neonates, children, and adolescents: an analysis of paediatric data from the European Centre for Disease Prevention and Control point-prevalence survey. Lancet Infect Dis. 2017;17(4):381–9.
6. Mermel LA, Allon M, Bouza E, et al. Clinical practice guidelines for the diagnosis and management of intravascular catheter-related infection: 2009 update by the Infectious Diseases Society of America. Clin Infect Dis. 2009;49(1):1–45.
7. Niedner MF, Huskins WC, Colantuoni E, et al. Epidemiology of central line-associated bloodstream infections in the pediatric intensive care unit. Infect Control Hosp Epidemiol. 2011;32(12):1200–8.
8. Lake JG, Weiner LM, Milstone AM, Saiman L, Magill SS, See I. Pathogen distribution and antimicrobial resistance among pediatric healthcare-associated infections reported to the National Healthcare Safety Network, 2011-2014. Infect Control Hosp Epidemiol. 2018;39(1):1–11.
9. O'Grady NP, Alexander M, Burns LA, et al. Guidelines for the prevention of intravascular catheter-related infections. Clin Infect Dis. 2011;52(9):e162–93.
10. Horan TC, Andrus M, Dudeck MA. CDC/NHSN surveillance definition of health care-associated infection and criteria for specific types of infections in the acute care setting. Am J Infect Control. 2008;36(5):309–32.
11. Gaur AH, Miller MR, Gao C, et al. Evaluating application of the National Healthcare Safety Network central line-associated bloodstream infection surveillance definition: a survey of pediatric intensive care and hematology/oncology units. Infect Control Hosp Epidemiol. 2013;34(7):663–70.
12. Weedon KM, Rupp AH, Heffron AC, et al. The impact of infection control upon hospital-acquired influenza and respiratory syncytial virus. Scand J Infect Dis. 2013;45(4):297–303.
13. Groothuis J, Bauman J, Malinoski F, Eggleston M. Strategies for prevention of RSV nosocomial infection. J Perinatol. 2008;28(5):319–23.

14. Valentini D, Ianiro G, Di Bartolo I, et al. Hospital-acquired rotavirus and norovirus acute gastroenteritis in a pediatric unit, in 2014-2015. J Med Virol. 2017;89(10):1768–74.
15. Sukhrie FH, Teunis P, Vennema H, et al. Nosocomial transmission of norovirus is mainly caused by symptomatic cases. Clin Infect Dis. 2012;54(7):931–7.
16. Siegel JD, Rhinehart E, Jackson M, Chiarello L, Health Care Infection Control Practices Advisory C. 2007 guideline for isolation precautions: preventing transmission of infectious agents in health care settings. Am J Infect Control. 2007;35(10 Suppl 2):S65–164.
17. Otter JA, Yezli S, French GL. The role played by contaminated surfaces in the transmission of nosocomial pathogens. Infect Control Hosp Epidemiol. 2011;32(7):687–99.
18. Weber DJ, Rutala WA, Miller MB, Huslage K, Sickbert-Bennett E. Role of hospital surfaces in the transmission of emerging health care-associated pathogens: norovirus, Clostridium difficile, and Acinetobacter species. Am J Infect Control. 2010;38(5 Suppl 1):S25–33.
19. Piedrahita CT, Cadnum JL, Jencson AL, Shaikh AA, Ghannoum MA, Donskey CJ. Environmental surfaces in healthcare facilities are a potential source for transmission of Candida auris and other Candida species. Infect Control Hosp Epidemiol. 2017;38(9):1107–9.
20. Lerner A, Adler A, Abu-Hanna J, Meitus I, Navon-Venezia S, Carmeli Y. Environmental contamination by carbapenem-resistant Enterobacteriaceae. J Clin Microbiol. 2013;51(1):177–81.
21. Boyce JM, Pittet D, Healthcare Infection Control Practices Advisory C, Force HSAIHHT. Guideline for hand hygiene in health-care settings. Recommendations of the Healthcare Infection Control Practices Advisory Committee and the HICPAC/SHEA/APIC/IDSA Hand Hygiene Task Force. Society for Healthcare Epidemiology of America/Association for Professionals in Infection Control/Infectious Diseases Society of America. MMWR Recomm Rep. 2002;51(RR-16):1–45, quiz CE1-4.
22. Allegranzi B, Pittet D. Role of hand hygiene in healthcare-associated infection prevention. J Hosp Infect. 2009;73(4):305–15.
23. Best M, Neuhauser D. Ignaz Semmelweis and the birth of infection control. Qual Saf Health Care. 2004;13(3):233–4.
24. Lane HJ, Blum N, Fee E. Oliver Wendell Holmes (1809-1894) and Ignaz Philipp Semmelweis (1818-1865): preventing the transmission of puerperal fever. Am J Public Health. 2010;100(6):1008–9.
25. Allegranzi B, Sax H, Pittet D. Hand hygiene and healthcare system change within multi-modal promotion: a narrative review. J Hosp Infect. 2013;83(Suppl 1):S3–10.
26. American Academy of Pediatrics. Infection control for hospitalized children. In: Kimberlin DW, Brady MT, Jackson MA, Long SS, editors. Red book: 2015 report of the Committee on Infectious Diseases. 30th ed. Elk Grove Village: American Academy of Pediatrics; 2015. p. 161–76.
27. Bidawid S, Malik N, Adegbunrin O, Sattar SA, Farber JM. Norovirus cross-contamination during food handling and interruption of virus transfer by hand antisepsis: experiments with feline calicivirus as a surrogate. J Food Prot. 2004;67(1):103–9.
28. Pittet D, Hugonnet S, Harbarth S, et al. Effectiveness of a hospital-wide programme to improve compliance with hand hygiene. Infection Control Programme. Lancet. 2000;356(9238):1307–12.
29. Pittet D. Promotion of hand hygiene: magic, hype, or scientific challenge? Infect Control Hosp Epidemiol. 2002;23(3):118–9.
30. Caris MG, Kamphuis PGA, Dekker M, de Bruijne MC, van Agtmael MA, Vandenbroucke-Grauls C. Patient safety culture and the ability to improve: a proof of concept study on hand hygiene. Infect Control Hosp Epidemiol. 2017;38(11):1277–83.
31. Kirkland KB, Homa KA, Lasky RA, Ptak JA, Taylor EA, Splaine ME. Impact of a hospital-wide hand hygiene initiative on healthcare-associated infections: results of an interrupted time series. BMJ Qual Saf. 2012;21(12):1019–26.
32. Lankford MG, Zembower TR, Trick WE, Hacek DM, Noskin GA, Peterson LR. Influence of role models and hospital design on hand hygiene of healthcare workers. Emerg Infect Dis. 2003;9(2):217–23.

33. Sax H, Allegranzi B, Uckay I, Larson E, Boyce J, Pittet D. 'My five moments for hand hygiene': a user-centred design approach to understand, train, monitor and report hand hygiene. J Hosp Infect. 2007;67(1):9–21.
34. Thirkell G, Chambers J, Gilbart W, Thornhill K, Arbogast J, Lacey G. Pilot study of digital tools to support multimodal hand hygiene in a clinical setting. Am J Infect Control. 2017;46(3):261–5.
35. Ward MA, Schweizer ML, Polgreen PM, Gupta K, Reisinger HS, Perencevich EN. Automated and electronically assisted hand hygiene monitoring systems: a systematic review. Am J Infect Control. 2014;42(5):472–8.
36. Bellissimo-Rodrigues F, Pires D, Zingg W, Pittet D. Role of parents in the promotion of hand hygiene in the paediatric setting: a systematic literature review. J Hosp Infect. 2016;93(2):159–63.
37. Siegel JD, Rhinehart E, Jackson M, Chiarello L, Healthcare Infection Control Practices Advisory C. Management of multidrug-resistant organisms in health care settings, 2006. Am J Infect Control. 2007;35(10 Suppl 2):S165–93.
38. Rubin LG, Kohn N, Nullet S, Hill M. Reduction in rate of nosocomial respiratory virus infections in a children's hospital associated with enhanced isolation precautions. Infect Control Hosp Epidemiol. 2018;39(2):152–6.
39. Garcia R, Raad I, Abi-Said D, et al. Nosocomial respiratory syncytial virus infections: prevention and control in bone marrow transplant patients. Infect Control Hosp Epidemiol. 1997;18(6):412–6.
40. Snydman DR, Greer C, Meissner HC, McIntosh K. Prevention of nosocomial transmission of respiratory syncytial virus in a newborn nursery. Infect Control Hosp Epidemiol. 1988;9(3):105–8.
41. Tan S, Clarkson M, Sharkey D. Variation in visiting and isolation policies in neonatal units: a U.K. nationwide survey. Pediatr Infect Dis J. 2018;37(1):e20–e2.
42. Washam M, Woltmann J, Ankrum A, Connelly B. Association of visitation policy and health care-acquired respiratory viral infections in hospitalized children. Am J Infect Control. 2018;46(3):353–5.
43. Storr J, Twyman A, Zingg W, et al. Core components for effective infection prevention and control programmes: new WHO evidence-based recommendations. Antimicrob Resist Infect Control. 2017;6:6.
44. Centers for Disease C. Antibiotic resistance threats in the United States, 2013. http://www.cdc.gov/drugresistance/threat-report-2013/pdf/ar-threats-2013-508.pdf. Accessed 27 Oct 2017.
45. Logan LK, Braykov NP, Weinstein RA, Laxminarayan R, Program CDCEP. Extended-spectrum beta-lactamase-producing and third-generation cephalosporin-resistant Enterobacteriaceae in children: trends in the United States, 1999-2011. J Pediatric Infect Dis Soc. 2014;3(4):320–8.
46. Logan LK, Gandra S, Mandal S, et al. Multidrug- and carbapenem-resistant Pseudomonas aeruginosa in children, United States, 1999-2012. J Pediatric Infect Dis Soc. 2017;6(4):352–9.
47. Brinsley K, Srinivasan A, Sinkowitz-Cochran R, et al. Implementation of the campaign to prevent antimicrobial resistance in healthcare settings: 12 steps to prevent antimicrobial resistance among hospitalized adults – experiences from 3 institutions. Am J Infect Control. 2005;33(1):53–4.
48. Septimus E, Yokoe DS, Weinstein RA, Perl TM, Maragakis LL, Berenholtz SM. Maintaining the momentum of change: the role of the 2014 updates to the compendium in preventing healthcare-associated infections. Infect Control Hosp Epidemiol. 2014;35(Suppl 2):S6–9.
49. Centers for Medicare and Medicaid Services. Medicare.gov: hospital compare. https://www.medicare.gov/hospitalcompare/search.html. Accessed 26 Oct 2017.
50. Rathore MH, Jackson MA, Committee on Infectious D. Infection prevention and control in pediatric ambulatory settings. Pediatrics. 2017; 140(5):pii: e20172857.

The Role of the Environment and Colonization in Healthcare-Associated Infections

Julie D. Wohrley and Allison H. Bartlett

Definition of Colonization

Colonization is the survival of a microorganism on an internal (gastrointestinal, respiratory, or genitourinary tract) or external (skin) surface of the host without causing disease. Different types of organisms colonize different surfaces. For example, skin and the mucous membranes of the nose may be colonized with gram-positive organisms, including *Staphylococcus aureus* and coagulase-negative staphylococci [1]. The pharynx is colonized with gram-positive and gram-negative organisms including *Streptococcus pneumoniae*, *Haemophilus influenzae*, and *Moraxella catarrhalis* [2]. Gram-negative aerobic and anaerobic organisms commonly found colonizing the gastrointestinal tract include gram-negative aerobic and anaerobic bacteria and gram-positive organisms including *Enterococcus* and *C. difficile*.

Hosts encounter microbes on a nearly constant basis from the environment around them. A patient's own colonizing flora can result in hospital-associated infections when host defenses are compromised by underlying disease, immune compromise, or invasive devices. Alternatively, the healthcare environment can provide a source of pathogens, either by indirect transmission on the hands of healthcare workers (HCWs) or by direct transfer from environmental contamination.

The outcome of human-microbe interactions depends on the complex interplay of host defenses against microbial invasion and microbial virulence factors. If microbes are not killed by the immune system, a commensal relationship between the colonizer and the host may develop; alternatively, this may be the first step in the process of infection, damaging the host as a result of multiplication of the microorganism. Prolonged illness leading to immunodeficiency and breaks in barriers

J. D. Wohrley · A. H. Bartlett (✉)
Department of Pediatrics, Section of Infectious Diseases, The University of Chicago Medicine, Chicago, IL, USA
e-mail: abartlett@peds.bsd.uchicago.edu

© Springer Nature Switzerland AG 2019
J. C. McNeil et al. (eds.), *Healthcare-Associated Infections in Children*,
https://doi.org/10.1007/978-3-319-98122-2_2

resulting from invasive devices or surgical procedures may be associated with a shift from colonization to infection.

A complex interaction occurs throughout the body between commensal organisms and the barriers they colonize, with research on the skin and gastrointestinal tract microbiome shedding light on these interactions. The skin is a protective barrier with large numbers of colonizing bacteria. The skin microbiome is inhabited by bacteria, fungi, viruses, archaea, and mites; however most research has focused on bacteria. The presence of various microbes may influence disease as evidenced by the shift from *Staphylococcus epidermidis* cultured from healthy skin in young children [3] to *Propionibacterium acnes* in teenagers with acne [4, 5]. Children with atopic dermatitis have a propensity to infection with *Staphylococcus aureus* [6]. Loss of skin integrity, as with wounds, burns, inflammation, or invasive devices, allows pathogens to enter.

The balance between host and flora is also important in the gut and is influenced by antibiotic usage, diarrheal diseases, and critical illness [7–9]. The gut provides both an essential immune response in maintaining health with normal flora stimulating proliferation of epithelial cells in small and large intestines, participating in development of competent gut-associated immune responses, as well as providing a physical barrier function against pathogen invasion through colonization resistance [10–12]. Inflammatory bowel disease is just one example of altered gut flora associated with a disease state.

The secretory antibody system is important in the defense against mucosal infections. Specific secretory immunoglobulin A (IgA), transported through secretory epithelia to the mucosal surface, inhibits pathogen colonization through microorganism entrapment in mucus and promotion of clearance of entrapped microbes via peristalsis or mucociliary movement [13]. IgA also plays a role in mucosal protection of the gut by binding to a mucous layer that separates commensal bacteria from the apical surface of intestinal epithelial cells [14].

The Role of Host Flora in Hospital-Acquired Infections

Patients admitted to the hospital bring with them their "normal" flora which may be very different in a previously healthy child than in a technology-dependent child who resides in a long-term care facility.

Colonization of children with organisms specific to their individual clinical conditions, such as *Pseudomonas aeruginosa* in a tracheostomy- and ventilator-dependent child, or multidrug-resistant *Enterobacteriaceae* in the GI tract of a neurologically impaired adolescent with neurogenic bladder and a history of frequent urinary tract infections, may lead to infection with these pathogens. These resident organisms may be transferred to the environment where they can be acquired directly by other patients or transmitted indirectly by HCW hands.

High-risk populations for acquisition of multidrug-resistant organisms include those who are critically ill, who are immunocompromised, or who have been hospitalized for long periods of time, either in acute care or long-term care settings.

Additional risk factors include prolonged use of antibiotics and contact with colonized patients or the colonized/contaminated hands of HCW.

Colonizing organisms may produce invasive infection whether or not colonization is acquired in the hospital or the community. Colonization with methicillin-resistant *Staphylococcus aureus* (MRSA) is a risk factor for subsequent invasive MRSA infection [15]. A study of relatedness between colonizing strains of *S. aureus* and those associated with invasive disease in adults found that more than 80% of *S. aureus* blood isolates were identical to those colonizing the patient's anterior nares [16]. Genotypes of *S. aureus* strains from surgical site infections were also noted to be identical to colonizing strains in more than 80% of surgical patients [17].

The Role of Environmental Flora in Hospital-Acquired Infections

The hospital environment represents a reservoir of organisms such as MRSA, vancomycin-resistant *Enterococcus* (VRE), and multidrug-resistant gram-negative pathogens as well as *Clostridium difficile*. Notably, these same drug-resistant organisms found on surfaces in acute care hospital settings can be found in outpatient settings [18–21].

Transmission between patients and the environment may occur directly from contaminated fomites, indirectly from fomites on HCW hands, or indirectly from patient to patient on HCW hands. *C. difficile* may be spread in this indirect fashion. For example, this organism may be first identified in the stool of hospitalized patients and then later found to be contaminating the hospital room and its contents, with spread to HCW hands and the hospital environment.

Surface as a Reservoir

Hospital surfaces may serve as both a reservoir and a vehicle of transmission for pathogens. Specific pathogens such as MRSA [22], *Pseudomonas aeruginosa* [23], *Acinetobacter* [24], and *C. difficile* can contaminate hospital surfaces because of their ability to survive in the environment. The amount of hospital surface contamination varies depending on body site of infection/colonization, patient type, and cleaning practices. VRE is commonly associated with environmental contamination, especially in the presence of diarrhea [25]. In a study of ICU patients, the rates of environmental contamination were higher for patients with more than one body site positive for VRE [26].

C. difficile is often identified from rooms of colonized and infected patients, proving difficult to eradicate due to resilience of the spores [27]. The frequency of positive environmental cultures for *C. difficile* is high; in one study 29% (11 of 38) of environmental cultures in rooms occupied by asymptomatic patients had positive cultures for *C. difficile*, and 49% (44 of 90) of cultures in rooms occupied by patients had *C. difficile*-associated diarrhea ($p = 0.014$) [25, 28]. Over 80% of the environmental isolates characterized in this study had an immunoblot type identical to that of the patient [28]. During an outbreak investigation in an adult long-term care facility, *C. difficile* skin isolates from asymptomatic patients and from environmental surfaces matched the source patient's isolate in 13/15 (87%) and 11/19 (58%) cases, respectively [29]. *C. difficile* has also been recovered from physician and nurse work areas [27, 30].

Contact with Contaminated Surfaces or Equipment Contaminating Gloves or Hands of HCWs

Given the potential for hospital surfaces to be contaminated with pathogens, it stands to reason that the hands, and even the gloves, of HCWs can become contaminated as well. Contamination of hands of HCWs occurs after direct patient care or contact with contaminated surfaces [31–33]. Positive environmental cultures were found to be a risk factor for development of hand/glove contamination [34]. Not surprisingly, the level of hand contamination has been shown to correlate with level of environmental contamination [35].

Transmission of HAI from Roommates and Associated with Prior Room Occupants

Prior room occupants infected with healthcare-associated (HCA) pathogens may provide a source of exposure to other patients [36, 37]. Admission to a room in which the prior occupant was infected or colonized with MRSA, VRE, *Acinetobacter*, or *C. difficile* is a risk factor for subsequent colonization or infection with these organisms [38–41].

Special terminal cleaning (after the patient has been discharged) of rooms previously occupied by patients with *C. difficile* infection, including the use of hydrogen peroxide vapor, has been implemented to reduce rates of subsequent infection [42]. These procedures have led to reduced rates of infection in patients subsequently admitted to a room where a prior room occupant was infected or colonized with *C. difficile* [43, 44].

The Role of Identifying Colonization

Since colonization may lead to infection, two basic strategies – horizontal and vertical – are employed to reduce HAIs. Horizontal strategies seek to broadly reduce the burden of common healthcare-associated pathogens including *S. aureus*, *Enterococcus*, gram-negative bacteria, and *Candida* through interventions such as hand hygiene and environmental cleaning. Vertical strategies target specific pathogens known to cause HAIs and utilize active surveillance testing as well as directed approaches to decrease colonization and prevent transmission and subsequent infection [45, 46].

General horizontal prevention strategies are approached elsewhere in this text and include hand hygiene, contact precautions, isolation, and PPE use (see Chap. 1, Principles of Infection Control).

Strategies applied to patients known or at risk for pathogen colonization when viewed from a vertical approach fall into three broad categories: active surveillance testing (AST), pathogen-specific isolation, and decolonization.

Active Surveillance Testing (Screening)

Screening (active surveillance testing, or AST) involves detection of colonized patients using culture or molecular methods and typically focuses on high-risk pathogens, including *S. aureus* (MRSA), *Enterococcus* (VRE), and *C. difficile*, that are transmitted from person-to-person from colonized or infected patients [45, 47, 48]. Some of the principles, strategies, challenges, and controversies of AST will be discussed below.

AST Samples

Optimal samples for AST vary by pathogen. Specimens for MRSA testing are most frequently obtained from nares; however *S. aureus* also colonizes the skin, perineum, pharynx [49–52], GI tract [49], vagina [53], and axillae [49, 50], and additional sites of screening may be indicated depending on the clinical scenario and potential consequences of infection. Specimens may undergo culture-based or molecular methods for detection of *S. aureus*/MRSA.

VRE colonization is based on samples from stool, rectal, and perirectal swabs, using both molecular methods and culture-based methods [54]. Rectal or stool samples are also used for detection of multidrug-resistant gram-negative organisms such as extended-spectrum β-lactamase-producing *Enterobacteriaceae*, as well as carbapenemase-producing *Enterobacteriaceae*. *Pseudomonas* and *Acinetobacter* may be detected in multiple sites, depending on clinical situation, including the rectum, skin, nares, pharynx, wounds, urine, and trachea if the patient is mechanically ventilated.

AST and Isolation (Screening and Isolation)

The use of AST without additional interventions to reduce risk for transmission has not proven effective. Universal screening effort for pathogens has been most widely studied for MRSA and is considered to be controversial due to questions regarding its effectiveness in controlling spread, as well as cost [45]. Screening alone has not shown to be effective in reducing colonization and infection for MRSA [55, 56]. Studies have failed to show benefit for a combination of AST and isolation in reducing VRE infection or colonization; however, outbreaks of VRE have been successfully controlled in hospital settings with use of active surveillance, contact precautions, patient isolation, and cohorting [57]. Similarly, active surveillance is most useful following outbreaks of MRSA [58].

A cluster randomized trial in intensive care units found that universal gown and glove use did not reduce overall acquisition of multidrug-resistant organisms (MDRO); there was, however, a small reduction in MRSA transmission noted as a secondary outcome [59]. Another prospective study of ICU patients failed to show a difference in MRSA transmission [60], with additional concerns for the psychosocial effect that isolation places on patients [61]. In observational studies, single room isolation was shown to reduce MRSA acquisition and infection among hospitalized patients [62, 63]. Current recommendations for MRSA colonized and infected patients include isolation in single rooms or cohorting [64, 65]. However, experts have called for a review of the current recommendations for contact precautions and isolation for MRSA colonization in view of the above stated concerns [66].

AST, Isolation, and Targeted Decolonization Using Mupirocin

The addition of targeted decolonization strategies to AST and isolation for control of spread of healthcare-associated pathogens has been most extensively studied to prevent MRSA spread in the hospital setting. Patients who are nasally colonized with *S. aureus* are more than twice as likely as non-colonized patients to develop *S. aureus* infection [1, 67, 68]. Carriage may be classified as persistent, intermittent, or non-carriage [69]. Persistent colonization is associated with an increased risk of infection compared with intermittent or non-carriers [70]. Carriers with high bacterial loads have a higher risk of infection and may be more likely to transmit the bacteria to their environment [70, 71]. Greater quantities of *S. aureus* are found in the nares of persistent *S. aureus* carriers compared with intermittent carriers [72, 73].

Much research exists regarding the efficacy of active surveillance cultures combined with decolonization to decrease *S. aureus* transmission and infection in adults, with growing literature in neonatal ICUs [74–76]. Intranasal antibiotics (mupirocin), with or without antibacterial skin washes (chlorhexidine), have been used in order to decrease the bacterial burden and prevent transmission and infection. Short-term nasal mupirocin has been demonstrated to be effective in eradicating MRSA nasal carriage, with up to 90% success after 1 week of treatment, and 30–60% efficacy for longer duration of follow-up, depending on patient profile and body sites colonized [77, 78]. Nasal mupirocin use in high-risk settings has been demonstrated to be effective in eradicating *S. aureus* nasal colonization and reducing the number of infections in ICU, hemodialysis, surgical, and long-term care settings [79–82].

In a study of nearly two million adult admissions, a significant reduction in the rate of MRSA transmission and infection was noted after introduction of an infection control bundle, which included decolonization of MRSA carriers and isolation [83, 84] as well as a hand hygiene program [84]. However, a crossover study of universal screening on surgical wards combined with targeted decolonization and contact precautions was unable to demonstrate reduction in MRSA infections despite high compliance with screening [85].

Nasal mupirocin decolonization of NICU infants with MRSA colonization in two units with high prevalence (>25%) of MRSA colonization decreased the rate of MRSA infections [86]. However, a retrospective study in the USA failed to demonstrate benefit when nasal mupirocin was used for 5 days in colonized neonates in a unit with a baseline prevalence of around 2% [87]. This study showed that some NICU infants develop infection prior to detection of colonization and infants who remain in the NICU can become recolonized over time [87]. Taken together, these data suggest that decolonization measures may be most beneficial when the baseline rate of colonization is high. Additional NICU studies have found a high correlation between colonizing strains and infecting strains and confirmed high rates (42%) of infections occurring before colonization is detected suggesting universal, rather than targeted, decolonization should be used to control the spread of MRSA [74]. Current recommendations suggest that decolonization may be considered in high-risk neonates during an MRSA outbreak or in cases of endemic MRSA when other measures are failing [88]. A recent Society for Hospital Epidemiology Association (SHEA) survey regarding practices for MRSA identification and eradication in NICUs noted that most (86%) performed surveillance screening (AST) for MRSA in neonates with variability in timing of samples, sites sampled, isolation protocols, and decolonization strategies employed [89].

Recommendations for MSSA are less clear. Invasive MSSA infections occur 2.5 times more frequently than invasive MRSA infections in neonates, leading to significant morbidity and mortality [90]. Targeted screening followed by MSSA decolonization in a single NICU reduced incidence rates of MSSA-positive clinical cultures and MSSA infections by more than 50% [91].

Mupirocin resistance among *S. aureus* isolates has been demonstrated in multiple studies, especially associated with prolonged use. High-level resistance has been associated with decolonization failure, and low-level resistance may be associated with early recolonization [71, 72]. Therefore, the long-term use of mupirocin is questioned, and alternatives to mupirocin for decolonization in those with mupirocin-resistant strains of MRSA are needed. However, in a long-term study examining use of mupirocin prophylaxis in the NICU over a 7-year period, the rate of *S. aureus* (MSSA and MRSA) infections decreased from 1.88 to 0.33 per 1000 patient days without any mupirocin-resistant isolates identified [92]. This finding is consistent with previous reports of low prevalence of resistance among *S. aureus* isolates from mupirocin-treated neonates [93].

The use of decolonization may be most effective for patients at risk of infection for short periods of time such as surgical patients, whose risk of infection may be less once the surgical site is closed, as well as ICU patients, whose risk may lower once they are discharged from the ICU [94, 95]. This is of import given that patients are recolonized within weeks or months following decolonization, and thus the effect is often short-lived [95, 96]. Mupirocin decolonization has been used specifically to reduce the risk of surgical site infections (SSIs) associated with gram-positive organisms. In a meta-analysis of 17 RCTs or quasi-experimental studies including adult cardiac and orthopedic surgery patients, mupirocin decolonization was found to be significantly protective against gram-positive SSIs, specifically *S. aureus* SSIs [46, 81, 97].

Preoperative *S. aureus* decolonization is not routinely recommended for most pediatric patients undergoing surgery, however the impact of preoperative colonization on risk of SSI in children has been examined in many small studies. Risk of SSI was not elevated in *S. aureus*-colonized children undergoing cardiac surgery [98]. Studies in adult cardiac surgery patients, however, suggest a benefit to mupirocin-based decolonization in prevention of SSI [99]; this topic as it pertains to cardiac surgery is discussed further in Chap. 11.

Use of Universal Decolonization Strategies: Chlorhexidine Bathing

Chlorhexidine (CHG) is a widely used broad-spectrum topical antimicrobial agent [100]. The Centers for Disease Control and Prevention recommend its use as a skin cleanser prior to insertion of central venous catheters (CVC) in both children and adults but do not recommend its use in infants less than 2 months of age due to lack of safety and efficacy data in this population [101].

In spite of these cautions, a national survey of neonatology training program directors indicates that most NICUs use chlorhexidine for CVC site prep and maintenance but restrict use based on gestational age, chronological age, and birth weight [102]. Risks to premature infants relate to the increased potential for chemical burns and contact dermatitis in the setting of underdeveloped skin [100] and the possibility of systemic absorption of CHG, although no adverse events have been reported despite demonstrable blood CHG levels [100, 103–105].

Chlorhexidine bathing has been suggested as another adjunct to decrease colonization and has been studied in adults and children, including neonates. An adult randomized controlled trial demonstrated that daily chlorhexidine bathing did not reduce HAI including central line-associated bloodstream infection (CLABSI), catheter-associated urinary tract infection (CAUTI), or ventilator-associated pneumonia (VAP) [106]. A number of other studies (including clinical trials) in adults, however, have shown positive benefits of chlorhexidine-containing products when used as part of a bundle approach for HAI prevention [107–109]. In the Pediatric SCRUB Trial, daily chlorhexidine bathing was compared with standard bathing practices to evaluate effect on incidence of bacteremia in critically ill children [110]. There was a non-statistically significant reduction in bacteremia in the CHG group in the intention-to-treat analysis and a 36% decrease in bacteremia in the per protocol arm [110].

The use of universal decolonization raises concerns about the possibility of chlorhexidine resistance. A study from Texas Children's Hospital found that nearly half of nosocomial *S. aureus* carried one or both genes associated with chlorhexidine tolerance (*qacA/qacB* and *smr*), noting that *smr*-positive isolates were more often resistant to methicillin, ciprofloxacin, or clindamycin as well [111]. Mupirocin resistance was also noted in 2.8% of the isolates in this study [111].

Vertical and horizontal approaches to infection prevention have been compared in two studies: Huang et al. compared three approaches to MRSA prevention among 74 adult ICU patients in the REDUCE-MRSA study [112]. Vertical approaches consisted of AST with and without targeted decolonization of MRSA carriers with CHG bathing and intranasal mupirocin compared with a horizontal approach involving universal decolonization of all ICU patients regardless of MRSA status. Universal decolonization was found to be associated with the largest reduction in all-cause BSI (44%) and MRSA clinical culture rates (37%) [112]. Another group showed that improved hand hygiene in addition to universal CHG bathing reduced overall infection rate and specific rates of *Candida* CAUTI and *Acinetobacter* VAP [113]. Additionally, when there is high adherence to CHG bathing and hand hygiene, there is no additional benefit to AST and isolation to reduce MDRO acquisition rates [114].

Digestive and Respiratory Tract Decolonization/ Decontamination Strategies

Selective digestive decontamination (SDD) and selective oral decontamination (SOD) are additional methods of universal decolonization employed in an effort to reduce colonization with gram-negative organisms, particularly in critically ill patients. Both methods use a polymyxin, an aminoglycoside, and an antifungal, applied to the oropharynx as a paste or gel (SOD) or in a liquid form administered per nasogastric or orogastric tube (SDD), paired with systemic antimicrobials, usually an intravenous third-generation cephalosporin. These two strategies have been studied in more than 50 RCTs and have been examined in 12 meta-analyses with demonstrated efficacy in reduction of colonization, morbidity, and mortality in adult ICU patients [115–117]. Widespread acceptance has been limited by concern over selecting for resistant organisms in universal applications, although long-term follow-up in units employing these strategies have not demonstrated an increase in resistant organisms [118]. Microbiome studies of adults undergoing SDD compared to healthy adults revealed dramatic shifts in the gastrointestinal microbiome of SDD recipients (as would be expected) as well as an increase in the relative abundance of organisms expressing antimicrobial resistance genes [119].

The pediatric experience with these strategies is limited. In a single meta-analysis of 4 RCTs including 335 children, ventilator-associated pneumonia rates were 69% lower in in those children receiving SDD [120]. The use in neonatal populations has not been studied.

Surgical Site Infections

The evidence for perioperative antimicrobial prophylaxis is well established, and the use of antimicrobials prior to incision reduces rates of SSI [121] by reducing the concentration of potential pathogens within or near the surgical incision. The basic tenets of antimicrobial use to prevent SSI include use of prophylaxis for all elective operations requiring entry into a hollow viscus, involving insertion of intravascular or orthopedic prosthetic devices or implants, or operations in which occurrence of SSI would pose catastrophic risk to the patient (e.g., sternotomy). The choice of antimicrobial is based upon a need for bactericidal activity against the expected pathogens for specific surgical procedures as well as agents which are known to be safe and cost-effective. The goal is to provide bactericidal concentrations in tissues and serum at the time of incision and to be continued throughout the entire operation until the wound is closed. Re-dosing of the antimicrobial agent may be required should the procedure last several hours or if there is significant blood loss.

An important risk factor contributing to SSI risk is the number of organisms which gain entry into the wound intraoperatively. The greater the burden, the greater the risk of infection. When appropriate antimicrobial prophylaxis has been administered, a bacterial burden of 10^5 is required to cause SSI; however if a foreign body is present, the threshold to cause infection may be significantly reduced. Virulence of the organism also contributes to SSI risk.

Pre- and perioperative antiseptics are utilized in order to decrease organism burden and thereby reduce the risk of SSI. Preoperative bathing with agents such as chlorhexidine has been shown to decrease the amount of endogenous flora on the skin but has not been shown to reduce rates of SSI in pooled analyses of adult surgical patients [122]. In certain very high-risk populations, however, such as cardiac and orthopedic surgery patients, preoperative chlorhexidine bathing has been associated with reduced rates of SSI (especially those due to *S. aureus* or MRSA) [123–125]. It is likely that the benefits of chlorhexidine bathing are influenced by the type of surgical procedure (i.e., high-risk vs. low-risk) as well as the baseline rate of SSI at a given institution. In spite of these controversies, the use of chlorhexidine body wash prior to surgery is routine.

There are several options for preoperative skin antisepsis with either chlorhexidine-alcohol or povidone-iodine as the active agent. The authors of a Cochrane Review conclude that other characteristics of skin prep agents such as potential side effects and cost should be taken into consideration as well until there are definitive data showing clinical superiority of one agent over another [126]. New CDC Guidelines for Prevention of SSI recommend an alcohol-based skin antiseptic, such as either chlorhexidine-alcohol or iodophor-alcohol products [127–129].

Surgical site infections generally arise from endogenous sources such as bacteria present on skin surfaces or in a viscus, with greatest risk occurring while the wound is open. In addition to skin surface, bacteria may be found in skin appendages, including sebaceous glands, hair follicles, and sweat glands [130]. When infections related to exogenous sources occur, they may be sporadic or related to an outbreak. Exogenous sources include contamination of the operating room environment, surgical instruments, equipment, or colonized or infected personnel [131, 132].

Environmental Contamination

Common nosocomial pathogens can persist for months on surfaces, contributing to transmission risk in the absence of regular and thorough cleaning and disinfection [133]. These pathogens importantly include gram-positive (*Enterococcus*, including VRE; *S. aureus*, including MRSA; and *Streptococcus pyogenes*) as well as gram-negative (*Acinetobacter* spp., *E. coli*, *Klebsiella* spp., *p. aeruginosa*, *Serratia marcescens*, or *Shigella*) organisms. Spore-forming bacteria, such as *Clostridium difficile*, can survive for months as can fungi and yeast. Viruses from the respiratory tract, such as coronavirus, influenza, coxsackie, and rhinovirus, survive a relatively short period of days, whereas viruses from the gastrointestinal tract, such as norovirus or rotavirus, may persist for up to 2 months [133].

Surfaces in rooms of patients infected or colonized with pathogens may (and frequently do) become contaminated. MRSA, VRE, *Acinetobacter* spp., norovirus, and *C. difficile* have been detected on environmental surfaces in rooms of infected or colonized patients, can colonize healthcare workers' hands, and can then be transmitted to others [134]. Contact with the environment is as likely as contact with the affected patient to result in contamination of HCW hands [32]. The presence of environmental contamination is a risk factor for HCW hand/glove contamination [33]. Admission to a room previously occupied by a patient colonized or infected with MRSA, VRE, *Acinetobacter* spp., or *C. difficile* has been shown to be a risk factor for subsequent development of colonization or infection by these pathogens [38, 40, 41].

Multiple studies have demonstrated that a lack of thorough cleaning [135, 136] contributes to persistence of environmental contamination. Assessing adequacy of cleaning can be performed using various methods including observation for visible soiling, culture-based colony counts, fluorescent dye, and ATP detection. For example, fluorescent dye can be applied as a dot to surfaces where it dries clear. If a surface was inadequately wiped, the area fluoresces when exposed to black light. ATP bioluminescence systems measure ATP, a marker for presence of residual organic material (e.g., human secretions or excretions and food). ATP, however, does not indicate presence of viable pathogens, and its absence does not rule out the presence of contamination, and as such, use of fluorescent dye correlates more closely with colony counts than does ATP bioluminescence [137].

Focused efforts to eradicate pathogens can improve cleaning efficacy, which may involve specialized teams [138] or through use of improved monitoring of cleaning practices with markers such as ATP and fluorescent dye [137, 139]. Feedback to environmental services (EVS) staff following use of enhanced methods has also been demonstrated to improve the frequency of achieving adequate cleaning [140, 141]. In a study of 36 acute care hospitals, only 48% (9910/20,646) of environmental surfaces were cleaned at baseline. After educational and procedural interventions combined with provision of objective performance feedback to EVS staff, 77% (7287/9464) of surfaces were cleaned ($p < 0.001$) [141].

In addition to ensuring each surface is cleaned, it is important to select the correct cleaning product as microorganisms vary in their resistance to disinfectants. For example, disinfection of a room potentially contaminated by *C. difficile* requires use of hypochlorite-based solutions [142] rather than phenols or quaternary ammonium compounds generally used for general hospital-based cleaning.

In spite of enhanced cleaning methods aimed at improving cleaning thoroughness and monitoring of cleaning practices, many surfaces remain inadequately cleaned. For this reason, no-touch room disinfection units that decontaminate environmental surfaces and objects utilizing either ultraviolet (UV) light or hydrogen peroxide (HP) vapor have been developed [143, 144]. These technologies are considered an adjunct to standard cleaning and disinfection since surfaces must be physically clean and the room must be emptied of people prior to use. UV irradiation with certain wavelengths breaks the molecular bond in DNA, thereby destroying the organism. This has been shown to be effective against MRSA, VRE, and *Acinetobacter baumannii*, in experimentally contaminated rooms [145]. Systems utilizing HP vapor have been found to be effective in eradicating pathogens such as MRSA, *Mycobacterium tuberculosis, Serratia,* and *C. difficile* spores from rooms and equipment [146]. Both of these methods have been found to be effective at reducing HAIs [146]. Their advantages include ability to substantially reduce *C. difficile* spores [147] as well as achieve substantial reductions in vegetative bacteria.

Failure to adequately clean and sterilize equipment may lead to transmission via contaminated equipment [148]. The level of disinfection or sterilization considered acceptable depends on the intended use of the object and is categorized as critical (items that come into contact with sterile tissue), semicritical (items contacting mucous membranes, such as endoscopes), and noncritical (items contacting skin, such as stethoscopes). These each require sterilization, high-level disinfection, or low-level disinfection, respectively. Cleaning should precede sterilization or disinfection.

Legionella and Other Water-Associated Infections

Among the many sources of infection within hospital environments, water remains of significant concern secondary to opportunity for exposure. Water is ubiquitous in its use throughout the hospital, not only for routine sanitation but also for air conditioning, mechanical ventilation, bathing, as well as the cleaning and processing of equipment. Certain organisms have special predilection for moist environments and include gram-negative bacilli, nontuberculous mycobacteria, fungi, and some viruses. In a recent review of waterborne healthcare-associated infections, 41 of 125 reports described hospitalized children [149]. The organisms primarily responsible included *Legionella* (hot water distribution systems), *Pseudomonas* (bottled water), and *Burkholderia* (distilled and sterile water contamination) [149]. Generally, tap water is the most frequently reported source of infection, with contamination at the sink, shower, and bathtub. *Legionella* was the primary cause of HAI among all the patients included in this review and was the predominant organism causing outbreaks [149]. *Legionella* outbreaks have been reported in premature neonates associated with the humidification trays of incubators [150] and in term neonates associated with cold mist humidifiers [151].

Environmental control measures are generally insufficient, and eradication requires use of a multistep control plan which includes education; use of sterile water for immunocompromised patients; use of periodic cleaning of showers, tubs, and sinks; and use of disinfection systems/filters on taps and shower heads. A team of specialists from all areas of infection control including engineers is required to eradicate contamination in the water system/supplies when it occurs [149].

Conclusion

Endogenous and exogenous microbes are a constant threat to hospitalized patients. Efforts to decrease endogenous pathogens via decolonization and skin antisepsis decrease the risk of infection in some settings. Controlling the spread of potential pathogens from the environment requires meticulous attention to cleaning and disinfection practices as well as hand hygiene.

References

1. Wertheim HF, Melles DC, Vos MC, van Leeuwen W, van Belkum A, Verbrugh HA, et al. The role of nasal carriage in Staphylococcus aureus infections. Lancet Infect Dis. 2005;5(12):751–62.
2. Bogaert D, Keijser B, Huse S, Rossen J, Veenhoven R, van Gils E, et al. Variability and diversity of nasopharyngeal microbiota in children: a metagenomic analysis. PLoS One. 2011;6(2):e17035.
3. Iwase T, Uehara Y, Shinji H, Tajima A, Seo H, Takada K, et al. Staphylococcus epidermidis Esp inhibits Staphylococcus aureus biofilm formation and nasal colonization. Nature. 2010;465(7296):346–9.
4. Grice EA, Segre JA. The skin microbiome. Nat Rev Microbiol. 2011;9(4):244–53.
5. Dessinioti C, Katsambas AD. The role of Propionibacterium acnes in acne pathogenesis: facts and controversies. Clin Dermatol. 2010;28(1):2–7.
6. Hanifin JM, Rogge JL. Staphylococcal infections in patients with atopic dermatitis. Arch Dermatol. 1977;113(10):1383–6.
7. Ferrer M, Mendez-Garcia C, Rojo D, Barbas C, Moya A. Antibiotic use and microbiome function. Biochem Pharmacol. 2017;134:114–26.
8. Young VB. The role of the microbiome in human health and disease: an introduction for clinicians. BMJ. 2017;356:j831.
9. Jacobs MC, Haak BW, Hugenholtz F, Wiersinga WJ. Gut microbiota and host defense in critical illness. Curr Opin Crit Care. 2017;23(4):257–63.
10. Singhi SC, Kumar S. Probiotics in critically ill children. F1000Res. 2016;5:F1000 Faculty Rev-407. https://doi.org/10.12688/f1000research.7630.1. eCollection 2016.
11. Huang XZ, Zhu LB, Li ZR, Lin J. Bacterial colonization and intestinal mucosal barrier development. World J Clin Pediatr. 2013;2(4):46–53.
12. Biedermann L, Rogler G. The intestinal microbiota: its role in health and disease. Eur J Pediatr. 2015;174(2):151–67.
13. Woof JM, Kerr MA. The function of immunoglobulin A in immunity. J Pathol. 2006;208(2):270–82.
14. Gutzeit C, Magri G, Cerutti A. Intestinal IgA production and its role in host-microbe interaction. Immunol Rev. 2014;260(1):76–85.
15. Huang YC, Chou YH, Su LH, Lien RI, Lin TY. Methicillin-resistant Staphylococcus aureus colonization and its association with infection among infants hospitalized in neonatal intensive care units. Pediatrics. 2006;118(2):469–74.
16. von Eiff C, Becker K, Machka K, Stammer H, Peters G. Nasal carriage as a source of Staphylococcus aureus bacteremia. Study Group. N Engl J Med. 2001;344(1):11–6.
17. Perl TM, Cullen JJ, Wenzel RP, Zimmerman MB, Pfaller MA, Sheppard D, et al. Intranasal mupirocin to prevent postoperative Staphylococcus aureus infections. N Engl J Med. 2002;346(24):1871–7.
18. Johnston CP, Cooper L, Ruby W, Carroll KC, Cosgrove SE, Perl TM. Epidemiology of community-acquired methicillin-resistant Staphylococcus aureus skin infections among healthcare workers in an outpatient clinic. Infect Control Hosp Epidemiol. 2006;27(10):1133–6.
19. Atta MG, Eustace JA, Song X, Perl TM, Scheel PJ Jr. Outpatient vancomycin use and vancomycin-resistant enterococcal colonization in maintenance dialysis patients. Kidney Int. 2001;59(2):718–24.
20. Otter JA. What's trending in the infection prevention and control literature? From HIS 2012 to HIS 2014, and beyond. J Hosp Infect. 2015;89(4):229–36.

21. Lin MY, Lyles-Banks RD, Lolans K, Hines DW, Spear JB, Petrak R, et al. The importance of long-term acute care hospitals in the regional epidemiology of Klebsiella pneumoniae carbapenemase-producing Enterobacteriaceae. Clin Infect Dis. 2013;57(9):1246–52.
22. Dancer SJ. Controlling hospital-acquired infection: focus on the role of the environment and new technologies for decontamination. Clin Microbiol Rev. 2014;27(4):665–90.
23. Nseir S, Blazejewski C, Lubret R, Wallet F, Courcol R, Durocher A. Risk of acquiring multidrug-resistant gram-negative bacilli from prior room occupants in the intensive care unit. Clin Microbiol Infect. 2011;17(8):1201–8.
24. Wendt C, Dietze B, Dietz E, Ruden H. Survival of Acinetobacter baumannii on dry surfaces. J Clin Microbiol. 1997;35(6):1394–7.
25. Drees M, Snydman DR, Schmid CH, Barefoot L, Hansjosten K, Vue PM, et al. Antibiotic exposure and room contamination among patients colonized with vancomycin-resistant enterococci. Infect Control Hosp Epidemiol. 2008;29(8):709–15.
26. Bonten MJ, Hayden MK, Nathan C, van Voorhis J, Matushek M, Slaughter S, et al. Epidemiology of colonisation of patients and environment with vancomycin-resistant enterococci. Lancet. 1996;348(9042):1615–9.
27. Kim KH, Fekety R, Batts DH, Brown D, Cudmore M, Silva J Jr, et al. Isolation of Clostridium difficile from the environment and contacts of patients with antibiotic-associated colitis. J Infect Dis. 1981;143(1):42–50.
28. McFarland LV, Mulligan ME, Kwok RY, Stamm WE. Nosocomial acquisition of Clostridium difficile infection. N Engl J Med. 1989;320(4):204–10.
29. Riggs MM, Sethi AK, Zabarsky TF, Eckstein EC, Jump RL, Donskey CJ. Asymptomatic carriers are a potential source for transmission of epidemic and nonepidemic Clostridium difficile strains among long-term care facility residents. Clin Infect Dis. 2007;45(8): 992–8.
30. Dumford DM 3rd, Nerandzic MM, Eckstein BC, Donskey CJ. What is on that keyboard? Detecting hidden environmental reservoirs of Clostridium difficile during an outbreak associated with North American pulsed-field gel electrophoresis type 1 strains. Am J Infect Control. 2009;37(1):15–9.
31. Huslage K, Rutala WA, Sickbert-Bennett E, Weber DJ. A quantitative approach to defining "high-touch" surfaces in hospitals. Infect Control Hosp Epidemiol. 2010;31(8):850–3.
32. Stiefel U, Cadnum JL, Eckstein BC, Guerrero DM, Tima MA, Donskey CJ. Contamination of hands with methicillin-resistant Staphylococcus aureus after contact with environmental surfaces and after contact with the skin of colonized patients. Infect Control Hosp Epidemiol. 2011;32(2):185–7.
33. Morgan DJ, Rogawski E, Thom KA, Johnson JK, Perencevich EN, Shardell M, et al. Transfer of multidrug-resistant bacteria to healthcare workers' gloves and gowns after patient contact increases with environmental contamination. Crit Care Med. 2012;40(4):1045–51.
34. Samore MH, Venkataraman L, DeGirolami PC, Arbeit RD, Karchmer AW. Clinical and molecular epidemiology of sporadic and clustered cases of nosocomial Clostridium difficile diarrhea. Am J Med. 1996;100(1):32–40.
35. Cohen B, Cohen CC, Loyland B, Larson EL. Transmission of health care-associated infections from roommates and prior room occupants: a systematic review. Clin Epidemiol. 2017;9:297–310.
36. Lemmen SW, Hafner H, Zolldann D, Stanzel S, Lutticken R. Distribution of multi-resistant gram-negative versus gram-positive bacteria in the hospital inanimate environment. J Hosp Infect. 2004;56(3):191–7.
37. Boyce JM, Potter-Bynoe G, Chenevert C, King T. Environmental contamination due to methicillin-resistant Staphylococcus aureus: possible infection control implications. Infect Control Hosp Epidemiol. 1997;18(9):622–7.
38. Huang SS, Datta R, Platt R. Risk of acquiring antibiotic-resistant bacteria from prior room occupants. Arch Intern Med. 2006;166(18):1945–51.
39. Rutala WA, Weber DJ. Disinfection and sterilization in health care facilities: an overview and current issues. Infect Dis Clin N Am. 2016;30(3):609–37.

40. Carling P. Methods for assessing the adequacy of practice and improving room disinfection. Am J Infect Control. 2013;41(5 Suppl):S20–5.
41. Shaughnessy MK, Micielli RL, DePestel DD, Arndt J, Strachan CL, Welch KB, et al. Evaluation of hospital room assignment and acquisition of Clostridium difficile infection. Infect Control Hosp Epidemiol. 2011;32(3):201–6.
42. Donskey CJ. Does improving surface cleaning and disinfection reduce health care-associated infections? Am J Infect Control. 2013;41(5 Suppl):S12–9.
43. Boyce JM, Havill NL, Otter JA, McDonald LC, Adams NM, Cooper T, et al. Impact of hydrogen peroxide vapor room decontamination on Clostridium difficile environmental contamination and transmission in a healthcare setting. Infect Control Hosp Epidemiol. 2008;29(8):723–9.
44. Passaretti CL, Otter JA, Reich NG, Myers J, Shepard J, Ross T, et al. An evaluation of environmental decontamination with hydrogen peroxide vapor for reducing the risk of patient acquisition of multidrug-resistant organisms. Clin Infect Dis. 2013;56(1):27–35.
45. Septimus E, Weinstein RA, Perl TM, Goldmann DA, Yokoe DS. Approaches for preventing healthcare-associated infections: go long or go wide? Infect Control Hosp Epidemiol. 2014;35(Suppl 2):S10–4.
46. Septimus EJ, Schweizer ML. Decolonization in prevention of health care-associated infections. Clin Microbiol Rev. 2016;29(2):201–22.
47. Wenzel RP, Edmond MB. Infection control: the case for horizontal rather than vertical interventional programs. Int J Infect Dis. 2010;14(Suppl 4):S3–5.
48. Wenzel RP, Bearman G, Edmond MB. Screening for MRSA: a flawed hospital infection control intervention. Infect Control Hosp Epidemiol. 2008;29(11):1012–8.
49. Williams RE. Healthy carriage of Staphylococcus aureus: its prevalence and importance. Bacteriol Rev. 1963;27:56–71.
50. Armstrong-Esther CA. Carriage patterns of Staphylococcus aureus in a healthy non-hospital population of adults and children. Ann Hum Biol. 1976;3(3):221–7.
51. Wertheim HF, Verveer J, Boelens HA, van Belkum A, Verbrugh HA, Vos MC. Effect of mupirocin treatment on nasal, pharyngeal, and perineal carriage of Staphylococcus aureus in healthy adults. Antimicrob Agents Chemother. 2005;49(4):1465–7.
52. Ridley M. Perineal carriage of Staph. aureus. Br Med J. 1959;1(5117):270–3.
53. Guinan ME, Dan BB, Guidotti RJ, Reingold AL, Schmid GP, Bettoli EJ, et al. Vaginal colonization with Staphylococcus aureus in healthy women: a review of four studies. Ann Intern Med. 1982;96(6 Pt 2):944–7.
54. Faron ML, Ledeboer NA, Buchan BW. Resistance mechanisms, epidemiology, and approaches to screening for vancomycin-resistant Enterococcus in the health care setting. J Clin Microbiol. 2016;54(10):2436–47.
55. Cooper BS, Stone SP, Kibbler CC, Cookson BD, Roberts JA, Medley GF, et al. Isolation measures in the hospital management of methicillin resistant Staphylococcus aureus (MRSA): systematic review of the literature. BMJ. 2004;329(7465):533.
56. Glick SB, Samson DJ, Huang ES, Vats V, Aronson N, Weber SG. Screening for methicillin-resistant Staphylococcus aureus: a comparative effectiveness review. Am J Infect Control. 2014;42(2):148–55.
57. Christiansen KJ, Tibbett PA, Beresford W, Pearman JW, Lee RC, Coombs GW, et al. Eradication of a large outbreak of a single strain of vanB vancomycin-resistant Enterococcus faecium at a major Australian teaching hospital. Infect Control Hosp Epidemiol. 2004;25(5):384–90.
58. Jernigan JA, Titus MG, Groschel DH, Getchell-White S, Farr BM. Effectiveness of contact isolation during a hospital outbreak of methicillin-resistant Staphylococcus aureus. Am J Epidemiol. 1996;143(5):496–504.
59. Harris AD, Pineles L, Belton B, Johnson JK, Shardell M, Loeb M, et al. Universal glove and gown use and acquisition of antibiotic-resistant bacteria in the ICU: a randomized trial. JAMA. 2013;310(15):1571–80.
60. Cepeda JA, Whitehouse T, Cooper B, Hails J, Jones K, Kwaku F, et al. Isolation of patients in single rooms or cohorts to reduce spread of MRSA in intensive-care units: prospective two-centre study. Lancet. 2005;365(9456):295–304.

61. Morgan DJ, Kaye KS, Diekema DJ. Reconsidering isolation precautions for endemic methicillin-resistant Staphylococcus aureus and vancomycin-resistant Enterococcus. JAMA. 2014;312(14):1395–6.

62. Bracco D, Dubois MJ, Bouali R, Eggimann P. Single rooms may help to prevent nosocomial bloodstream infection and cross-transmission of methicillin-resistant Staphylococcus aureus in intensive care units. Intensive Care Med. 2007;33(5):836–40.

63. Gastmeier P, Schwab F, Geffers C, Ruden H. To isolate or not to isolate? Analysis of data from the German Nosocomial Infection Surveillance System regarding the placement of patients with methicillin-resistant Staphylococcus aureus in private rooms in intensive care units. Infect Control Hosp Epidemiol. 2004;25(2):109–13.

64. Coia JE, Duckworth GJ, Edwards DI, Farrington M, Fry C, Humphreys H, et al. Guidelines for the control and prevention of meticillin-resistant Staphylococcus aureus (MRSA) in healthcare facilities. J Hosp Infect. 2006;63(Suppl 1):S1–44.

65. Calfee DP, Salgado CD, Milstone AM, Harris AD, Kuhar DT, Moody J, et al. Strategies to prevent methicillin-resistant Staphylococcus aureus transmission and infection in acute care hospitals: 2014 update. Infect Control Hosp Epidemiol. 2014;35(7):772–96.

66. Fatkenheuer G, Hirschel B, Harbarth S. Screening and isolation to control meticillin-resistant Staphylococcus aureus: sense, nonsense, and evidence. Lancet. 2015;385(9973):1146–9.

67. Russell DL, Flood A, Zaroda TE, Acosta C, Riley MM, Busuttil RW, et al. Outcomes of colonization with MRSA and VRE among liver transplant candidates and recipients. Am J Transplant. 2008;8(8):1737–43.

68. Kluytmans J, van Belkum A, Verbrugh H. Nasal carriage of Staphylococcus aureus: epidemiology, underlying mechanisms, and associated risks. Clin Microbiol Rev. 1997;10(3):505–20.

69. VandenBergh MF, Yzerman EP, van Belkum A, Boelens HA, Sijmons M, Verbrugh HA. Follow-up of Staphylococcus aureus nasal carriage after 8 years: redefining the persistent carrier state. J Clin Microbiol. 1999;37(10):3133–40.

70. Nouwen JL, Fieren MW, Snijders S, Verbrugh HA, van Belkum A. Persistent (not intermittent) nasal carriage of Staphylococcus aureus is the determinant of CPD-related infections. Kidney Int. 2005;67(3):1084–92.

71. Kalmeijer MD, van Nieuwland-Bollen E, Bogaers-Hofman D, de Baere GA. Nasal carriage of Staphylococcus aureus is a major risk factor for surgical-site infections in orthopedic surgery. Infect Control Hosp Epidemiol. 2000;21(5):319–23.

72. Mermel LA, Eells SJ, Acharya MK, Cartony JM, Dacus D, Fadem S, et al. Quantitative analysis and molecular fingerprinting of methicillin-resistant Staphylococcus aureus nasal colonization in different patient populations: a prospective, multicenter study. Infect Control Hosp Epidemiol. 2010;31(6):592–7.

73. Cheng VC, Li IW, Wu AK, Tang BS, Ng KH, To KK, et al. Effect of antibiotics on the bacterial load of meticillin-resistant Staphylococcus aureus colonisation in anterior nares. J Hosp Infect. 2008;70(1):27–34.

74. Milstone AM, Budd A, Shepard JW, Ross T, Aucott S, Carroll KC, et al. Role of decolonization in a comprehensive strategy to reduce methicillin-resistant Staphylococcus aureus infections in the neonatal intensive care unit: an observational cohort study. Infect Control Hosp Epidemiol. 2010;31(5):558–60.

75. Khoury J, Jones M, Grim A, Dunne WM Jr, Fraser V. Eradication of methicillin-resistant Staphylococcus aureus from a neonatal intensive care unit by active surveillance and aggressive infection control measures. Infect Control Hosp Epidemiol. 2005;26(7):616–21.

76. Huang YC, Lien RI, Su LH, Chou YH, Lin TY. Successful control of methicillin-resistant Staphylococcus aureus in endemic neonatal intensive care units – a 7-year campaign. PLoS One. 2011;6(8):e23001.

77. Harbarth S, Dharan S, Liassine N, Herrault P, Auckenthaler R, Pittet D. Randomized, placebo-controlled, double-blind trial to evaluate the efficacy of mupirocin for eradicating carriage of methicillin-resistant Staphylococcus aureus. Antimicrob Agents Chemother. 1999;43(6):1412–6.

78. Ammerlaan HS, Kluytmans JA, Wertheim HF, Nouwen JL, Bonten MJ. Eradication of methicillin-resistant Staphylococcus aureus carriage: a systematic review. Clin Infect Dis. 2009;48(7):922–30.
79. Tacconelli E, Carmeli Y, Aizer A, Ferreira G, Foreman MG, D'Agata EM. Mupirocin prophylaxis to prevent Staphylococcus aureus infection in patients undergoing dialysis: a meta-analysis. Clin Infect Dis. 2003;37(12):1629–38.
80. van Rijen MM, Bonten M, Wenzel RP, Kluytmans JA. Intranasal mupirocin for reduction of Staphylococcus aureus infections in surgical patients with nasal carriage: a systematic review. J Antimicrob Chemother. 2008;61(2):254–61.
81. Kallen AJ, Wilson CT, Larson RJ. Perioperative intranasal mupirocin for the prevention of surgical-site infections: systematic review of the literature and meta-analysis. Infect Control Hosp Epidemiol. 2005;26(12):916–22.
82. van Rijen M, Bonten M, Wenzel R, Kluytmans J. Mupirocin ointment for preventing Staphylococcus aureus infections in nasal carriers. Cochrane Database Syst Rev. 2008;4:CD006216.
83. Robicsek A, Beaumont JL, Paule SM, Hacek DM, Thomson RB Jr, Kaul KL, et al. Universal surveillance for methicillin-resistant Staphylococcus aureus in 3 affiliated hospitals. Ann Intern Med. 2008;148(6):409–18.
84. Jain R, Kralovic SM, Evans ME, Ambrose M, Simbartl LA, Obrosky DS, et al. Veterans Affairs initiative to prevent methicillin-resistant Staphylococcus aureus infections. N Engl J Med. 2011;364(15):1419–30.
85. Harbarth S, Fankhauser C, Schrenzel J, Christenson J, Gervaz P, Bandiera-Clerc C, et al. Universal screening for methicillin-resistant Staphylococcus aureus at hospital admission and nosocomial infection in surgical patients. JAMA. 2008;299(10):1149–57.
86. Huang YC, Lien RI, Lin TY. Effect of mupirocin decolonization on subsequent methicillin-resistant Staphylococcus aureus infection in infants in neonatal intensive care units. Pediatr Infect Dis J. 2015;34(3):241–5.
87. Popoola VO, Budd A, Wittig SM, Ross T, Aucott SW, Perl TM, et al. Methicillin-resistant Staphylococcus aureus transmission and infections in a neonatal intensive care unit despite active surveillance cultures and decolonization: challenges for infection prevention. Infect Control Hosp Epidemiol. 2014;35(4):412–8.
88. Calfee DP, Salgado CD, Milstone AM, Harris AD, Kuhar DT, Moody J, et al. Strategies to prevent methicillin-resistant Staphylococcus aureus transmission and infection in acute care hospitals: 2014 update. Infect Control Hosp Epidemiol. 2014;35(Suppl 2):S108–32.
89. Milstone AM, Song X, Coffin S, Elward A, Society for Healthcare Epidemiology of America's Pediatric Special Interest G. Identification and eradication of methicillin-resistant Staphylococcus aureus colonization in the neonatal intensive care unit: results of a national survey. Infect Control Hosp Epidemiol. 2010;31(7):766–8.
90. Ericson JE, Popoola VO, Smith PB, Benjamin DK, Fowler VG, Benjamin DK Jr, et al. Burden of invasive Staphylococcus aureus infections in hospitalized infants. JAMA Pediatr. 2015;169(12):1105–11.
91. Popoola VO, Colantuoni E, Suwantarat N, Pierce R, Carroll KC, Aucott SW, et al. Active surveillance cultures and decolonization to reduce Staphylococcus aureus infections in the neonatal intensive care unit. Infect Control Hosp Epidemiol. 2016;37(4):381–7.
92. Delaney HM, Wang E, Melish M. Comprehensive strategy including prophylactic mupirocin to reduce Staphylococcus aureus colonization and infection in high-risk neonates. J Perinatol. 2013;33(4):313–8.
93. Hitomi S, Kubota M, Mori N, Baba S, Yano H, Okuzumi K, et al. Control of a methicillin-resistant Staphylococcus aureus outbreak in a neonatal intensive care unit by unselective use of nasal mupirocin ointment. J Hosp Infect. 2000;46(2):123–9.
94. Lee BY, Wiringa AE, Bailey RR, Goyal V, Lewis GJ, Tsui BY, et al. Screening cardiac surgery patients for MRSA: an economic computer model. Am J Manag Care. 2010;16(7):e163–73.
95. Holton DL, Nicolle LE, Diley D, Bernstein K. Efficacy of mupirocin nasal ointment in eradicating Staphylococcus aureus nasal carriage in chronic haemodialysis patients. J Hosp Infect. 1991;17(2):133–7.

96. Immerman I, Ramos NL, Katz GM, Hutzler LH, Phillips MS, Bosco JA 3rd. The persistence of Staphylococcus aureus decolonization after mupirocin and topical chlorhexidine: implications for patients requiring multiple or delayed procedures. J Arthroplast. 2012;27(6):870–6.
97. Schweizer M, Perencevich E, McDanel J, Carson J, Formanek M, Hafner J, et al. Effectiveness of a bundled intervention of decolonization and prophylaxis to decrease gram positive surgical site infections after cardiac or orthopedic surgery: systematic review and meta-analysis. BMJ. 2013;346:f2743.
98. Silvetti S, Ranucci M, Isgro G, Villa V, Costa E. Preoperative colonization in pediatric cardiac surgery and its impact on postoperative infections. Paediatr Anaesth. 2017;27(8):849–55.
99. Bode LG, Kluytmans JA, Wertheim HF, Bogaers D, Vandenbroucke-Grauls CM, Roosendaal R, et al. Preventing surgical-site infections in nasal carriers of Staphylococcus aureus. N Engl J Med. 2010;362(1):9–17.
100. Chapman AK, Aucott SW, Milstone AM. Safety of chlorhexidine gluconate used for skin antisepsis in the preterm infant. J Perinatol. 2012;32(1):4–9.
101. O'Grady NP, Alexander M, Burns LA, Dellinger EP, Garland J, Heard SO, et al. Summary of recommendations: guidelines for the prevention of intravascular catheter-related infections. Clin Infect Dis. 2011;52(9):1087–99.
102. Tamma PD, Aucott SW, Milstone AM. Chlorhexidine use in the neonatal intensive care unit: results from a national survey. Infect Control Hosp Epidemiol. 2010;31(8):846–9.
103. Aggett PJ, Cooper LV, Ellis SH, McAinsh J. Percutaneous absorption of chlorhexidine in neonatal cord care. Arch Dis Child. 1981;56(11):878–80.
104. Cowen J, Ellis SH, McAinsh J. Absorption of chlorhexidine from the intact skin of newborn infants. Arch Dis Child. 1979;54(5):379–83.
105. Garland JS, Alex CP, Uhing MR, Peterside IE, Rentz A, Harris MC. Pilot trial to compare tolerance of chlorhexidine gluconate to povidone-iodine antisepsis for central venous catheter placement in neonates. J Perinatol. 2009;29(12):808–13.
106. Noto MJ, Domenico HJ, Byrne DW, Talbot T, Rice TW, Bernard GR, et al. Chlorhexidine bathing and healthcare-associated infections: a randomized clinical trial. JAMA. 2015;313(4):369–78.
107. Frost SA, Alogso MC, Metcalfe L, Lynch JM, Hunt L, Sanghavi R, et al. Chlorhexidine bathing and health care-associated infections among adult intensive care patients: a systematic review and meta-analysis. Crit Care. 2016;20(1):379.
108. Bleasdale SC, Trick WE, Gonzalez IM, Lyles RD, Hayden MK, Weinstein RA. Effectiveness of chlorhexidine bathing to reduce catheter-associated bloodstream infections in medical intensive care unit patients. Arch Intern Med. 2007;167(19):2073–9.
109. Climo MW, Yokoe DS, Warren DK, Perl TM, Bolon M, Herwaldt LA, et al. Effect of daily chlorhexidine bathing on hospital-acquired infection. N Engl J Med. 2013;368(6):533–42.
110. Milstone AM, Elward A, Song X, Zerr DM, Orscheln R, Speck K, et al. Daily chlorhexidine bathing to reduce bacteraemia in critically ill children: a multicentre, cluster-randomised, crossover trial. Lancet. 2013;381(9872):1099–106.
111. McNeil JC, Kok EY, Vallejo JG, Campbell JR, Hulten KG, Mason EO, et al. Clinical and molecular features of decreased chlorhexidine susceptibility among nosocomial Staphylococcus aureus isolates at Texas Children's Hospital. Antimicrob Agents Chemother. 2016;60(2):1121–8.
112. Huang SS, Septimus E, Kleinman K, Moody J, Hickok J, Avery TR, et al. Targeted versus universal decolonization to prevent ICU infection. N Engl J Med. 2013;368(24):2255–65.
113. Martinez-Resendez MF, Garza-Gonzalez E, Mendoza-Olazaran S, Herrera-Guerra A, Rodriguez-Lopez JM, Perez-Rodriguez E, et al. Impact of daily chlorhexidine baths and hand hygiene compliance on nosocomial infection rates in critically ill patients. Am J Infect Control. 2014;42(7):713–7.
114. Derde LPG, Cooper BS, Goossens H, Malhotra-Kumar S, Willems RJL, Gniadkowski M, et al. Interventions to reduce colonisation and transmission of antimicrobial-resistant bacteria in intensive care units: an interrupted time series study and cluster randomised trial. Lancet Infect Dis. 2014;14(1):31–9.

115. Price R, MacLennan G, Glen J. Selective digestive or oropharyngeal decontamination and topical oropharyngeal chlorhexidine for prevention of death in general intensive care: systematic review and network meta-analysis. BMJ. 2014;348:g2197.
116. Zhao D, Song J, Gao X, Gao F, Wu Y, Lu Y, et al. Selective oropharyngeal decontamination versus selective digestive decontamination in critically ill patients: a meta-analysis of randomized controlled trials. Drug Des Devel Ther. 2015;9:3617–24.
117. Plantinga NL, de Smet A, Oostdijk EAN, de Jonge E, Camus C, Krueger WA, et al. Selective digestive and oropharyngeal decontamination in medical and surgical ICU patients: individual patient data meta-analysis. Clin Microbiol Infect. 2017;24(5):505–13.
118. Houben AJ, Oostdijk EA, van der Voort PH, Monen JC, Bonten MJ, van der Bij AK. Selective decontamination of the oropharynx and the digestive tract, and antimicrobial resistance: a 4 year ecological study in 38 intensive care units in the Netherlands. J Antimicrob Chemother. 2014;69(3):797–804.
119. Buelow E, Bello Gonzalez TDJ, Fuentes S, de Steenhuijsen Piters WAA, Lahti L, Bayjanov JR, et al. Comparative gut microbiota and resistome profiling of intensive care patients receiving selective digestive tract decontamination and healthy subjects. Microbiome. 2017;5(1):88.
120. Petros A, Silvestri L, Booth R, Taylor N, van Saene H. Selective decontamination of the digestive tract in critically ill children: systematic review and meta-analysis. Pediatr Crit Care Med. 2013;14(1):89–97.
121. Classen DC, Evans RS, Pestotnik SL, Horn SD, Menlove RL, Burke JP. The timing of prophylactic administration of antibiotics and the risk of surgical-wound infection. N Engl J Med. 1992;326(5):281–6.
122. Franco LM, Cota GF, Pinto TS, Ercole FF. Preoperative bathing of the surgical site with chlorhexidine for infection prevention: systematic review with meta-analysis. Am J Infect Control. 2017;45(4):343–9.
123. Kapadia BH, Elmallah RK, Mont MA. A randomized, clinical trial of preadmission chlorhexidine skin preparation for lower extremity total joint arthroplasty. J Arthroplasty. 2016;31(12):2856–61.
124. Saraswat MK, Magruder JT, Crawford TC, Gardner JM, Duquaine D, Sussman MS, et al. Preoperative Staphylococcus Aureus screening and targeted decolonization in cardiac surgery. Ann Thorac Surg. 2017;104(4):1349–56.
125. Wang Z, Zheng J, Zhao Y, Xiang Y, Chen X, Zhao F, et al. Preoperative bathing with chlorhexidine reduces the incidence of surgical site infections after total knee arthroplasty: a meta-analysis. Medicine (Baltimore). 2017;96(47):e8321.
126. Dumville JC, McFarlane E, Edwards P, Lipp A, Holmes A, Liu Z. Preoperative skin antiseptics for preventing surgical wound infections after clean surgery. Cochrane Database Syst Rev. 2015;4:CD003949.
127. Berrios-Torres SI, Umscheid CA, Bratzler DW, Leas B, Stone EC, Kelz RR, et al. Centers for Disease Control and Prevention guideline for the prevention of surgical site infection, 2017. JAMA Surg. 2017;152(8):784–91.
128. Darouiche RO, Wall MJ Jr, Itani KM, Otterson MF, Webb AL, Carrick MM, et al. Chlorhexidine-alcohol versus povidone-iodine for surgical-site antisepsis. N Engl J Med. 2010;362(1):18–26.
129. Thom KA, Escobar D, Boutin MA, Zhan M, Harris AD, Johnson JK. Frequent contamination of nursing scrubs is associated with specific care activities. Am J Infect Control. 2018;46(5):503–6.
130. Tuazon CU. Skin and skin structure infections in the patient at risk: carrier state of Staphylococcus aureus. Am J Med. 1984;76(5A):166–71.
131. Crusz SA, Yates C, Holden S, Kearns A, Boswell T. Prolonged outbreak of Staphylococcus aureus surgical site infection traced to a healthcare worker with psoriasis. J Hosp Infect. 2014;86(1):42–6.
132. van Ingen J, Kohl TA, Kranzer K, Hasse B, Keller PM, Katarzyna Szafranska A, et al. Global outbreak of severe Mycobacterium chimaera disease after cardiac surgery: a molecular epidemiological study. Lancet Infect Dis. 2017;17(10):1033–41.

133. Kramer A, Schwebke I, Kampf G. How long do nosocomial pathogens persist on inanimate surfaces? A systematic review. BMC Infect Dis. 2006;6:130.
134. Otter JA, Yezli S, French GL. The role played by contaminated surfaces in the transmission of nosocomial pathogens. Infect Control Hosp Epidemiol. 2011;32(7):687–99.
135. Carling PC, Parry MF, Von Beheren SM, Healthcare Environmental Hygiene Study G. Identifying opportunities to enhance environmental cleaning in 23 acute care hospitals. Infect Control Hosp Epidemiol. 2008;29(1):1–7.
136. Carling PC, Von Beheren S, Kim P, Woods C, Healthcare Environmental Hygiene Study G. Intensive care unit environmental cleaning: an evaluation in sixteen hospitals using a novel assessment tool. J Hosp Infect. 2008;68(1):39–44.
137. Boyce JM, Havill NL, Havill HL, Mangione E, Dumigan DG, Moore BA. Comparison of fluorescent marker systems with 2 quantitative methods of assessing terminal cleaning practices. Infect Control Hosp Epidemiol. 2011;32(12):1187–93.
138. Eckstein BC, Adams DA, Eckstein EC, Rao A, Sethi AK, Yadavalli GK, et al. Reduction of Clostridium difficile and vancomycin-resistant Enterococcus contamination of environmental surfaces after an intervention to improve cleaning methods. BMC Infect Dis. 2007;7:61.
139. Boyce JM, Havill NL, Dumigan DG, Golebiewski M, Balogun O, Rizvani R. Monitoring the effectiveness of hospital cleaning practices by use of an adenosine triphosphate bioluminescence assay. Infect Control Hosp Epidemiol. 2009;30(7):678–84.
140. Goodman ER, Platt R, Bass R, Onderdonk AB, Yokoe DS, Huang SS. Impact of an environmental cleaning intervention on the presence of methicillin-resistant Staphylococcus aureus and vancomycin-resistant enterococci on surfaces in intensive care unit rooms. Infect Control Hosp Epidemiol. 2008;29(7):593–9.
141. Carling PC, Parry MM, Rupp ME, Po JL, Dick B, Von Beheren S, et al. Improving cleaning of the environment surrounding patients in 36 acute care hospitals. Infect Control Hosp Epidemiol. 2008;29(11):1035–41.
142. McDonnell G, Russell AD. Antiseptics and disinfectants: activity, action, and resistance. Clin Microbiol Rev. 1999;12(1):147–79.
143. Rutala WA, Weber DJ. Are room decontamination units needed to prevent transmission of environmental pathogens? Infect Control Hosp Epidemiol. 2011;32(8):743–7.
144. Davies A, Pottage T, Bennett A, Walker J. Gaseous and air decontamination technologies for Clostridium difficile in the healthcare environment. J Hosp Infect. 2011;77(3):199–203.
145. Rutala WA, Gergen MF, Weber DJ. Room decontamination with UV radiation. Infect Control Hosp Epidemiol. 2010;31(10):1025–9.
146. Weber DJ, Rutala WA, Anderson DJ, Chen LF, Sickbert-Bennett EE, Boyce JM. Effectiveness of ultraviolet devices and hydrogen peroxide systems for terminal room decontamination: focus on clinical trials. Am J Infect Control. 2016;44(5 Suppl):e77–84.
147. Rutala WA, Weber DJ. Selection of the ideal disinfectant. Infect Control Hosp Epidemiol. 2014;35(7):855–65.
148. 2018. Available from: https://www.cdc.gov/infectioncontrol/pdf/guidelines/disinfection-guidelines.pdf.
149. Ferranti G, Marchesi I, Favale M, Borella P, Bargellini A. Aetiology, source and prevention of waterborne healthcare-associated infections: a review. J Med Microbiol. 2014;63(Pt 10):1247–59.
150. Verissimo A, Vesey G, Rocha GM, Marrao G, Colbourne J, Dennis PJ, et al. A hot water supply as the source of Legionella pneumophila in incubators of a neonatology unit. J Hosp Infect. 1990;15(3):255–63.
151. Yiallouros PK, Papadouri T, Karaoli C, Papamichael E, Zeniou M, Pieridou-Bagatzouni D, et al. First outbreak of nosocomial Legionella infection in term neonates caused by a cold mist ultrasonic humidifier. Clin Infect Dis. 2013;57(1):48–56.

Role of Antimicrobial Stewardship

3

Sarah Kubes and Luis A. Castagnini

Introduction

The introduction and innovation of antibiotics has drastically improved current medical practice and made once untreatable infections curable today. Prompt administration of antibiotics to treat infections reduces morbidity and mortality [1]; however, overuse and inappropriate use of antibiotics can result in the emergence of antibiotic-resistant bacteria. Studies report between 20 and 50% of all antibiotics prescribed in the United States are unnecessary or inappropriate [2–5]. Furthermore, antibiotics are commonly prescribed in pediatric practice, with about 60% of inpatient visits and nearly 20% of outpatient visits resulting in at least one prescribed antibiotic [6–8].

The Centers for Disease Control and Prevention (CDC) report over 23,000 deaths and more than two million infections attributable to antibiotic-resistant bacteria in the United States each year. As a result, the CDC and Centers for Medicare and Medicaid Services (CMS) collaborated to promote the implementation of antibiotic stewardship programs (ASP) in healthcare centers that receive funding from CMS or accreditation by the Joint Commission [9]. Effective January 1, 2017, the Joint Commission required that all acute care hospitals, nursing homes, and outpatient facilities have an ASP in place [10, 11].

Antimicrobial stewardship is a coordinated effort to optimize antimicrobial choice, dose, route, and duration of therapy appropriate for the type and location of infection [12, 13]. The primary goal of ASPs is to improve clinical outcomes while preventing unintended consequences of antimicrobial prescribing,

L. A. Castagnini (✉)
Department of Pediatrics, Section of Infectious Diseases, Baylor College of Medicine and The Children's Hospital of San Antonio, San Antonio, TX, USA
e-mail: Luis.castagnini@bcm.edu

S. Kubes
Pharmacy, The Children's Hospital of San Antonio, San Antonio, TX, USA

© Springer Nature Switzerland AG 2019
J. C. McNeil et al. (eds.), *Healthcare-Associated Infections in Children*,
https://doi.org/10.1007/978-3-319-98122-2_3

including adverse drug reactions, *Clostridium difficile* infections, and the emergence of multidrug-resistant organisms (MDROs). Through this multifaceted effort, many programs report improvements in their local bacterial resistance patterns, as well as a decrease in antimicrobial spending [13]. It is in this regard that ASPs provide an essential role in infection prevention. The basic principles of antimicrobial stewardship and their relationship to prevention of MDROs will be discussed in this chapter.

Mechanisms of Antibiotic Resistance

Bacteria can have intrinsic or acquired resistance to antibiotics depending on whether all members of the species display such resistance or not. Different types of mechanisms account for phenotypic resistance to antibiotics, some of which will be discussed here (Table 3.1) [14]:

1. Enzymatic inactivation of the antibiotic
2. Decreased penetration (or increased efflux) of the antibiotic to the target site
3. Alteration of the antibiotic binding site

Resistance to β-lactam antibiotics most commonly is caused by the production of enzymes that inactivates the drug (β-lactamases) or by alteration of the binding site (penicillin-binding proteins, or PBPs). Most resistant gram-negative organisms produce β-lactamases as their primary resistance mechanism, whereas gram-positive organisms usually manifest their β-lactam resistance through the alteration of PBPs.

Table 3.1 Mechanisms of resistance in classes of antibiotics used to treat resistant pathogens. Examples of resistance mechanisms are also provided

	Permeability	Enzymatic destruction	Altered binding sites	Efflux pumps
β-lactams	X	X β-lactamases	X Penicillin-binding proteins	X
Fluoroquinolones	X		X Alteration in DNA gyrase and topoisomerase IV. Protection by plasmid-mediated Qnr protein	X
Aminoglycosides	X	X Adenolyating and acetylating enzymes	X 30S ribosomal subunit	X
Tetracyclines	X	X Modification enzymes	X 70S ribosomal unit	X

Reproduced from Karam et al. [14]

Occasionally, some organisms harbor both mechanisms of resistance, for example, methicillin-resistant *Staphylococcus aureus* (MRSA) possesses altered PBP2 and a β-lactamase [15]. As β-lactamase-producing gram-negative organisms emerged, new enzyme inhibitors were developed to overcome this resistance mechanism. These enzyme inhibitors include clavulanic acid, sulbactam, and tazobactam. However, over the last few decades, an increasing number of MDROs with the ability to hydrolyze these enzyme inhibitors are being reported among community-acquired infections [16].

Such multidrug-resistant gram-negative pathogens commonly express extended-spectrum β-lactamases (ESBLs) as their primary resistance mechanism and are phenotypically resistant to benzylpenicillin, cephalosporins, and monobactams while maintaining susceptibilities to carbapenems and cephamycins [17]. An emerging group of β-lactamases called carbapenemases are plasmid-encoded and can now be found in many species of Enterobacteriaceae. These organisms are particularly worrisome because, in addition to degrading penicillin and cephalosporins, they are also capable of hydrolyzing carbapenems [18]. Another type of β-lactamase called Ambler class C (or simply AmpC) is a chromosomally or plasmid-encoded enzyme that has the potential to be "induced" during β-lactam therapy, especially is the organism is exposed to ampicillin, cefoxitin, or imipenem [19]. The AmpC enzyme is most commonly found in *Enterobacter*, *Citrobacter*, and *Serratia* species [20]. Organisms carrying the plasmid containing AmpC are frequently resistant to penicillins (including those in combination with a β-lactamase inhibitor) and third-generation cephalosporins but are usually susceptible to cefepime and carbapenems [20]. Another mechanism of resistance involves efflux pumps, which are specific proteins capable of removing the antibiotic from inside the cell, rendering them ineffective. Most macrolide-resistant *Streptococcus pneumoniae* express a macrolide efflux pump [21].

Benefits of ASP

Minimizing the Risk of Multidrug-Resistant Pathogens

The emergence of multidrug-resistant organisms is one of the biggest threats the healthcare system faces today. Several strategies have been described to curb the emergence of resistance, including preventing infections, understanding and minimizing risk factors in individual patients, developing new antimicrobials and modern technologies for rapid and accurate diagnosis, and improving antibiotic prescribing by the implementation of ASPs. Multiple studies show a significant reduction in the prevalence of MDROs in institutions where an ASP is in place [22–25], underscoring stewardship's place in infection prevention. In March 2015, the National Action Plan for Combating Antibiotic-Resistant Bacteria issued by the White House called for the establishment of an ASP in all acute care facilities throughout the United States by the year 2020 to halt the threat of antibiotic resistance throughout the nation [3, 13].

Decrease in Inappropriate Antimicrobials

Improving antibiotic use is a patient safety and quality of care priority, and therefore healthcare organizations should make every effort to institute policies and procedures to optimize their use and track changes over time. There is large variation in antibiotic use among pediatric hospitals across the United States [7]. Inappropriate or unnecessary use of antimicrobials is estimated to account for approximately 25–30% of all prescriptions in pediatric settings [5]. Agwu et al. demonstrated a reduction of 15% in antibiotic use and a decrease in antibiotic-related costs of more than 20% after the implementation of an ASP; moreover, the authors reported an increase in provider satisfaction from 22% to 68% after ASP implementation [26]. Other studies report similar findings [27–29]. Inappropriate antibiotic use has been linked to adverse outcomes, including toxicity, the selection of pathogenic organisms such as *C. difficile*, and the emergence of organisms resistant to broad-spectrum antimicrobial agents [23, 30, 31], highlighting the potential benefits of an ASP.

Many ASP strategies have been proposed to augment reductions in resistance and assist in inappropriate use. The most effective strategies to decrease the inappropriate use of antimicrobials are the prospective audit with feedback and preauthorization. These approaches will be discussed below. Antibiotic cycling (also called antibiotic rotation) is a strategy in which an antibiotic (or antibiotic class) is substituted with a different antibiotic (or antibiotic class) with a similar spectrum of activity for a defined period of time. This practice has not demonstrated to be effective in reducing the emergence of resistance, and, thus, this strategy is not routinely recommended [13, 32].

Components of an ASP

The CDC outlines the seven core elements of a successful hospital antibiotic stewardship program as leadership commitment, accountability, drug expertise, action, tracking, reporting, and education (Table 3.2) [9].

Table 3.2 Core elements of an effective antimicrobial stewardship program

Core elements
Leadership support
Formal statement of support
Support training and education
Assure ASP personnel has time, authority, and accountability
Accountability/drug expertise
Appointment of a single leader who will be responsible for program outcomes
Key supporters: infection preventionists, quality improvement staff, clinicians and department heads, laboratory staff, information technology staff, and nurses
Identify a single pharmacy leader who will co-lead the program
Formal training in infectious diseases and/or antibiotic stewardship is beneficial

Table 3.2   (continued)

Core elements
Action
Develop guidelines, policies, and protocols to support optimal prescribing
Establish pharmacy-driven interventions (automatic intravenous to oral change, dose adjustments for organ dysfunction, dose optimization, detection of antibiotic-related drug-drug interactions, automatic stop orders, and alerts for duplicative therapy)
Provide real-time interventions through prospective audit with feedback and/or preauthorization
Improve prescribing for specific syndromes
Tracking/reporting
Monitor antibiotic prescribing
Measure antibiotic use as either days of therapy (DOT) or defined daily dose (DDD)
Track clinical outcomes to measure the impact of interventions to improve antibiotic use
Assessment of antibiotic use process measures through periodic assessments of the quality of antibiotic use
Education
ASP should provide regular updates on antibiotic prescribing, resistance, and infectious diseases management
Web-based educational resources can help facilities develop educational content
Education may be communicated via didactic lectures, posters, educational flyers, and/or newsletters

Adapted from Pollack and Srinivasan [9]

Leadership Commitment

Leadership commitment and support is imperative for the success of ASPs. Resources must be allocated to staff, pharmacy, laboratory, and information technology as needed by the program. A formal statement of support from leadership, supporting training and education, and participation from many departments within the hospital are examples of leadership support [9]. The staff from relevant departments that actively participate in the ASP should be given sufficient time to successfully perform their stewardship activities. An Internet-based survey of pediatric hospitals estimated the median annual cost for a pediatric ASP as $187,400 [33]. Funding and financial support can vastly influence the success of stewardship programs; however, this investment can ultimately lead to reduced expenditures in other areas [26, 34–38]. Stewardship programs will often pay for themselves during the first year of implementation though indirect cost savings and decreased antibiotic expenditures [36, 38].

Accountability

In addition to leadership commitment, the CDC recommends identifying a single physician leader as responsible for the program implementation and outcomes. Some institutions appoint a pharmacist to co-lead the program [39, 40]. The co-leaders should have formal training in infectious diseases and/or antibiotic stewardship and should have enough time allotted to develop and manage stewardship programs [40]. Large institutions usually implement successful programs by hiring full-time staff to develop the program, while smaller institutions employ part-time or off-site personnel [41]. Studies do acknowledge that hospitalists may be a reasonable option as a physician leader [42, 43]; however, infectious diseases physicians may be the ideal physician champion to lead multidisciplinary ASP teams given their additional training [44]. Additionally, the CDC recommends that local Pharmacy and Therapeutics committees, if serving as the stewardship team, should participate in activities beyond only formulary management and patient safety issues [41, 45, 46]. Furthermore, ASPs are most successful when key personnel, such as prescribers from different departments, infection preventionists, quality improvement personnel, laboratory staff, nurses, and information technology personnel, play an active role in the program [47–51].

Expertise

The established leaders and key support members of the team should develop and implement policies and interventions to improve antibiotic use [9]. The development of a facility-specific formulary, antibiograms, and evidence-based treatment guidelines and pathways can help to standardize care and ensure optimal antibiotic selection, duration, and dose [4, 52, 53]. Programs should choose interventions based on the needs of the facility and implement them progressively to ensure staff acceptance and adequate data collection over time [54].

General interventions include antibiotic "time-outs" [55–58], prior authorization [59], and prospective audit and feedback [60, 61]. Automatic intravenous to oral interchange [62, 63], dose adjustments based on renal and hepatic dysfunction, dose optimization [64, 65], prevention of duplication of therapy [66], time-sensitive automatic stop orders, and assessing antibiotic-associated drug-drug interactions are examples of pharmacy-driven ASP initiatives. Furthermore, facility-specific guidelines for common conditions, including community-acquired pneumonia [67–70], urinary tract infections [71–73], skin and soft tissue infections [62, 74], *C. difficile* infections [75, 76], invasive bacterial infections [77], and empiric coverage for MRSA infections [78, 79], should be created to guide practice and improve prescribing.

After the establishment of clinical pathways and guidelines, the ASP should monitor antimicrobial use and track resistance patterns, as well as report data trends to respective committees. Finally, the ASP should provide formative feedback and education to prescribers and other clinical staff [3, 9].

ASP Strategies

Many different antibiotic stewardship strategies have been shown to be effective together or apart [28, 80]. Strategies that are utilized by ASPs are based on local utilization patterns, pharmacy formulary, available resources, and expertise. When initiating a program, it is important to focus on key issues, rather than implementing multiple different interventions at a time [13, 54].

Antibiotic use oversight is one of the major functions that ASPs play. Both prospective audit and feedback and preauthorization are approaches of antibiotic oversight. A newer method coined "the handshake method," developed at the Children's Hospital of Colorado, is a rounding-based, in-person approach to feedback by a co-led pharmacist and physician team, which has been found to be very effective at reducing antimicrobial use and subsequent antibiotic costs [81].

Prospective Audit and Feedback

Prospective audit and feedback utilizes trained staff, such as an antibiotic stewardship pharmacist or a physician expert in antibiotic use, to provide daily reviews of all antimicrobial orders and strive to optimize their use based on drug, dose, and route of administration [82]. Furthermore, the ASP team provides verbal or written recommendations to providers regarding their prescribing practices. This approach does not delay the first dose of an antibiotic to the patient and recommendation acceptance is voluntary by the prescriber. This strategy allows for provider autonomy when making prescribing choices and can increase the visibility of the ASP with the focus on collegial relationships [13]. Advantages of this approach include reduction of inappropriate use of antibiotics in multiple settings (i.e., inpatient, nursing homes, and outpatient), cost savings, and decrease in hospital-acquired infections [26, 28, 29, 78, 83–85]. Acceptance of recommendations improves when they come from an established program [83]. This strategy, however, is labor and time intensive and greatly depends on available resources – such as a full-time pharmacist or infectious disease physician and information technology support/surveillance systems. Furthermore, agreement with ASP recommendations is voluntary and success often depends on the method of delivering feedback. As a result, many programs focus their efforts around specific groups of patients (e.g., intensive care and neonatal units), targeted antibiotics, high-cost antibiotics, or antibiotics with higher risk of toxic side effects (e.g., vancomycin and aminoglycosides) [86]. Overall interventions are more frequently accepted when formative feedback is given on a regular basis [87].

Preauthorization

Preauthorization is another strategy that is often utilized by ASPs in conjunction with prospective audit and feedback or as a sole means of antibiotic oversight. This strategy focuses on requiring approval by an infectious disease physician or ASP team member prior to administration of restricted antibiotics. Some antibiotics may be restricted to certain indications or patient populations [13]. This approach allows for optimization of initial antibiotic selection and allows the ASP to provide education to prescribers regarding antibiotic choice. Preauthorization has been shown to be effective in reducing costs of antibiotic use and decreasing the utilization of targeted antibiotics (e.g., carbapenems) [88], which suggests that preauthorization is a passive barrier to prescribing. There are conflicting data regarding the impact of preauthorization on improvement of local antibiotic susceptibility patterns – some studies suggest improvements, while others do not. Preauthorization programs may be perceived as intrusive with prescriber autonomy [89], which may limit its successful implementation and acceptance; furthermore, prescribers may feel this approach results in a delay of therapy. It is also a time and labor-intensive process, requiring full-time coverage or a provider on call. Many programs with limited resources may allow for initiation of the restricted antibiotic therapy during off hours and review the following day for appropriateness and approval. Finally, preauthorization may cause an inadvertent increase in utilization of nonrestricted antibiotics, which would diminish the intended clinical effect [13].

Clinical Guidelines

In addition to antibiotic oversight, ASPs should play an active role in developing hospital-specific clinical guidelines and algorithms centered on antibiotic susceptibilities and formulary. Clinical pathways guide prescribers when selecting empiric therapy and promote de-escalation of treatment, shorter duration of therapy, and conversion to oral alternatives earlier in the course of treatment [13, 90]. Programs should focus on common pediatric infections such as community-acquired pneumonia, urinary tract infections, musculoskeletal infections, febrile neutropenia, and complicated appendicitis [91–94]. Lee et al. utilized guideline implementation as their means for stewardship and found a significant reduction in the use of targeted broad-spectrum antibiotics and pharmacy acquisition costs [92]. Additionally, Willis et al. reported that implementation of both an ASP and clinical practice guidelines decreased the use of unnecessary antibiotics and surgical site infections in patients diagnosed with complicated appendicitis [93], again suggesting the value of ASPs in infection prevention. The development of clinical guidance pathways has improved clinical outcomes in patients by decreasing mortality, length of stay, adverse events from antibiotics, readmission rates, and cost of therapy [13].

Pharmacy-Led Initiatives

Pharmacy-driven interventions may be utilized to optimize antibiotic therapy; examples include streamlining and de-escalation of therapy, intravenous to oral conversions, dosing adjustments for renal or hepatic dysfunction, and therapeutic drug monitoring.

De-escalation and Antimicrobial Streamlining

Antimicrobial streamlining and de-escalation play a major role in ASPs, especially among programs that utilize the prospective audit with feedback method. Antibiotic streamlining is the practice of converting a broad-spectrum empirical regimen to directed therapy with either a single, narrow-spectrum parenteral agent, an oral agent based on cultures and susceptibilities, or discontinuing all therapy based on negative cultures when appropriate [95]. De-escalating therapy can result in a decrease in antibiotic expenditures, antibiotic-related adverse events, and unnecessary antibiotic exposure [40, 96, 97]. De-escalation of therapy may come with challenges, as recommendations to de-escalate treatment may not be accepted because of physicians' reluctance to change therapy if the patient is improving regardless of culture results. Additionally, if initial cultures were obtained after the initiation of antibiotics or cultures were not obtained, the ASP may have limited ability to assess a patient's therapy for de-escalation [40].

Intravenous to Oral Transition
Transition from intravenous (IV) to orally (PO) administered therapy is another important modality by which ASPs de-escalate therapy. ASPs should work closely with the pharmacy team to develop policies and protocols to transition patients from IV to PO preparations of antibiotics when clinically appropriate [13]. Programs that aim to increase the use of oral antibiotics and early transition for IV to PO in select conditions demonstrate a decrease in length of stay and drug costs without compromising safety [13, 98, 99]. When developing this type of policy, it is important to outline patients who would benefit from it and determine the most appropriate timing to do so. Some key factors to consider in pediatric patients include indication of therapy, bioavailability of the drug, penetration of the agent into the infected site, targeted microbes, ability to tolerate an enteral diet, and compliance with the treatment regimen [13].

Pharmacokinetic Drug Monitoring
Another pharmacy-driven intervention is pharmacokinetic drug monitoring, which utilizes personalized dosing based on the patient's absorption, distribution, and clearance, to ensure optimal outcomes and minimize toxicity [100]. Individualized monitoring and adjustment of both aminoglycosides and vancomycin have been shown to increase the chance of attaining appropriate therapeutic drug levels while also reducing the risk of toxicity [101–104]. Additionally, studies have reported an overall decrease in costs, hospital length of stay, and mortality when these interventions are in place [105–108]. Pharmacists also play a key role in dose optimization for end-organ dysfunction on an ongoing basis to ensure an adequate dose is utilized in cases where renal and/or hepatic dysfunction may occur [100].

Education

ASPs should aim to provide routine education to many targeted disciplines such as pharmacy personnel, nursing, students, and prescribers [13]. Timely education and feedback should focus on antibiotic prescribing, resistance patterns, and infectious disease-related updates on current national and local practices [3]. Additionally, benchmarking current prescribing to that of other facilities has been found to be an effective method to improve variable prescribing practices between institutions [109]. Education through lectures, posters, flyers, and newsletters are also key aspects of the program to ensure the most current recommendations and guidelines are being implemented, as well as updating the hospital staff on the successes and opportunities for improvement of the program. Furthermore, Web-based educational activities are valuable resources to assist in an educational curriculum [110, 111]. The combination of education and antibiotic oversight is the most effective way to sustain appropriate prescribing [40, 112].

ASP Metrics

While the optimal metrics for monitoring and reporting have not been established, ongoing measurements are imperative, as they help the ASP to identify areas to allocate resources and efforts to improve the quality and success of the program [113, 114]. ASPs should utilize local and national benchmark data, where available, to assess their own improvement opportunities. The two main measures of antibiotic usage are the defined daily dose (DDD) and the number of days of therapy (DOT). The Infectious Diseases Society of America (IDSA)/Society of Healthcare Epidemiology of America (SHEA) guidelines suggest using DOT as the preferred method to evaluate ASPs [13].

DOT is the number of days a patient receives antibiotics and is calculated as the total number of days any antibiotic agent is administered to a patient, divided by a census-based denominator (usually 1000 patient-days), regardless of the number of daily doses or the strength of the dose [113, 115]. For example, if a patient receives one antibiotic for 4 days, the DOT would be 4; however, the data can be skewed by patients receiving more than one antibiotic per day (e.g., if a patient receives two antibiotics for 4 days, the DOT would be 8) or patients receiving antibiotics every other day (e.g., if a patient receives one antibiotic every other day for 4 days, the DOT would be 2). Additionally, cost savings cannot be easily calculated because the dose is not included in DOT calculations. (Note: cost savings should be determined based off administration data and not purchasing data [13, 90].) However, DOT is the standard method used to collect antibiotic use (AU) data to report to the National Healthcare Safety Network (NHSN) [13, 90].

DDD summates the total number of grams of each antibiotic administered over a period of time divided by a standard DDD per the World Health Organization. This value is easy to calculate but underestimates exposure in patients with renal dysfunction and does not account for weight-based dosing; thus it is not the preferred modality for pediatric patients [13, 90, 116].

Stewardship programs should perform reviews of antibiotic use to determine appropriateness of prescribing. Drug utilization evaluations, as well as assessing the appropriateness of orders, should be conducted on a routine basis. Antibiotic use should be assessed for the following [13]:

- The frequency of appropriate diagnostic testing utilization and if they were conducted prior to treatment
- The frequency of documenation of appropriate duration of and indication for antimicrobials
- The rate at which antibiotics are tailored to final cultures
- The rate of "drug-bug" mismatches
- The rate of intravenous to oral switch when appropriate
- The frequency of clinical practice guideline utilization

Furthermore, ASPs should evaluate the effectiveness of antibiotic oversight. For the prospective audit and feedback method, the number of documented interventions and the proportion of accepted recommendations should be assessed. Facilities utilizing the preauthorization method should evaluate the overall adherence to implemented policies or protocols [13].

Outcome measures should be determined for patients who receive antibiotics to quantify the impact of ASP interventions. These outcome measures include [13]:

- Hospital length of stay
- Rate or number of patients with infections caused by multidrug-resistant organisms
- Readmission rates
- Mortality rates attributed to infections
- *Clostridium difficile* infections rates
- Time to administration of first dose of antibiotics in identified sepsis patients

An antibiogram is a summative representation of antibiotic susceptibility data for bacterial isolates over a specified period and has an important role in ASPs and infection control. Antibiograms provide prescribers with a starting point to select empiric antibiotics for the likely bacteria causing the infection. Some hospitals report an annual antibiogram of the entire facility, while other hospitals may report quarterly and unit-specific or infection site-specific data. For facilities in a multiple hospital system or a pediatric hospital within an adult hospital, data should be stratified and specific to the population of interest [13]. The antibiogram should follow guidelines set by the Clinical and Laboratory Standards Institute (CLSI), which recommend cumulative reporting at least annually with finalized cultures, including data on organisms with greater than 30 unique isolates per reporting period, and including only susceptibility data for antibiotics utilized at the facility with selective reporting.

Future Directions of ASP Programs

Broad-spectrum antibiotics are given empirically during the period of time when awaiting an organism identification and susceptibility information. However, with the new implementation of rapid diagnostics, microbiology laboratories are able to provide accurate identification of organisms and their susceptibilities faster, allowing the ASP to streamline therapy earlier in the course of illness [117]. Molecular and gene-based resistance detection platforms are rapidly being taken to market, in hopes to improve infectious disease-related outcomes. Recent data show improved all-cause 30-day mortality, decreased length of stay, and significant cost reduction when rapid diagnostic methods are integrated with ASPs [118]. New technologies include nucleic acid-based diagnostics (i.e., monoplex and multiplex PCR testing) [119–121], microarray panels [122], matrix-assisted laser desorption-ionization time-of-flight mass spectrometry (MALDI-TOF MS) [123], peptide nucleic acid fluorescent in situ hybridization (FISH) [124], and next-generation sequencing [125]. While these new innovative platforms can rapidly detect and identify an organism, they cannot definitively rule out an infection [117]. Additionally, improper utilization of these new diagnostic modalities can drive up hospital-related costs [126]. As such, ASPs may also have a role in providing guidance on which patients may benefit most from these potentially helpful but costly technologies.

In addition to the diagnostic stewardship with innovative technology, ASPs are branching to other care areas. Currently, hospital-based ASPs focus primarily on inpatient antibiotic prescribing during a patient's hospitalization, rarely assessing discharge prescribing or even outpatient antibiotic management [127]. Antibiotic prescribing at the time of discharge is often inappropriate and may be associated with unnecessary outpatient parenteral antibiotic therapy, which can result in adverse outcomes such as catheter infections, intravascular clots, and increased incurred costs [128]. A mandatory ASP review of discharge parenteral antibiotics can reduce the unnecessary use of outpatient parenteral antibiotic therapy, likely due to a transition to oral therapy [129].

In addition to targeting discharge parenteral antibiotics, stewardship programs should strive to reduce outpatient antibiotic use by branching into the community. Since the majority of antibiotic prescribing is done in outpatient settings, ASPs should target these patients [130–132]. Audit and feedback has been found to be an effective method, in an outpatient setting, to reduce antibiotic prescribing through ongoing provider feedback and education [133, 134]. Such interventions when performed on a large scale could conceivably reduce the incidence of community-acquired antibiotic-resistant infections, although data for this are lacking.

Conclusion

Antimicrobial stewardship is a coordinated effort to optimize antimicrobial therapy for patients. Implementation of facility-specific formularies and clinical guidance pathways coupled with prospective audit and feedback and preauthorization are effective techniques to improve antibiotic use. From a global perspective, ASP interventions have been shown to result in decreased antimicrobial use, reduced antimicrobial costs, fewer prescribing errors, and overall improvements in local susceptibility patterns. Finally, ASP interventions improve patient outcomes with reported reductions in mortality, length of stay, adverse drug events, and readmissions.

References

1. Dellinger RP, et al. Surviving Sepsis Campaign: international guidelines for management of severe sepsis and septic shock, 2012. Intensive Care Med. 2013;39(2):165–228.
2. Ingram PR, et al. Point-prevalence study of inappropriate antibiotic use at a tertiary Australian hospital. Intern Med J. 2012;42(6):719–21.
3. Camins BC, et al. Impact of an antimicrobial utilization program on antimicrobial use at a large teaching hospital: a randomized controlled trial. Infect Control Hosp Epidemiol. 2009;30(10):931–8.
4. Levin PD, et al. Antimicrobial use in the ICU: indications and accuracy – an observational trial. J Hosp Med. 2012;7(9):672–8.
5. Patel SJ, et al. Antibiotic use in neonatal intensive care units and adherence with Centers for Disease Control and Prevention 12 step campaign to prevent antimicrobial resistance. Pediatr Infect Dis J. 2009;28(12):1047–51.
6. Nichols K, et al. Pediatric antimicrobial stewardship programs. J Pediatr Pharmacol Ther. 2017;22(1):77–80.
7. Gerber JS, et al. Variability in antibiotic use at children's hospitals. Pediatrics. 2010;126(6):1067–73.
8. Hersh AL, et al. Antibiotic prescribing in ambulatory pediatrics in the United States. Pediatrics. 2011;128(6):1053–61.
9. Pollack LA, Srinivasan A. Core elements of hospital antibiotic stewardship programs from the Centers for Disease Control and Prevention. Clin Infect Dis. 2014;59(Suppl 3):S97–100.
10. Goff DA, et al. Eight habits of highly effective antimicrobial stewardship programs to meet the Joint Commission standards for hospitals. Clin Infect Dis. 2017;64(8):1134–9.
11. Joint Commission on Hospital, A. Approved: new antimicrobial stewardship standard. Jt Comm Perspect. 2016;36(7):1, 3–4, 8.
12. Society for Healthcare Epidemiology of, A, A. Infectious Diseases Society of, S. Pediatric Infectious Diseases. Policy statement on antimicrobial stewardship by the Society for Healthcare Epidemiology of America (SHEA), the Infectious Diseases Society of America (IDSA), and the Pediatric Infectious Diseases Society (PIDS). Infect Control Hosp Epidemiol. 2012;33(4):322–7.
13. Barlam TF, et al. Executive summary: implementing an antibiotic stewardship program: guidelines by the Infectious Diseases Society of America and the Society for Healthcare Epidemiology of America. Clin Infect Dis. 2016;62(10):1197–202.
14. Karam G, et al. Antibiotic strategies in the era of multidrug resistance. Crit Care. 2016;20(1):136.
15. Tenover FC. Mechanisms of antimicrobial resistance in bacteria. Am J Infect Control. 2006;34(5 Suppl 1):S3–10; discussion S64–73.
16. Mirelis B, et al. Community transmission of extended-spectrum beta-lactamase. Emerg Infect Dis. 2003;9(8):1024–5.
17. Paterson DL, et al. International prospective study of Klebsiella pneumoniae bacteremia: implications of extended-spectrum beta-lactamase production in nosocomial infections. Ann Intern Med. 2004;140(1):26–32.
18. Bradford PA, et al. Emergence of carbapenem-resistant Klebsiella species possessing the class A carbapenem-hydrolyzing KPC-2 and inhibitor-resistant TEM-30 beta-lactamases in New York City. Clin Infect Dis. 2004;39(1):55–60.

19. Chow JW, et al. Enterobacter bacteremia: clinical features and emergence of antibiotic resistance during therapy. Ann Intern Med. 1991;115(8):585–90.
20. Jacoby GA. AmpC beta-lactamases. Clin Microbiol Rev. 2009;22(1):161–82, Table of Contents.
21. Sutcliffe J, Tait-Kamradt A, Wondrack L. Streptococcus pneumoniae and Streptococcus pyogenes resistant to macrolides but sensitive to clindamycin: a common resistance pattern mediated by an efflux system. Antimicrob Agents Chemother. 1996;40(8):1817–24.
22. Pakyz AL, Oinonen M, Polk RE. Relationship of carbapenem restriction in 22 university teaching hospitals to carbapenem use and carbapenem-resistant Pseudomonas aeruginosa. Antimicrob Agents Chemother. 2009;53(5):1983–6.
23. White AC Jr, et al. Effects of requiring prior authorization for selected antimicrobials: expenditures, susceptibilities, and clinical outcomes. Clin Infect Dis. 1997;25(2):230–9.
24. Rahal JJ, et al. Class restriction of cephalosporin use to control total cephalosporin resistance in nosocomial Klebsiella. JAMA. 1998;280(14):1233–7.
25. Buising KL, et al. Electronic antibiotic stewardship – reduced consumption of broad-spectrum antibiotics using a computerized antimicrobial approval system in a hospital setting. J Antimicrob Chemother. 2008;62(3):608–16.
26. Agwu AL, et al. A world wide web-based antimicrobial stewardship program improves efficiency, communication, and user satisfaction and reduces cost in a tertiary care pediatric medical center. Clin Infect Dis. 2008;47(6):747–53.
27. Metjian TA, et al. Evaluation of an antimicrobial stewardship program at a pediatric teaching hospital. Pediatr Infect Dis J. 2008;27(2):106–11.
28. Newland JG, et al. Impact of a prospective-audit-with-feedback antimicrobial stewardship program at a children's hospital. J Pediatric Infect Dis Soc. 2012;1(3):179–86.
29. Di Pentima MC, Chan S, Hossain J. Benefits of a pediatric antimicrobial stewardship program at a children's hospital. Pediatrics. 2011;128(6):1062–70.
30. Harbarth S, et al. Epidemiology and prognostic determinants of bloodstream infections in surgical intensive care. Arch Surg. 2002;137(12):1353–9; discussion 1359.
31. Ibrahim EH, et al. The influence of inadequate antimicrobial treatment of bloodstream infections on patient outcomes in the ICU setting. Chest. 2000;118(1):146–55.
32. Brown EM, Nathwani D. Antibiotic cycling or rotation: a systematic review of the evidence of efficacy. J Antimicrob Chemother. 2005;55(1):6–9.
33. Zachariah P, et al. Costs of antimicrobial stewardship programs at US children's hospitals. Infect Control Hosp Epidemiol. 2016;37(7):852–4.
34. Davey P, et al. Interventions to improve antibiotic prescribing practices for hospital inpatients. Cochrane Database Syst Rev. 2013;4:CD003543.
35. Griffith M, Postelnick M, Scheetz M. Antimicrobial stewardship programs: methods of operation and suggested outcomes. Expert Rev Anti-Infect Ther. 2012;10(1):63–73.
36. Roberts RR, et al. Hospital and societal costs of antimicrobial-resistant infections in a Chicago teaching hospital: implications for antibiotic stewardship. Clin Infect Dis. 2009;49(8):1175–84.
37. Sick AC, et al. Sustained savings from a longitudinal cost analysis of an internet-based preapproval antimicrobial stewardship program. Infect Control Hosp Epidemiol. 2013;34(6):573–80.
38. Standiford HC, et al. Antimicrobial stewardship at a large tertiary care academic medical center: cost analysis before, during, and after a 7-year program. Infect Control Hosp Epidemiol. 2012;33(4):338–45.
39. Laible BR, et al. Implementation of a pharmacist-led antimicrobial management team in a community teaching hospital: use of pharmacy residents and pharmacy students in a prospective audit and feedback approach. J Pharm Pract. 2010;23(6):531–5.
40. Dellit TH, et al. Infectious Diseases Society of America and the Society for Healthcare Epidemiology of America guidelines for developing an institutional program to enhance antimicrobial stewardship. Clin Infect Dis. 2007;44(2):159–77.

41. Yam P, et al. Implementation of an antimicrobial stewardship program in a rural hospital. Am J Health Syst Pharm. 2012;69(13):1142–8.
42. Rohde JM, Jacobsen D, Rosenberg DJ. Role of the hospitalist in antimicrobial stewardship: a review of work completed and description of a multisite collaborative. Clin Ther. 2013;35(6):751–7.
43. Srinivasan A. Engaging hospitalists in antimicrobial stewardship: the CDC perspective. J Hosp Med. 2011;6(Suppl 1):S31–3.
44. Ostrowsky B, et al. Infectious diseases physicians: leading the way in antimicrobial stewardship. Clin Infect Dis. 2018;66(7):995–1003.
45. Goff DA, et al. Is the "low-hanging fruit" worth picking for antimicrobial stewardship programs? Clin Infect Dis. 2012;55(4):587–92.
46. Ohl CA, Dodds Ashley ES. Antimicrobial stewardship programs in community hospitals: the evidence base and case studies. Clin Infect Dis. 2011;53(Suppl 1):S23–8; quiz S29–30.
47. Moody J, et al. Antimicrobial stewardship: a collaborative partnership between infection preventionists and healthcare epidemiologists. Infect Control Hosp Epidemiol. 2012;33(4):328–30.
48. Pestotnik SL. Expert clinical decision support systems to enhance antimicrobial stewardship programs: insights from the society of infectious diseases pharmacists. Pharmacotherapy. 2005;25(8):1116–25.
49. Kullar R, et al. The "epic" challenge of optimizing antimicrobial stewardship: the role of electronic medical records and technology. Clin Infect Dis. 2013;57(7):1005–13.
50. Edwards R, et al. Covering more territory to fight resistance: considering nurses' role in antimicrobial stewardship. J Infect Prev. 2011;12(1):6–10.
51. Cheng VC, et al. Antimicrobial stewardship program directed at broad-spectrum intravenous antibiotics prescription in a tertiary hospital. Eur J Clin Microbiol Infect Dis. 2009;28(12):1447–56.
52. Braxton CC, Gerstenberger PA, Cox GG. Improving antibiotic stewardship: order set implementation to improve prophylactic antimicrobial prescribing in the outpatient surgical setting. J Ambul Care Manage. 2010;33(2):131–40.
53. Malcolm W, et al. From intermittent antibiotic point prevalence surveys to quality improvement: experience in Scottish hospitals. Antimicrob Resist Infect Control. 2013;2(1):3.
54. Morris AM, et al. Establishing an antimicrobial stewardship program. Healthc Q. 2010;13(2):64–70.
55. Bornard L, et al. Impact of an assisted reassessment of antibiotic therapies on the quality of prescriptions in an intensive care unit. Med Mal Infect. 2011;41(9):480–5.
56. Kaye KS. Antimicrobial de-escalation strategies in hospitalized patients with pneumonia, intra-abdominal infections, and bacteremia. J Hosp Med. 2012;7(Suppl 1):S13–21.
57. Pardo J, et al. Time to positivity of blood cultures supports antibiotic de-escalation at 48 hours. Ann Pharmacother. 2014;48(1):33–40.
58. Stocker M, et al. Antibiotic surveillance on a paediatric intensive care unit: easy attainable strategy at low costs and resources. BMC Pediatr. 2012;12:196.
59. Dancer SJ, et al. Approaching zero: temporal effects of a restrictive antibiotic policy on hospital-acquired Clostridium difficile, extended-spectrum beta-lactamase-producing coliforms and meticillin-resistant Staphylococcus aureus. Int J Antimicrob Agents. 2013;41(2):137–42.
60. DiazGranados CA. Prospective audit for antimicrobial stewardship in intensive care: impact on resistance and clinical outcomes. Am J Infect Control. 2012;40(6):526–9.
61. Toth NR, Chambers RM, Davis SL. Implementation of a care bundle for antimicrobial stewardship. Am J Health Syst Pharm. 2010;67(9):746–9.
62. Jenkins TC, et al. Skin and soft-tissue infections requiring hospitalization at an academic medical center: opportunities for antimicrobial stewardship. Clin Infect Dis. 2010;51(8):895–903.
63. McCallum AD, Sutherland RK, Mackintosh CL. Improving antimicrobial prescribing: implementation of an antimicrobial i.v.-to-oral switch policy. J R Coll Physicians Edinb. 2013;43(4):294–300.

64. Canton R, Bryan J. Global antimicrobial resistance: from surveillance to stewardship. Part 2: stewardship initiatives. Expert Rev Anti-Infect Ther. 2012;10(12):1375–7.
65. Avdic E, et al. Impact of an antimicrobial stewardship intervention on shortening the duration of therapy for community-acquired pneumonia. Clin Infect Dis. 2012;54(11):1581–7.
66. Rattanaumpawan P, et al. Impact of antimicrobial stewardship programme changes on unnecessary double anaerobic coverage therapy. J Antimicrob Chemother. 2011;66(11):2655–8.
67. Ostrowsky B, et al. Antimicrobial stewardship and automated pharmacy technology improve antibiotic appropriateness for community-acquired pneumonia. Infect Control Hosp Epidemiol. 2013;34(6):566–72.
68. Bosso JA, Drew RH. Application of antimicrobial stewardship to optimise management of community acquired pneumonia. Int J Clin Pract. 2011;65(7):775–83.
69. Mandell LA, et al. Infectious Diseases Society of America/American Thoracic Society consensus guidelines on the management of community-acquired pneumonia in adults. Clin Infect Dis. 2007;44(Suppl 2):S27–72.
70. Bradley JS, et al. Executive summary: the management of community-acquired pneumonia in infants and children older than 3 months of age: clinical practice guidelines by the Pediatric Infectious Diseases Society and the Infectious Diseases Society of America. Clin Infect Dis. 2011;53(7):617–30.
71. Slekovec C, et al. Impact of a region wide antimicrobial stewardship guideline on urinary tract infection prescription patterns. Int J Clin Pharm. 2012;34(2):325–9.
72. Hermanides HS, et al. Development of quality indicators for the antibiotic treatment of complicated urinary tract infections: a first step to measure and improve care. Clin Infect Dis. 2008;46(5):703–11.
73. Nicolle LE. Asymptomatic bacteriuria. Curr Opin Infect Dis. 2014;27(1):90–6.
74. Stevens DL, et al. Practice guidelines for the diagnosis and management of skin and soft-tissue infections. Clin Infect Dis. 2005;41(10):1373–406.
75. Drekonja DM, et al. Antimicrobial use and risk for recurrent Clostridium difficile infection. Am J Med. 2011;124(11):1081. e1–7.
76. Mullane KM, et al. Efficacy of fidaxomicin versus vancomycin as therapy for Clostridium difficile infection in individuals taking concomitant antibiotics for other concurrent infections. Clin Infect Dis. 2011;53(5):440–7.
77. Garnacho-Montero J, et al. De-escalation of empirical therapy is associated with lower mortality in patients with severe sepsis and septic shock. Intensive Care Med. 2014;40(1):32–40.
78. Di Pentima MC, Chan S. Impact of antimicrobial stewardship program on vancomycin use in a pediatric teaching hospital. Pediatr Infect Dis J. 2010;29(8):707–11.
79. Johannsson B, et al. Antimicrobial therapy for bloodstream infection due to methicillin-susceptible Staphylococcus aureus in an era of increasing methicillin resistance: opportunities for antimicrobial stewardship. Ann Pharmacother. 2012;46(6):904–5.
80. Newland JG, et al. Antimicrobial stewardship in pediatric care: strategies and future directions. Pharmacotherapy. 2012;32(8):735–43.
81. Hurst AL, et al. Handshake stewardship: a highly effective rounding-based antimicrobial optimization service. Pediatr Infect Dis J. 2016;35(10):1104–10.
82. Lighter-Fisher J, et al. Implementing an inpatient pediatric prospective audit and feedback antimicrobial stewardship program within a larger medical center. Hosp Pediatr. 2017;7(9):516–22.
83. Cosgrove SE, et al. Evaluation of postprescription review and feedback as a method of promoting rational antimicrobial use: a multicenter intervention. Infect Control Hosp Epidemiol. 2012;33(4):374–80.
84. LaRocco A Jr. Concurrent antibiotic review programs – a role for infectious diseases specialists at small community hospitals. Clin Infect Dis. 2003;37(5):742–3.
85. Vettese N, et al. Outcomes associated with a thrice-weekly antimicrobial stewardship programme in a 253-bed community hospital. J Clin Pharm Ther. 2013;38(5):401–4.
86. Gillon J, et al. Vancomycin use: room for improvement among hospitalized children. J Pharm Pract. 2017;30(3):296–9.

87. Willis ZI, et al. Reducing antimicrobial use in an academic pediatric institution: evaluation of the effectiveness of a prospective audit with real-time feedback. J Pediatric Infect Dis Soc. 2017;6(4):339–45.
88. Seah VXF, et al. Impact of a carbapenem antimicrobial stewardship program on patient outcomes. Antimicrob Agents Chemother. 2017; 61(9):pii: e00736-17.
89. Flannery DD, et al. Prescriber perceptions of a pediatric antimicrobial stewardship program. Clin Pediatr (Phila). 2014;53(8):747–50.
90. Smith MJ, Gerber JS, Hersh AL. Inpatient antimicrobial stewardship in pediatrics: a systematic review. J Pediatric Infect Dis Soc. 2015;4(4):e127–35.
91. Newman RE, et al. Impact of a guideline on management of children hospitalized with community-acquired pneumonia. Pediatrics. 2012;129(3):e597–604.
92. Lee KR, Bagga B, Arnold SR. Reduction of broad-spectrum antimicrobial use in a tertiary children's hospital post antimicrobial stewardship program guideline implementation. Pediatr Crit Care Med. 2016;17(3):187–93.
93. Willis ZI, et al. Improvements in Antimicrobial Prescribing and Outcomes in Pediatric Complicated Appendicitis. Pediatr Infect Dis J. 2018;37(5):429–35.
94. Wolf J, et al. Antimicrobial stewardship barriers and goals in pediatric oncology and bone marrow transplantation: a survey of antimicrobial stewardship practitioners. Infect Control Hosp Epidemiol. 2016;37(3):343–7.
95. Briceland LL, et al. Streamlining antimicrobial therapy through pharmacists' review of order sheets. Am J Hosp Pharm. 1989;46(7):1376–80.
96. Masterton RG. Antibiotic de-escalation. Crit Care Clin. 2011;27(1):149–62.
97. Garnacho-Montero J, Escoresca-Ortega A, Fernandez-Delgado E. Antibiotic de-escalation in the ICU: how is it best done? Curr Opin Infect Dis. 2015;28(2):193–8.
98. Jones M, et al. Parenteral to oral conversion of fluoroquinolones: low-hanging fruit for antimicrobial stewardship programs? Infect Control Hosp Epidemiol. 2012;33(4):362–7.
99. Sevinc F, et al. Early switch from intravenous to oral antibiotics: guidelines and implementation in a large teaching hospital. J Antimicrob Chemother. 1999;43(4):601–6.
100. Owens RC Jr, Ambrose PG. Antimicrobial stewardship and the role of pharmacokinetics-pharmacodynamics in the modern antibiotic era. Diagn Microbiol Infect Dis. 2007;57(3 Suppl):77S–83S.
101. Kemme DJ, Daniel CI. Aminoglycoside dosing: a randomized prospective study. South Med J. 1993;86(1):46–51.
102. Leehey DJ, et al. Can pharmacokinetic dosing decrease nephrotoxicity associated with aminoglycoside therapy. J Am Soc Nephrol. 1993;4(1):81–90.
103. Streetman DS, et al. Individualized pharmacokinetic monitoring results in less aminoglycoside-associated nephrotoxicity and fewer associated costs. Pharmacotherapy. 2001;21(4):443–51.
104. Iwamoto T, Kagawa Y, Kojima M. Clinical efficacy of therapeutic drug monitoring in patients receiving vancomycin. Biol Pharm Bull. 2003;26(6):876–9.
105. Bond CA, Raehl CL. Clinical and economic outcomes of pharmacist-managed aminoglycoside or vancomycin therapy. Am J Health Syst Pharm. 2005;62(15):1596–605.
106. Whipple JK, et al. Effect of individualized pharmacokinetic dosing on patient outcome. Crit Care Med. 1991;19(12):1480–5.
107. Welty TE, Copa AK. Impact of vancomycin therapeutic drug monitoring on patient care. Ann Pharmacother. 1994;28(12):1335–9.
108. Jiang SP, et al. Impact of pharmacist antimicrobial dosing adjustments in septic patients on continuous renal replacement therapy in an intensive care unit. Scand J Infect Dis. 2013;45(12):891–9.
109. Patel SJ, et al. Development of an antimicrobial stewardship intervention using a model of actionable feedback. Interdiscip Perspect Infect Dis. 2012;2012:150367.
110. Rocha-Pereira N, Lafferty N, Nathwani D. Educating healthcare professionals in antimicrobial stewardship: can online-learning solutions help? J Antimicrob Chemother. 2015;70(12):3175–7.

111. Gauthier TP, et al. Internet-based institutional antimicrobial stewardship program resources in leading US academic medical centers. Clin Infect Dis. 2014;58(3):445–6.
112. Landgren FT, et al. Changing antibiotic prescribing by educational marketing. Med J Aust. 1988;149(11–12):595–9.
113. Morris AM, et al. Use of a structured panel process to define quality metrics for antimicrobial stewardship programs. Infect Control Hosp Epidemiol. 2012;33(5):500–6.
114. Morris AM. Antimicrobial stewardship programs: appropriate measures and metrics to study their impact. Curr Treat Options Infect Dis. 2014;6(2):101–12.
115. Polk RE, et al. Measurement of adult antibacterial drug use in 130 US hospitals: comparison of defined daily dose and days of therapy. Clin Infect Dis. 2007;44(5):664–70.
116. Gravatt LA, Pakyz AL. Challenges in measuring antibiotic consumption. Curr Infect Dis Rep. 2013;15(6):559–63.
117. Messacar K, et al. Implementation of rapid molecular infectious disease diagnostics: the role of diagnostic and antimicrobial stewardship. J Clin Microbiol. 2017;55(3):715–23.
118. Perez KK, et al. Integrating rapid diagnostics and antimicrobial stewardship improves outcomes in patients with antibiotic-resistant gram-negative bacteremia. J Infect. 2014;69(3):216–25.
119. Poritz MA, et al. FilmArray, an automated nested multiplex PCR system for multi-pathogen detection: development and application to respiratory tract infection. PLoS One. 2011;6(10):e26047.
120. Blaschke AJ, et al. Rapid identification of pathogens from positive blood cultures by multiplex polymerase chain reaction using the FilmArray system. Diagn Microbiol Infect Dis. 2012;74(4):349–55.
121. Leber AL, et al. Multicenter evaluation of BioFire FilmArray meningitis/encephalitis panel for detection of bacteria, viruses, and yeast in cerebrospinal fluid specimens. J Clin Microbiol. 2016;54(9):2251–61.
122. Buchan BW, et al. Multiplex identification of gram-positive bacteria and resistance determinants directly from positive blood culture broths: evaluation of an automated microarray-based nucleic acid test. PLoS Med. 2013;10(7):e1001478.
123. Seng P, et al. Ongoing revolution in bacteriology: routine identification of bacteria by matrix-assisted laser desorption ionization time-of-flight mass spectrometry. Clin Infect Dis. 2009;49(4):543–51.
124. Stender H. PNA FISH: an intelligent stain for rapid diagnosis of infectious diseases. Expert Rev Mol Diagn. 2003;3(5):649–55.
125. Naccache SN, et al. A cloud-compatible bioinformatics pipeline for ultrarapid pathogen identification from next-generation sequencing of clinical samples. Genome Res. 2014;24(7):1180–92.
126. Caliendo AM, et al. Better tests, better care: improved diagnostics for infectious diseases. Clin Infect Dis. 2013;57(Suppl 3):S139–70.
127. Hersh AL, Newland JG, Gerber JS. Pediatric antimicrobial discharge stewardship: an unmet need. JAMA Pediatr. 2016;170(3):191–2.
128. Knackstedt ED, et al. Outpatient parenteral antimicrobial therapy in pediatrics: an opportunity to expand antimicrobial stewardship. Infect Control Hosp Epidemiol. 2015;36(2):222–4.
129. Shrestha NK, et al. Antimicrobial stewardship at transition of care from hospital to community. Infect Control Hosp Epidemiol. 2012;33(4):401–4.
130. Hicks LA, et al. US outpatient antibiotic prescribing variation according to geography, patient population, and provider specialty in 2011. Clin Infect Dis. 2015;60(9):1308–16.
131. Hicks LA, Blaser MJ. Variability in antibiotic prescribing: an inconvenient truth. J Pediatric Infect Dis Soc. 2015;4(1):e136–8.
132. Gerber JS, et al. Variation in antibiotic prescribing across a pediatric primary care network. J Pediatric Infect Dis Soc. 2015;4(4):297–304.

133. Gerber JS, et al. Durability of benefits of an outpatient antimicrobial stewardship intervention after discontinuation of audit and feedback. JAMA. 2014;312(23):2569–70.
134. Gerber JS, et al. Effect of an outpatient antimicrobial stewardship intervention on broad-spectrum antibiotic prescribing by primary care pediatricians: a randomized trial. JAMA. 2013;309(22):2345–52.

Infection Control and the Need for Family-/Child-Centered Care

4

John Darby and Carla Falco

Introduction

Patient- and family-centered care (FCC) has been considered an important aspect of medical care over the last 20 years. FCC is focused on the mutually beneficial partnership and relationship between medical provider, patients, and families with an emphasis on collaboration [1]. This change in perspective to focus on patient- and family-centered care includes a shift away from the concept of families, especially parents and legal guardians, as visitors [2–6]. The key tenants of FCC include dignity and respect of the patient and family, information sharing, participation by the patient and family in the care and decision-making at the level they choose, and collaboration. FCC has been shown to improve patient outcomes [1, 7–13].

In the hospital setting, FCC espouses that family members are accepted as the ones who both know the patient best and are the primary support for the patient. Parents and legal guardians are treated as an extension of the patient; their importance is underscored frequently in the literature on visitation policies by the lack of limitations implemented for parents, legal guardians, or siblings [14]. Family presence at the bedside has been increasingly recognized as crucial for patient well-being [15]. More flexible visiting hours have been shown to improve patient outcomes in adult intensive care unit (ICU) patients [2, 16–21]. For example, visitation policies for family members have been a focus for change in ICUs with the advancement of FCC, including advocating for open visitation, i.e., visitation

J. Darby, MD (✉)
Department of Pediatrics, Wake Forest School of Medicine,
Winston-Salem, NC, USA
e-mail: jdarby@wakehealth.edu

C. Falco
Department of Pediatrics, Section of Hospital Medicine, Baylor College of Medicine,
Houston, TX, USA

© Springer Nature Switzerland AG 2019
J. C. McNeil et al. (eds.), *Healthcare-Associated Infections in Children*,
https://doi.org/10.1007/978-3-319-98122-2_4

without restrictions [22–26]. Private rooms within ICUs have also been cited to both support FCC and infection control [23].

Infection control within the hospital setting prioritizes patient safety from transmissible diseases. Infection control practices have the potential to greatly influence family centeredness because isolation practices can affect the ways that patient families are supported and affect how patients cope with hospitalization. Approaching infection control through the lens of FCC requires balancing patient safety and overall patient well-being through bonding with caregivers, family members, and visitors and engaging in activities to encourage normalcy during their hospitalization, including participating in play and pet therapy [27]. In this chapter, we explore this balance and will also address the psychosocial impact of isolation policies.

Isolation Practices and Family Members

FCC encourages the presence of family members, especially caregivers, to be at the bedside to participate in clinical decision-making because of their role as the primary support and strength for the patient [27]. FCC also regards caregivers as experts on their child with invaluable knowledge that is critical to excellent medical care; healthcare professionals are also called to support families in their caregiving and decision-making. The physical presence of family members is a consolation for patients and is essential for young children, but their presence can also pose a risk of transmissible disease at the same time. Isolation practices, including personal protective equipment (PPE) and limitation of visitation, are ways to mitigate that risk for patients, family members, and healthcare workers.

Evidence that visitors and family members pose a health risk to hospitalized patients is overall equivocal except in the case of childhood tuberculosis. Caregivers of pediatric patients with tuberculosis are the highest-risk population for transmitting infection within the hospital since they can be the child's primary source of disease [28–31]. Two studies in a pediatric hospital found that 15–17% of patients who were treated for tuberculosis had caregivers who received a new diagnosis of tuberculosis [29, 32]. Outbreaks have been traced back to adults caring or visiting children with tuberculosis (see section below). The infection control aproach recommended is to address the family as a unit and not simply isolate the patient individually [31]. Appropriate screening measures for tuberculosis include having parents wear a surgical mask until a chest x-ray can be performed; the use of N95 masks is not recommended since fit testing is not practical for visitors. These measures were shown to be cost-effective as screening tools [32].

More broadly, visitation policies, which do not include caregivers, have been examined to see how they affect hospital-acquired infections. One recent study by Washam et al. demonstrated that during the winter respiratory viral season, visitors were a source of infection; creating a standardized, visitation restriction policy decreased hospital-acquired viral pathogens on non-ICU floors and influenza infections overall [14]. Hospital-acquired infections were decreased by 37% through limiting visitation by nonsiblings and ill visitors. In the ICUs, only four nonparent, nonlegal guardian persons on a fixed list were permitted to visit; later in the study, they changed this policy to apply hospital-wide and to allow six persons on a fixed list to visit. Restricting visitors was also shown to decrease respiratory syncytial virus (RSV) infection in an open-room neonatal intensive care unit (NICU). Peluso et al. in 2015 published RSV surveillance data from 2001–2010 in their NICU [33]. In 2007, they restricted the visitation of children less than 13 years old during RSV season (October–March); they found less frequent RSV infections, both asymptomatic and symptomatic, with the more restrictive policy. The groups before and after 2007 were similar in characteristics, and the disease prevalence of RSV in the region remained constant during the study time period. Other studies in special units have examined the restriction of ill visitors and children as part of infection control bundles and seen a reduction in infections, for example, in adult bone marrow transplant (BMT) units and NICUs during RSV season [33, 34]. Some studies in adult ICUs have shown an increase in environmental contamination and even bioaerosols but no effect on the rate of hospital-acquired infections with liberalizing visitation policies; the same has been shown for NICUs [16, 35–39]. The bulk of research on infections via hand transmission has focused on healthcare workers [28, 40]. Yet, visitors have also been implicated in outbreaks of various pathogens (see section below).

Given the limited data available, guidelines for isolation practices and visitors have been published using expert consensus and take into account the specific pathogen, the disease manifestation of the infection, and the endemicity of the pathogen in both the hospital and community [14, 28, 41]. General recommendations for visitors have been published by the Society for Healthcare Epidemiology of America (SHEA) and recommend that all visitors should perform hand hygiene before entering and directly after leaving the patient's room, which has been shown to decrease pathogenic organisms [42, 43]. Some institutions apply transmission-based precautions only for healthcare workers where others include visitors in these policies. In a survey of SHEA members in 2014, 57% of over 250 respondents indicated that they had the same requirements for isolation precautions (primarily in contact isolation) for visitors as for healthcare providers; however, this practice was not closely monitored for visitors. Until appropriate studies are performed, isolation precautions among visitors should be considered based upon pathogens, infectious condition, patient population, and local epidemiology in the hospital and community. Furthermore, hospitals should have specific policies regarding visitation that are feasible and can be enforced [28]. Other tenants of the SHEA Guidance are outlined in Table 4.1.

In the pediatric hospital setting, it is important to distinguish between visitors that have been exposed to the patient as household contacts and those who have less intense contact with the patient. Parents and caregivers are frequently exposed to the patient at home and often continue their vigil to care for their child in the hospital at the bedside overnight or for prolonged periods of time. Given the high likelihood of exposure that these parent caregivers have experienced and will continue to experience, it is not practical for caregivers to use PPE other than for standard precautions [14, 28]. In addition, concerns about bonding between caregivers and children have been cited as reasons to not fully enforce PPE use in parent caregivers; the psychosocial impact of isolation practices remains a topic for future research.

Table 4.1 Transmission-based precautions for visitors [14, 28, 41]

Isolation practice	Who should use
Contact precautions: *gowns and gloves*	Visitors to patients with enteric pathogens (e.g., *C. difficile*, norovirus) Visitors to patient(s) with MRSA or VRE if they will be visiting multiple patients (i.e., clergy) *Consider with:* Visitors to patients who are either colonized or infected with extensively drug-resistant gram-negative organisms Outbreaks Visitors to a single patient with MRSA or VRE who are immunocompromised or are unable to perform good hand hygiene
Droplet precautions: *surgical mask*	All visitors, except for those with extensive exposure to the patient before admission (i.e., member of the patient's household)
Airborne precautions: *surgical mask*[a]	Visitors to patients who are on airborne precautions, except for those with extensive exposure to the patient before admission
Restricted visitation[b]	Any visitor who is ill (e.g., active cough, fever, vomiting, and/or diarrhea) Outbreak or increased baseline rates *Consider with:* Nonsibling children during respiratory viral season Consider limiting visitation to a fixed list of nonparent, nonlegal guardian persons during winter respiratory viral season

[a]Caregivers of children with suspected tuberculosis should wear a surgical mask until a chest x-ray is performed and reported as negative
[b]In cases of emerging pathogens that are highly contagious (e.g., Severe Acute Respiratory Virus Syndrome[SARS], Middle East Respiratory Syndrome Coronavirus [MERS-CoV], Ebola, etc.), guidance from updated health authorities (CDC and state health departments) is essential in developing specific visitation policies in those special circumstances. We would highly recommend consulting these authorities if a patient is suspected of having one of these pathogens.

Family members and other visitors are likely to have a variable compliance rate with infection control measures. Research shows that hand hygiene compliance is highly variable (from <1% to 57%) among visitors. At least two studies have shown that visitors only partially comply with contact precautions; most visitors who don gown and gloves neglect to perform hand hygiene [44, 45]. Efforts that improve hand hygiene practices of visitors include signs that accompany readily available alcohol hand rub and, in more extreme cases, a motion detection sensor [43, 46, 47]. Visitors' use of gown and gloves for contact precautions and the addition of masks for respiratory isolation are also highly variable: 40–60% and 23%, respectively [44, 48]. No studies have examined education of visitors regarding good hand hygiene or gown and glove use; in addition, no studies on isolation practices have distinguished between visitors and parents or caregivers at the bedside.

Outbreaks

There are select cases where visitors to patients have been cited as sources for the transmission of pathogens including tuberculosis, RSV, norovirus, and SARS [28, 49]. Outbreaks are defined by the Centers for Disease Control as the occurrence of more cases of a disease than expected in a given area or among a specific group of people over a particular period of time [50]. The screening and restriction of visitors, especially symptomatic visitors, is essential to prevent or control an outbreak. First, caregivers and adult visitors of pediatric patients with tuberculosis must be screened as described above. One report describes a tuberculosis outbreak that involved 24 children, including some immunocompromised patients, who had contact with a patient's mother with cavitary tuberculosis [51, 52]. An adult visitor was a source of two cases of latent tuberculosis infection in hospital staff members in another report [53]. Second, a report in 2005 of an RSV outbreak in a NICU suspected a sibling visitor to be the initial source which resulted in RSV infection in nine babies in open bassinets, five of whom required intubation and one required ECMO for 9 days [54]. The total hospital charge of the outbreak was $1.15 M. In response, control measures included limiting all visitors to those older than 13 years old who had no respiratory symptoms, contact precautions, and cohorting the infants infected with RSV. They also tested all NICU infants and administered palivizumab to uninfected infants, although the latter practice has since been discouraged by the AAP [55]. Third, norovirus, a highly contagious enteropathogen, frequently requires some type of visitor restriction [56, 57]. At a minimum, symptomatic visitors should be restricted, which has shown to aid in outbreak control [56]. One report of a large outbreak involving more than 500 patients and staff resorted to restricting all visitors after the limitation of symptomatic visitors did not curb a norovirus outbreak [57]. The limitation of symptomatic visitors has been used to prevent the outbreak of respiratory viruses, including influenza [53, 58, 59]. Finally, during the 2003–2004 epidemic of severe acute respiratory syndrome (SARS), visitors to the hospital were a significant part of the transmission cycle, including transmission to hospital staff, other patients, and the community [60–63]. The control measures used first included using PPE for symptomatic visitors; later, visitor restriction and quarantine of both symptomatic individuals in their homes and of entire hospitals were used [63]. Screening measures of visitors and staff were also implemented, including body temperature screening and questionnaires.

Even in extreme circumstances such as outbreaks of highly contagious or novel infections, including but not limited to SARS, Middle East respiratory syndrome coronavirus (MERS-CoV), and novel-H1N1 influenza, when visitor restriction is in place, parents and caregivers of hospitalized children typically remain at the bedside. Their bonding with and support for the patient, combined with the likelihood that they were exposed previously to the infectious agent before admission, supports continued caregiver presence [28, 41]. Indeed, many of the recommendations by SHEA are intended to be adjusted for parents and caregivers. A case-by-case analysis should be made in situations where the patient contracts an infection after admission; usually caregivers still remain at the bedside unless they themselves are immunocompromised. Visitation by other family members besides parents or caregivers depends on the infectious organism, the timing of illness, and the degree of contact that the family member had with the patient before and after admission. Those with less frequent contact with the patient should follow the isolation guidance outlined in Table 4.1.

Sibling Visitation

In pediatrics, while parents have transitioned from being visitors to being an extension of the patient themselves and are indispensable to care and medical decision-making, siblings are still considered visitors. Yet, hospitals can offer a more family-centered environment by supporting the attachment between pediatric patients and their siblings [64]. The American Academy of Pediatrics shifted the perspective on sibling visitation in the 1980s by encouraging restrictions to be liberalized to allow children and siblings less than 12 years old to visit hospitalized children. They stated that concerns over infection control were not evidence-based [64, 65]. Hospitals then started to encourage sibling presence in the hospital [66]. Since then, a small body of literature has shown that in certain areas of the hospital or during certain times of year, for example, RSV and influenza season, restrictions on child and sibling visitation remain an important tool in infection control and prevention [14, 34, 67]. Each hospital should consider the necessary balance between family-centered care and sibling visitation with the importance of infection control measures to prevent transmission of pathogenic organisms and outbreaks.

With a focus on family-centered care, sibling visitation facilitates the entire family's adaptation to a child's hospitalization [68]. The limited research available on the effect of sibling separation in the setting of hospitalization suggests that it is stressful to both the patient and well sibling and disrupts the family structure [69–72]. Well siblings experience a change in family routine and in family focus and separation from their parents [73–75]. As a result, they can experience loneliness, worry, and decreased sleep [75–79]. Siblings of hospitalized children tend to have more emotional and behavioral problems, which are similar to the effects on siblings of children with a chronic illness or disability [75]. The anxiety that parents and siblings feel can then be transferred to the hospitalized child [80]. Sibling visitation in the hospital mitigates the disruption the family experiences and supports the family unit and family continuity [68]. Sibling visitation is also a way to diminish the negative emotional and behavioral effects on well siblings [68, 81, 82]. Child life programs within the hospital often provide education to siblings while also caring for the hospitalized child [80, 83, 84]. Sibling visitation also encourages the hospital staff to view the family as a unit, which enhances family-centered care [68, 85].

Since the AAP's statement encouraging sibling visitation, there has been more literature published about the most significant balancing measure for sibling visitation: infection control, especially with newborns and NICU patients. It is known that younger children have a "relatively high frequency of asymptomatic viral shedding and difficulties adhering to basic respiratory etiquette and hand hygiene practices" [67, 86]. Initially, studies examined the bacterial colonization of healthy newborns who were visited by a sibling as a marker for risk of infection and found no cause for concern. In 1980, Umphenour examined nasal and umbilical swabs of newborns at admission and discharge in both a control group ($N = 214$) and intervention group ($N = 182$) with sibling visitation [87]. Of note, siblings who were obviously ill were asked to not come to the hospital; children that did visit underwent hand hygiene with an iodine scrub before interacting with the newborns who were rooming-in with their mothers. There was no difference in the two groups in terms of bacterial colonization in the newborn. Similar studies yielded the same results in support of well siblings visiting well newborns assuming aggressive hand hygiene is adhered to [82, 88, 89]. A survey of 69 hospitals showed that the majority of hospitals have an open visitation policy for siblings of newborns; however, rarely do hospitals observe visiting siblings for signs of illness [90]. Furthermore, more recent studies have shown that siblings can be a source of infection in the NICU. A report in 2005 of an RSV outbreak in a NICU suspected a visiting sibling as being the source of RSV that infected nine babies with serious consequences (as discussed above) [54]. In 2015, Peluso published data from their own NICU surveillance practices from 2001–2010 [33]. During the 2001–2002 season, they noted an increase in RSV infections after they heeded the AAP's encouragement to liberalize sibling visitation [65]. After they implemented age-based restrictions during RSV season (October–March), they found less frequent RSV infections, both asymptomatic and symptomatic. They suggest that applying visitation restriction can prevent RSV infection in open-room design NICUs but that it should be applied carefully so as to support families as much as possible. Studies examining the infection risk to hospitalized patients with sibling visitation outside the NICU are lacking. However, restriction of children, both siblings and nonsiblings, visiting the hospital remains a resource for infection control in times of outbreak [91].

Currently, there are no universal standards for sibling visitation in the NICU or hospital-wide [14, 82]. The American Academy of Pediatrics' Committee on Infectious Diseases (AAP Red Book) recommends that siblings be screened for infection by a healthcare professional and that the appropriate documentation should be made [67]. If a sibling was known to be exposed to communicable disease, then their visit should be postponed. They also recommend that all vaccines be up to date, including influenza vaccine, and that these visiting well children should only visit their sibling and not be in contact with other patients. Each institution must evaluate the feasibility and process for these recommendations as they develop policies and procedures for their hospitals. The most important recommendation for all visitors, but especially siblings, is proper hand hygiene prior to and after visiting. One recent study at a quaternary children's hospital on healthcare-acquired respiratory infections found a 37% reduction in infections with a standardized visitation policy [14]. The policy did not limit sibling visitation but did exclude nonsibling children during the winter respiratory viral season. An informal review of the visiting policies listed on the websites of children's hospitals across the USA shows that parents have no restrictions on visitation. Siblings under 12–14 years old must be well to visit. Some hospitals limit sibling visitation depending on different factors, including specific visiting hours, contact isolation, influenza season, and location in the hospital [92, 93]. Special units like NICUs, BMT units, and PICUs have more restrictive policies; there, well siblings under the ages of 3–5 years old are usually prohibited from visiting [14]. Some special units require evidence of adequate of vaccination [94]. Research on ICU visitation has found that there is benefit to family and sibling visitation [85]. We recommend facilities review or draft sibling visitation policies with the perspective of the benefits of FCC while incorporating

Table 4.2 Sibling visitation policy recommendations

Hospital unit	Sibling visitation recommendation[a]	Recommendation during influenza season or outbreak[a]
Acute care floor, including patients with contact precautions	Open sibling visitation	Open sibling visitation
NICU	Siblings older than 3 years old	Siblings older than 13 years old
PICU	Siblings older than 3 years old	Siblings older than 13 years old
BMT or immunocompromised patients	Siblings older than 3 years old	Siblings older than 13 years old

[a]Screening measures should be implemented and monitored for compliance to identify visitors with cough, rhinorrhea, fever, rash, vomiting, and diarrhea. Siblings who are ill should not visit the hospital

infection control considerations. Suggestion of a framework for these discussions with key stakeholders, including patient advocacy councils, is outlined in Table 4.2. Policies need to include who conducts the screening and training for those staff. Any ill siblings should not visit the hospital, and well siblings who do visit should perform standard hand hygiene.

Sibling visitation is a means to promote family-centered care by honoring the family unit; this worthwhile focus of medical care must remain in balance with concerns for infection control. The safety of the hospitalized child remains the ultimate goal such that, whether siblings have visited or not, a healthy reunion of the family can occur at discharge.

Pet Therapy

Overview

Animals in pediatric healthcare facilities have become commonplace and pose important infection control considerations. The following subchapter will outline some of the proposed benefits of animals on pediatric health, potential infection risks, and outline recommendations for infection control.

Children come into contact with animals outside of healthcare facilities on a regular basis. A national poll conducted in 2017 found that 68% of households contain a pet with 48% of households containing a dog and 38% containing a cat [95]. Inside healthcare facilities, there has been increased presence of animals with the growth of animal-assisted activities (AAA) and service animals. Additionally, some facilities may allow visitation from personal pets to hospitalized patients, especially in chronic care or end-of-life situations. AAA, animal-assisted therapy (AAT), pet therapy, and pet volunteer programs are all terms that have been used to describe various healthcare animal programs. AAT specifically refers to sessions conducted by trained therapists, typically the handler and animal, and are structured, organized visits with individualized patient goals. For the purpose of this discussion, the term animal-assisted interventions (AAI) will be used to encompass activities and therapies conducted with animals in the healthcare setting. Animals in healthcare (AHC) is a broad term that encompasses personal pet visitation as well.

Benefits of Animals in Healthcare

The benefits of animals in healthcare facilities are many. Studies conducted in adult psychiatric patients have shown that the use of AAI leads to an increase in self-esteem, self-determination, and a decrease in positive psychiatric symptoms and emotional symptoms [96]. The use of AAI in elderly patients in healthcare facilities has also shown positive impacts including a decrease in depressive symptoms, significant decreases in systolic blood pressure, and decreases in anxiety [97, 98]. Specifically in pediatric patients, a range of positive benefits have been observed including decreased anxiety, lower pain scores, and positive parental perceptions of child confidence, mood, and happiness [99–101]. Despite a lack of high-quality randomized controlled trials, the pediatric medical community has been accepting of AAI. Hospital staff members, as well as parents of patients, are generally very receptive to animals in healthcare facilities. This trend is consistent with the overall FCC movement and attempts to address the stresses of hospitalization for children and families. The use of AAI can make the hospital environment seem more familiar, provide distraction, enhance quality of life, and, in some cases, achieve specific therapy goals including promoting improvements in physical, social, emotional, or cognitive function. Consistent with the concepts of FCC, AAI takes a humanistic approach to patient care. With the growing presence of AHC however, there comes some degree of risk.

Risks of Animals in Healthcare

Studies and discussions surrounding the risk of animals in healthcare facilities have focused on the risk of infection, allergies, and bodily injury from bites and scratches. With specific regard to infection risk, many published studies have focused on the potential for animal to human transmission of diseases. Swabs taken from dogs used in pet visitation programs have isolated many transmissible bacteria including toxigenic *Clostridium difficile*, *Salmonella*, *Toxocara canis*, *Ancylostoma caninum*, *Giardia*, *Escherichia coli*, *Malassezia pachydermatis*, *Pasteurella* spp., and *Trichophyton mentagrophytes* [102]. Other reports have found the presence of healthcare-associated strains of methicillin-resistant *Staphylococcus aureus* (MRSA) in several species including dogs and cats. Additionally, there have been reports of hospital outbreaks of zoonoses although most occur when hospital personnel, such as nurses or operating room staff, are colonized or infected by pets or working animals kept in the home environment [103–107]. One notable exception is a described MRSA outbreak, which occurred in a geriatric rehabilitation ward and was traced to a cat that roamed freely inside the hospital [108].

Despite the cited infection concerns, the overall risk of zoonosis transmission from animals to humans in healthcare facilities is likely very low, albeit the literature is rather sparse in this area. In part the low risk of transmission from animals to humans in the healthcare setting may be a reflection of dogs being used primarily in AAI as opposed to other animals with a higher risk of transmission of zoonotic infections (such as reptiles). Given the high prevalence of animals in American households, many patients will return to animal contact after leaving the hospital. Additionally, rates of zoonotic infections in the general American public are also relatively low. One study noted no increase in hospital infections after the introduction of AAI [100]. Additionally, a review of the literature published in 2016 noted that with appropriate screening precautions, risks could be effectively mitigated [109]. Many of these risks may be effectively prevented with appropriate selection of patients and animals along with adherence to published guidelines and implementation of local facility protocols. With these preventative measures, the benefits of animals in healthcare facilities likely greatly outweigh risks.

Guidelines to Minimize Infection Risk in Animals in Healthcare

Several published guidelines exist to guide facilities in establishing precautions and security measures for minimizing risk from AAI and animals in healthcare facilities. Notably, in 2008, the *American Journal of Infection Control* published a set of guidelines established through a working group of expert stakeholders and including evidence-based statements [102]. Additionally, in 2015, the SHEA published recommendations to minimize risks of animals in healthcare [110]. The Centers for Disease Control (CDC) has published recommendations and so has the AAP Red Book [111, 112]. Some of the basic principles of animals in healthcare facilities and AAI are discussed in Table 4.3.

Table 4.3 Recommendations related to animal-assisted interventions

Stakeholders	Recommendation
Prior to hospital visit	
Hospital or healthcare facilities	Individual facilities should develop guidelines and policies to minimize the risks of injury or transmission of pathogens from animals to humans in the healthcare setting. Policies should be developed in consultation with physicians, nursing staff, infection control specialists, risk management, and veterinarians
Medical providers	Animal visits to patients should be approved by the primary medical provider after consideration of the risks and benefits. A history of allergic reactions with animal contact, a fear of animals, and the patient's medical condition should be part of this consideration Verbal or written consent should be obtained from patients or caretakers prior to visitation from facility animals and their handlers

Table 4.3 (continued)

Stakeholders	Recommendation
Animal handlers and veterinarians	Visiting animals should have veterinary documentation of good health including a certificate of immunization from a licensed veterinarian and an annual fecal exam for enteric parasites. The animal should be checked for any skin infections, including those caused by bacteria, ectoparasites such as fleas and ticks, or superficial dermatophytes Animals used in AAT and volunteer pet programs should have documentation of temperament testing or prior behavior assessment by a trained volunteer or employee Animals should be well groomed and recently bathed prior to facility visitation
Precautions and visitation exclusions	
Hospital or healthcare facilities, medical providers, animal handlers	Patients should be excluded if there are isolation restrictions, undressed wounds, and/or burns, if there is a sterile field present, or if there is a severe immunodeficiency Animal interaction in high-risk patient areas such as the intensive care units (including cardiac intensive care), hematology-oncology unit, and transplant units should be considered cautiously and approved by medical leadership
Medical providers	Patients with medical devices including indwelling catheters, feeding tubes, tracheostomy tubes, or oxygen delivery devices should undergo preparation to secure and cover devices prior to animal visits in order to prevent body or mouth contact and/or dislodgement of the device
Hospital or healthcare facilities, animal handlers	Animals excluded from visitation should include reptiles and amphibians, nonhuman primates, hamsters, gerbils, mice, rats or other rodents, and other animals that have not been litter trained, such as birds. Fish may be considered on a case-by-case basis
During animal visit	
Animal handlers	Animals should be transported around the facility by a trained handler or employee familiar with the animal. Pet carriers or a short leash (4 feet or less) should be used. In the cases of personal pet visitation, it may be appropriate that a family member carries or walks the animal with direct facility employee supervision Contact with animal dander, saliva, urine, or feces should be minimized
Medical providers	Facility personnel should supervise all animal visits. Child life staff may be trained in patient-animal interactions and may provide guidance and oversight. Supervisors should be trained in facility policies including how to respond to cases of animal bites or animal defecation or vomiting
Medical providers and animal handlers	Before and after animal contact, patients, staff, and visitors should perform hand hygiene with facility-approved alcohol-based foams or gels or wash their hands with soap and water if their hands are visibility soiled. Areas of the facility with animal contact should be cleaned and disinfected after the animal visit is complete Take prompt action if an animal bite or scratch occurs. The animal should be removed from the facility, and the event should be reported to appropriate authorities including infection control staff and animal program coordinators. The bite or scratch should be quickly treated according to medical best practices

Play Areas

Family-centered care at its core is patient-centered care. In pediatric hospitals, normalization of an unfamiliar environment is a critical part of supporting hospitalized children [80]. The importance of play and child life programs that facilitate and participate in patient play has grown with the shift toward family- and patient-centered care [80]. Play has shown to promote child development and create a sense of normalcy [80, 113]. Play can also be a means for expression and learning about the hospital environment. Playrooms are "an essential part of creating a normal childhood environment for ill children" since they bring an outside, familiar habitat into the hospital [113]. Some hospitals welcome siblings in the playroom to further enhance the family-centered care although this is not universally accepted. Playrooms universally include toys, which have been shown to decrease the anxiety hospitalized children experience [114].

Playrooms can also be a source of infection as research has shown that children that congregate often spread communicable diseases [115–118]. Specifically, studies of daycare and hospital toys have shown that they can be a source of pathogens [119, 120]. Contamination with pathogenic organisms can happen within a week of a toy being introduced into the hospital environment, as demonstrated by a study of sterilized teddy bears that were given to hospitalized children [121]. The teddy bears were originally part of a campaign to promote hand hygiene within the hospital. Hospital toys have also been the source of rare outbreaks. For example, an outbreak of *Pseudomonas* occurred in a pediatric oncology unit related to bath toys and their container [122]. On another oncology ward, an outbreak of rotavirus was related to lack of regular cleaning of playroom toys [123]. The material of the toys affects the likelihood that they will contain bacteria, with plastic being the most prevalent followed by metal and other materials [124]. In a study in an Argentinian children's hospital, the toys that were handled by patients in a playroom were contaminated 87% of the time by bacteria from the *Staphylococcus* genus [125]. Playroom toys have been noted to be colonized with coagulase-negative staphylococci in 38.8–45.5% of cases [124, 125]. *S. aureus* are also found on toys with one study showing 28.8% of toys contaminated by this organism. Of all the *S. aureus* strains found in that study of playroom toys, 21.4% were resistant to oxacillin. In a study in a Peruvian pediatric hospital, of 40 toys that were tested, 20% had *S. aureus* recovered in culture [126]. These percentages of *S. aureus* are not unexpected, however, since between 20 and 40% of the general population are colonized and this organism is known to be prevalent in the environment [125]. While these studies examine the level of contamination with *S. aureus*, they make no mention of the prevalence of *S. aureus* infections or any relationship of infections to contact with the contaminated toys. For both bacteria and viruses, the presence of contamination does not always correlate with the risk of infection since the exact infectious doses of each organism are difficult to determine [86].

Playroom surfaces can also harbor pathogens, including bacteria and viruses. A number of clinically important viruses can survive for prolonged periods of time, especially on doors, high hand-touch sites, and work surfaces [86]. Viruses like norovirus, rotavirus, and astrovirus have been found in pediatric hospital wards [42, 86]. Surface contamination with rotavirus, adenovirus, and norovirus are frequently associated with healthcare settings [127]. In one study, viral contamination within a hospital unit was associated with areas trafficked by parents of hospitalized children [42]. This suggests that playrooms, where parents and hospitalized children frequent, are more likely to have viral contamination. Again, the exact level at which contamination leads to infection, however, is difficult to determine.

Mitigating the risk of infection from the playroom is crucial to the safety of hospitalized children. Our recommendations are that all children's hospitals should have a playroom that is readily accessible to patients. In addition, no one who is on airborne, droplet, or contact precautions should visit the playroom. The AAP Committee on Infectious Diseases recommends that siblings should not visit the playroom, albeit there is no robust evidence to support this recommendation [67]. If family members are allowed in the playroom, screening of siblings or adult caretakers for acute illness (fever, cough, vomiting, diarrhea, or rash) is advised prior to entering the playroom. Notably, one study focusing on family-centered care argues for including siblings in the playroom as long as they are screened appropriately [67, 113]. Regular cleaning of toys and hard surfaces inside the playroom are important to break the chain of transmission of pathogenic organisms [128]. We recommend the selection of toys and containers for toys made from material that are amenable to washing with soap and water as well as 70% alcohol, like plastic, acrylic, rubber, and metal [125]. Regular cleaning of the toys is recommended, whether it be after each use or calendar-based (e.g., daily). Cleaning and/or disinfecting surfaces within the playroom should also be on a schedule and tailored to the individual playroom with a focus on high-touch surfaces [119, 128]. One study demonstrated a decrease in surface viral contamination with daily floor cleaning with surface cleaning twice daily while glass screens and windows were cleaned weekly [42].

Adverse Impacts of Contact Precautions on Patient Care

Since the onset of infection control practices, concerns have been raised about the potential impact to patient care. Historically, much of the concern centered on the social stigma that comes along with isolation. In the current hospital environment however, and specifically within pediatrics, isolation precautions are commonplace and may occur in a large percentage of patients. As previously noted, infection control decisions require a balance between patient safety and the need for FCC and patient well-being. Research to date examining the potential negative impacts of isolation practices has largely been conducted in adult patients and has sought to investigate if isolated patients, when compared to non-isolated patients, experience the following negative effects: a decrease in the quality of care, fewer interactions with healthcare workers, delays in care and adverse events, the presence of symptoms of depression and anxiety, and lower satisfaction with their care. Providers and families of hospitalized children have also worried about the psychosocial impacts of isolation practices. The following subchapter outlines some of the conflicting reports regarding the potential for untoward effects.

The Impact of Contract Precautions on the Quality of Care

For decades, a principal concern has been that patients isolated for infection control, in addition to social stigmatization, may receive lower quality care. Several studies conducted in adult populations have documented that providers spent less time in patient rooms when patients were on isolation precautions regardless of the setting (wards or intensive care unit) and were less likely to enter the rooms of isolated patients when compared to non-isolated patients [129–131]. Another report published in 2003 noted that adult patients isolated for MRSA colonization or infection were less likely to have vital signs documented, had fewer daily physician progress notes, had twice as many preventable adverse events, and were more likely to formally complain about their care to the hospital when compared to control (non-isolated) patients [132].

These reports are balanced, however, by two other studies conducted in pediatric settings which showed no differences in the quality of care or direct patient contact between isolated and non-isolated patients. The first, published in 1989, was conducted prospectively in a pediatric intensive care setting and demonstrated no difference in the frequency of contact by hospital personnel or family members between patients receiving isolation precautions and those receiving standard precautions [133]. Additionally, it was reported that patients tolerated contact isolation well, and there was no increase in adverse events between groups. The second study published in 2008 was a blinded prospective observational study and additionally reported no differences in time spent with isolated vs non-isolated patients on an acute care, general pediatrics service [134]. Study investigators reported on other quantitative measures including the number of organ systems examined, vital signs recorded, and other balance measures. Parent satisfaction questionnaires showed no differences in the caregiver perceived quality of care between isolated and non-isolated patients. These two studies cast doubt on the theory that the quality of care and patient satisfaction may be negatively impacted by the use of contact precautions, especially in pediatric care. Larger, multicenter studies focusing on pediatric inpatient care are needed however to better understand the true impacts of contact precautions on children's care and caregiver satisfaction.

The Psychosocial and Behavioral Impacts of Contact Precautions

Isolation practices can have profound psychosocial and behavioral impacts, however, and providers should strive to understand the implications of placing a patient on contact isolation. A hospital can be a frightening and anxiety-producing place for pediatric patients. To add to this, when a physician or hospital staff member enters a patient room dressed in a mask, gown, gloves, and/or other personal protective equipment (PPE), this will likely only worsen a sense of fear in a child. Contact precautions often may preclude the patient from leaving the room or moving to other areas of the hospital. A child's reaction to infection control practices is influenced by their age, development, and potentially parental or caretaker reaction to the measures.

In adult studies, the data is again mixed. Higher depressions scores, anxiety scores, and anger-hostility scores have all been reported in isolated patients when compared to non-isolated patients suggesting that infection prevention measures have negative impacts on patient psychological well-being. [135] Patients have reported increased fear and loneliness while in isolation for infection reasons as well. It is worth noting that many of these symptoms seem to increase as the length of time in the hospital increased and short-term isolation practices may be less associated with increased depression and anxiety [136]. Other studies, however, have shown no differences in development of increased depression, anxiety, or other negative emotions such as sadness, anger, and worry [137, 138].

In children, the psychological and behavioral effects of isolation practices are perhaps harder to quantify, and there is lack of recent literature in this area. A review published in 2013 draws attention to the lack of current literature examining the pediatric patient experience while in hospital isolation [139]. This review notes that much of the research conducted on the developmental impacts of source isolation is dated, occurring in the 1970s and 1980s, and often involves single patients, with a single disease process such as severe combined immunodeficiency, who were isolated for prolonged periods (months to years). More recent literature has examined patient and caretaker perspectives during outbreaks such as the 2003 SARS outbreak [140, 141]. These studies provide examples of extreme infection prevention precautions including complete separation of the child from the caregiver. Not unexpectedly, this form of isolation was associated with significant emotional distress including reported feelings of sadness, loneliness, worry, and fear among both patients and their caretakers. More common reasons for patient isolation, including upper and lower respiratory track viral infections, gastroenteritis, draining lesions and wounds, and MRSA infections to name a few, may affect a wide range of patients of different ages and cultures and may result in a range of time in the hospital. The psychosocial impact of contact precautions on this patient group deserves further investigation.

More has been written about the fear children experience when hospitalized or facing medical care. Forsner et al. comment that medical care may cause profound fear and is even perceived as threatening to the very existence of the child [142]. School-age children often use magical and fantastical thinking to interpret the world around them, and medical care may be perceived as a danger or a "monster" that threatens to destroy the child, according to Forsner and colleagues. It is easy to see that the use of PPE may only worsen this perception by pediatric patients. Forsner reports as well that children under 7 years of age rely heavily on appearances when making assessments of potential threats. PPE can distort normal human appearance and prevent the ability of a child to interpret who is friendly and who is threatening. Children have expressed a sense of feeling overpowered and helpless in the medical environment. Hospital staff entering a room may outnumber the child and his or her parents or caretakers and this contributes to a sense of powerlessness. Medical environments include equipment necessary for providing care that may be perceived by a young child as being designed to cause harm including needles, other sharp objects, and even blood pressure cuffs. The addition of PPE can only add to this feeling that the intent of medical personnel is to harm the child. Children's narratives, as studied by Forsner, suggest that fear experienced is magnified when children feel objectified and their own feelings are not validated by those performing a procedure or examination. PPE may obscure the child's ability to see a provider smile, express empathy, or convey comforting gestures [142].

Confinement to a space due to isolation precautions is potentially detrimental situation for a child as well. Isolation may prevent normalization activities such as trips to a playroom, library, or social events with other children. Especially in younger children, confinement to an area may be perceived as punishment. In the home environment, children may be punished by being told to stand in a corner or being sent to their room. Inability to leave a hospital room likely triggers strong associations to punishment for young children. [142] Even in older children, the inability to socialize and leave a confined space may negatively affect self-esteem.

Mitigation of the Negative Effects of Contact Precautions

Medical providers should make every effort to minimize the potential for negative effects of isolation precautions. The first step toward reducing untoward effects is simply to avoid overuse. Providers should be cognizant of the potential for negative impacts and work closely with hospital infection control departments to effectively identify patients who are appropriate for contact precautions and appropriate timing for discontinuation of these precautions. National guidelines and recommendations (as outlined in this text) serve to guide practitioners toward the judicious use of these precautions. For patients on contact precautions, there should also be a daily reassessment by the medical team to determine if precautions can be removed. In the busy clinical environment, it is easy to overlook details such as contact precautions, and diligence in this area is necessary for all providers involved in the care of the child. The presence or absence of isolation precautions may be a memorable experience for families and patients and influence their perceived care. In the many instances, when contact precautions cannot be avoided, however, physicians and staff should consider bundling care and minimizing interruptions to the patient's day as well as minimizing the number of care providers in the room at a given time.

Adequate communication regarding the reasons for contact precautions is another important step to minimizing the negative effects. In a study published in 2000 in *Nursing Standard*, study authors note that clear and frequent communication about the need for contact precautions was highly impactful on patient satisfaction [143]. Similarly, in children, age appropriate communication and explanations regarding the reasons for contact isolation is very important. When speaking to a young school-aged child, for example, using the words, "since you have the flu, when you cough, you could spread germs to other children and adults and make them sick too, and for this reason, we need you to stay in this room right now," is preferable to "you have to stay in your room because you are sick." In the first example, specific language is used to clearly state why precautions are necessary.

Many pediatric facilities have access to child life trained staff who can be an invaluable resource to aiding the child and family with normalization activities, developing a routine, and integrating the "outside" into the patient's room. Decorating the room, bringing developmental activities to the patient room, and familiarizing the child with the hospital environment and equipment are all key strategies that can help with coping and anxiety relief especially in the setting of isolation practices. Familiarity with PPE may help decrease anxiety and fear, and when possible, care providers can allow children to touch and, when appropriate, play with equipment such as gloves and gowns. The use of technology can be highly effective in confronting the challenges of isolation practices as well. Teenagers and young children are increasingly engaged in social media, texting, and using video conferences with friends and family members, and the use of these technologies can help with social stimulation and relieve boredom. Cystic fibrosis patients, for example, are a particular group of patients who are often isolated in the hospital environment and have limited contact with peers who also have cystic fibrosis so as to decrease the bacterial and fungal pulmonary colonization risk. Texting, online chat rooms, and social media can all be very beneficial in connecting these teenage patients at an age when social connectedness and normalization can be very important to self-image.

References

1. Patient- and family-centered care. http://www.ipfcc.org/about/pfcc.html. Accessed 15 Jan 2018.
2. Adams S, Herrera A, Miller L, Soto R. Visitation in the intensive care unit: impact on infection prevention and control. Crit Care Nurs Q. 2011;34(1):3–10.
3. Dingeman RS, Mitchell EA, Meyer EC, Curley MA. Parent presence during complex invasive procedures and cardiopulmonary resuscitation: a systematic review of the literature. Pediatrics. 2007;120(4):842–54.
4. Dokken D, Parent K, Ahmann E. Family presence and participation: pediatrics leading the way … and still evolving. Pediatr Nurs. 2015;41(4):204–6.
5. Institute for Patient- and Family-Centered Care. Changing hospital "visiting" policies and practices: supporting family presence and participation. 2010. http://www.ipfcc.org/resources/visiting.pdf. Accessed 16 Jan 2010.
6. Muething SE, Kotagal UR, Schoettker PJ, Gonzalez del Rey J, TG DW. Family-centered bedside rounds: a new approach to patient care and teaching. Pediatrics. 2007;119(4):829–32.
7. Bertakis KD, Azari R. Patient-centered care is associated with decreased health care utilization. J Am Board Fam Med. 2011;24(3):229–39.
8. Bertakis KD, Azari R. Determinants and outcomes of patient-centered care. Patient Educ Couns. 2011;85(1):46–52.
9. Goldfarb MJ, Bibas L, Bartlett V, Jones H, Khan N. Outcomes of patient- and family-centered care interventions in the ICU: a systematic review and meta-analysis. Crit Care Med. 2017;45(10):1751–61.
10. Stewart M, Brown JB, Donner A, et al. The impact of patient-centered care on outcomes. J Fam Pract. 2000;49(9):796–804.
11. Sweeney L, Halpert A, Waranoff J. Patient-centered management of complex patients can reduce costs without shortening life. Am J Manag Care. 2007;13(2):84–92.
12. Wolff JL, Roter DL. Family presence in routine medical visits: a meta-analytical review. Soc Sci Med. 2011;72(6):823–31.

13. Anonymous. Data trends. Measuring the cost benefits of family-centered care. Healthc Financ Manage. 2003;57(9):118.
14. Washam M, Woltmann J, Ankrum A, Connelly B. Association of visitation policy and health care-acquired respiratory viral infections in hospitalized children. Am J Infect Control. 2017;46(3):353–5.
15. Slota M, Shearn D, Potersnak K, Haas L. Perspectives on family-centered, flexible visitation in the intensive care unit setting. Crit Care Med. 2003;31(5 Suppl):S362–6.
16. Fumagalli S, Boncinelli L, Lo Nostro A, et al. Reduced cardiocirculatory complications with unrestrictive visiting policy in an intensive care unit: results from a pilot, randomized trial. Circulation. 2006;113(7):946–52.
17. Usher BM, Hill KM. Family visitation in the adult intensive care unit. Crit Care Nurse. 2016;36(1):e15–8.
18. Berwick DM, Kotagal M. Restricted visiting hours in ICUs: time to change. JAMA. 2004;292(6):736–7.
19. Simpson T, Shaver J. Cardiovascular responses to family visits in coronary care unit patients. Heart Lung. 1990;19(4):344–51.
20. Kleman M, Bickert A, Karpinski A, et al. Physiologic responses of coronary care patients to visiting. J Cardiovasc Nurs. 1993;7(3):52–62.
21. Ramsey P, Cathelyn J, Gugliotta B, Glenn LL. Visitor and nurse satisfaction with a visitation policy change in critical care units. Dimens Crit Care Nurs. 1999;18(5):42–8.
22. Davidson JE, Powers K, Hedayat KM, et al. Clinical practice guidelines for support of the family in the patient-centered intensive care unit: American College of Critical Care Medicine Task Force 2004-2005. Crit Care Med. 2007;35(2):605–22.
23. Davidson JE, Aslakson RA, Long AC, et al. Guidelines for family-centered care in the neonatal, pediatric, and adult ICU. Crit Care Med. 2017;45(1):103–28.
24. Sims JM, Miracle VA. A look at critical care visitation: the case for flexible visitation. Dimens Crit Care Nurs. 2006;25(4):175–80.
25. Hupcey JE. Looking out for the patient and ourselves – the process of family integration into the ICU. J Clin Nurs. 1999;8(3):253–62.
26. Chapman DK, Collingridge DS, Mitchell LA, et al. Satisfaction with elimination of all visitation restrictions in a mixed-profile intensive care unit. Am J Crit Care. 2016;25(1):46–50.
27. Committee on Hospital Care, Institute for Patient- and Family-Centered Care. Patient- and family-centered care and the pediatrician's role. Pediatrics. 2012;129(2):394–404.
28. Munoz-Price LS, Banach DB, Bearman G, et al. Isolation precautions for visitors. Infect Control Hosp Epidemiol. 2015;36(7):747–58.
29. Munoz FM, Ong LT, Seavy D, Medina D, Correa A, Starke JR. Tuberculosis among adult visitors of children with suspected tuberculosis and employees at a children's hospital. Infect Control Hosp Epidemiol. 2002;23(10):568–72.
30. Jensen PA, Lambert LA, Iademarco MF, Ridzon R, Centers for Disease Control and Prevention. Guidelines for preventing the transmission of Mycobacterium tuberculosis in health-care settings, 2005. MMWR Recomm Rep. 2005;54(RR-17):1–141.
31. Cruz AT, Starke JR. A current review of infection control for childhood tuberculosis. Tuberculosis. 2011;91(Suppl 1):S11–5.
32. Cruz AT, Medina D, Whaley EM, Ware KM, Koy TH, Starke JR. Tuberculosis among families of children with suspected tuberculosis and employees at a children's hospital. Infect Control Hosp Epidemiol. 2011;32(2):188–90.
33. Peluso AM, Harnish BA, Miller NS, Cooper ER, Fujii AM. Effect of young sibling visitation on respiratory syncytial virus activity in a NICU. J Perinatol. 2015;35(8):627–30.
34. Garcia R, Raad I, Abi-Said D, et al. Nosocomial respiratory syncytial virus infections: prevention and control in bone marrow transplant patients. Infect Control Hosp Epidemiol. 1997;18(6):412–6.
35. Rosa RG, Tonietto TF, da Silva DB, et al. Effectiveness and safety of an extended ICU visitation model for delirium prevention: a before and after study. Crit Care Med. 2017;45(10):1660–7.

36. Malacarne P, Pini S, De Feo N. Relationship between pathogenic and colonizing microorganisms detected in intensive care unit patients and in their family members and visitors. Infect Control Hosp Epidemiol. 2008;29(7):679–81.
37. Malacarne P, Corini M, Petri D. Health care-associated infections and visiting policy in an intensive care unit. Am J Infect Control. 2011;39(10):898–900.
38. Tang CS, Chung FF, Lin MC, Wan GH. Impact of patient visiting activities on indoor climate in a medical intensive care unit: a 1-year longitudinal study. Am J Infect Control. 2009;37(3):183–8.
39. Polak J, Ringler N, Daugherty B. Unit based procedures: impact on the incidence of nosocomial infections in the newborn intensive care unit. Newborn Infant Nurs Rev. 2004;4(1):38–45.
40. Lofgren ET. Estimating the impact post randomization changes in staff behavior in infection prevention trials: a mathematical modeling approach. BMC Infect Dis. 2017;17(1):539.
41. Banach DB, Bearman GM, Morgan DJ, Munoz-Price LS. Infection control precautions for visitors to healthcare facilities. Expert Rev Anti-Infect Ther. 2015;13(9):1047–50.
42. Gallimore CI, Taylor C, Gennery AR, et al. Contamination of the hospital environment with gastroenteric viruses: comparison of two pediatric wards over a winter season. J Clin Microbiol. 2008;46(9):3112–5.
43. Birnbach DJ, Rosen LF, Fitzpatrick M, Arheart KL, Munoz-Price LS. An evaluation of hand hygiene in an intensive care unit: are visitors a potential vector for pathogens? J Infect Public Health. 2015;8(6):570–4.
44. Clock SA, Cohen B, Behta M, Ross B, Larson EL. Contact precautions for multidrug-resistant organisms: current recommendations and actual practice. Am J Infect Control. 2010;38(2):105–11.
45. Afif W, Huor P, Brassard P, Loo VG. Compliance with methicillin-resistant Staphylococcus aureus precautions in a teaching hospital. Am J Infect Control. 2002;30(7):430–3.
46. Nishimura S, Kagehira M, Kono F, Nishimura M, Taenaka N. Handwashing before entering the intensive care unit: what we learned from continuous video-camera surveillance. Am J Infect Control. 1999;27(4):367–9.
47. Fakhry M, Hanna GB, Anderson O, Holmes A, Nathwani D. Effectiveness of an audible reminder on hand hygiene adherence. Am J Infect Control. 2012;40(4):320–3.
48. Kellerman SE, Saiman L, San Gabriel P, Besser R, Jarvis WR. Observational study of the use of infection control interventions for Mycobacterium tuberculosis in pediatric facilities. Pediatr Infect Dis J. 2001;20(6):566–70.
49. Said MA, Perl TM, Sears CL. Healthcare epidemiology: gastrointestinal flu: norovirus in health care and long-term care facilities. Clin Infect Dis. 2008;47(9):1202–8.
50. Centers for Disease Control and Prevention. Principles of epidemiology in public health practice, third edition: an introduction to applied epidemiology and biostatistics. 2016. https://www.cdc.gov/ophss/csels/dsepd/ss1978/lesson6/section2.html#step2. Accessed 15 Jan 2018.
51. George RH, Gully PR, Gill ON, Innes JA, Bakhshi SS, Connolly M. An outbreak of tuberculosis in a children's hospital. J Hosp Infect. 1986;8(2):129–42.
52. Bosley AR, George G, George M. Outbreak of pulmonary tuberculosis in children. Lancet. 1986;1(8490):1141–3.
53. Weinstein JW, Barrett CR, Baltimore RS, Hierholzer WJ Jr. Nosocomial transmission of tuberculosis from a hospital visitor on a pediatrics ward. Pediatr Infect Dis J. 1995;14(3):232–4.
54. Halasa NB, Williams JV, Wilson GJ, Walsh WF, Schaffner W, Wright PF. Medical and economic impact of a respiratory syncytial virus outbreak in a neonatal intensive care unit. Pediatr Infect Dis J. 2005;24(12):1040–4.
55. Committee on Infectious Diseases. From the American Academy of Pediatrics: policy statements – modified recommendations for use of palivizumab for prevention of respiratory syncytial virus infections. Pediatrics. 2009;124(6):1694–701.
56. Friesema IH, Vennema H, Heijne JC, et al. Norovirus outbreaks in nursing homes: the evaluation of infection control measures. Epidemiol Infect. 2009;137(12):1722–33.
57. Johnston CP, Qiu H, Ticehurst JR, et al. Outbreak management and implications of a nosocomial norovirus outbreak. Clin Infect Dis. 2007;45(5):534–40.

58. Buchbinder N, Dumesnil C, Pinquier D, et al. Pandemic A/H1N1/2009 influenza in a paediatric haematology and oncology unit: successful management of a sudden outbreak. J Hosp Infect. 2011;79(2):155–60.
59. Munoz FM, Campbell JR, Atmar RL, et al. Influenza A virus outbreak in a neonatal intensive care unit. Pediatr Infect Dis J. 1999;18(9):811–5.
60. Centers for Disease Control and Prevention. Revised U.S. surveillance case definition for severe acute respiratory syndrome (SARS) and update on SARS cases – United States and worldwide, December 2003. MMWR Morb Mortal Wkly Rep. 2003;52(49):1202–6.
61. Mukhopadhyay A, Tambyah PA, Singh KS, Lim TK, Lee KH. SARS in a hospital visitor and her intensivist. J Hosp Infect. 2004;56(3):249–50.
62. Gopalakrishna G, Choo P, Leo YS, et al. SARS transmission and hospital containment. Emerg Infect Dis. 2004;10(3):395–400.
63. Dwosh H, Hong H, Austgarden D, Herman S, Schabas R. Identification and containment of an outbreak of SARS in a community hospital. CMAJ. 2003;168(11):1415–20.
64. Shuler SN, Reich CA. Sibling visitation in pediatric hospitals: policies, opinions, and issues. Child Health Care. 1982;11(2):54–60.
65. Moore KA, Coker K, DuBuisson AB, Swett B, Edwards WH. Implementing potentially better practices for improving family-centered care in neonatal intensive care units: successes and challenges. Pediatrics. 2003;111(4 Pt 2):e450–60.
66. Meyer EC, Kennally KF, Zika-Beres E, Cashore WJ, Oh W. Attitudes about sibling visitation in the neonatal intensive care unit. Arch Pediatr Adolesc Med. 1996;150(10):1021–6.
67. Committee on Infectious Diseases, American Academy of Pediatrics. Infection Control and Prevention for Hospitalized Children: Sibling Visitation. In: Kimberlin DW, Brady MT, Jackson MA, Long SS, editors. Red Book. 30th ed. Elk Grove Village: American Academy of Pediatrics; 2015. p. 173.
68. Poster EC, Betz CL. Survey of sibling and peer visitation policies in southern California hospitals. Child Health Care. 1987;15(3):166–71.
69. Simon K. Perceived stress of nonhospitalized children during the hospitalization of a sibling. J Pediatr Nurs. 1993;8(5):298–304.
70. Cairns NU, Clark GM, Smith SD, Lansky SB. Adaptation of siblings to childhood malignancy. J Pediatr. 1979;95(3):484–7.
71. Meyendorf R. Infant depression due to separation from siblings: syndrome of depression, retardation, starvation, and neurological symptoms. A re-evaluation of the concept of maternal deprivation. Psychiatr Clin (Basel). 1971;4(5):321–35.
72. Petrillo M. Preparing children and parents for hospitalization and treatment. Pediatr Ann. 1972;1(3):24–41.
73. Craft MJ, Wyatt N, Sandell B. Behavior and feeling changes in siblings of hospitalized children. Clin Pediatr (Phila). 1985;24(7):374–8.
74. Knafl KA. Parents' views of the response of siblings to a pediatric hospitalization. Res Nurs Health. 1982;5(1):13–20.
75. Hartling L, Milne A, Tjosvold L, Wrightson D, Gallivan J, Newton AS. A systematic review of interventions to support siblings of children with chronic illness or disability. J Paediatr Child Health. 2014;50(10):E26–38.
76. Youngblut JM, Shiao SY. Child and family reactions during and after pediatric ICU hospitalization: a pilot study. Heart Lung. 1993;22(1):46–54.
77. Rozdilsky JR. Enhancing sibling presence in pediatric ICU. Crit Care Nurs Clin North Am. 2005;17(4):451–61, xii.
78. Craft MJ. Validation of responses reported by school-aged siblings of hospitalized children. Child Health Care. 1986;15(1):6–13.
79. Craft MJ, Craft JL. Perceived changes in siblings of hospitalized children: a comparison of sibling and parent reports. Child Health Care. 1989;18(1):42–8.
80. Committee on Hospital Care, Child Life Council. Child life services. Pediatrics. 2014;133(5):e1471–8.
81. Oehler JM, Vileisis RA. Effect of early sibling visitation in an intensive care nursery. J Dev Behav Pediatr. 1990;11(1):7–12.

82. Montgomery LA, Kleiber C, Nicholson A, Craft-Rosenberg M. A research-based sibling visitation program for the neonatal ICU. Crit Care Nurse. 1997;17(2):29–35, 38-40.
83. Gursky B. The effect of educational interventions with siblings of hospitalized children. J Dev Behav Pediatr. 2007;28(5):392–8.
84. Beickert K, Mora K. Transforming the pediatric experience: the story of child life. Pediatr Ann. 2017;46(9):e345–51.
85. Smith L, Medves J, Harrison MB, Tranmer J, Waytuck B. The impact of hospital visiting hour policies on pediatric and adult patients and their visitors. JBI Libr Syst Rev. 2009;7(2):38–79.
86. D'Arcy N, Cloutman-Green E, Klein N, Spratt DA. Environmental viral contamination in a pediatric hospital outpatient waiting area: implications for infection control. Am J Infect Control. 2014;42(8):856–60.
87. Umphenour JH. Bacterial colonization in neonates with sibling visitation. JOGN Nurs. 1980;9(2):73–5.
88. Wranesh BL. The effect of sibling visitation on bacterial colonization rate in neonates. JOGN Nurs. 1982;11(4):211–3.
89. Solheim K, Spellacy C. Sibling visitation: effects on newborn infection rates. J Obstet Gynecol Neonatal Nurs. 1988;17(1):43–8.
90. Spear HJ. Child visitation policy and practice for maternity units. MCN Am J Matern Child Nurs. 2009;34(6):372–7.
91. Gupta M, Pursley DM. A survey of infection control practices for influenza in mother and newborn units in US hospitals. Am J Obstet Gynecol. 2011;204(6 Suppl):S77–83.
92. Visiting hours. 2018. https://www.childrensomaha.org/visiting-hours. Accessed 15 Jan 2018.
93. For vistors: visiting and deliveries. 2018. http://www.seattlechildrens.org/visitors/visiting/. Accessed 15 Jan 2018.
94. Visiting hours and policies. 2018. https://www.urmc.rochester.edu/childrens-hospital/visitor-information/visiting-hours.aspx. Accessed 15 Jan 2018.
95. 2017 – 2018 APPA national pet owners survey. 2017. http://www.americanpetproducts.org/pubs_survey.asp.
96. Chu CI, Liu CY, Sun CT, Lin J. The effect of animal-assisted activity on inpatients with schizophrenia. J Psychosoc Nurs Ment Health Serv. 2009;47(12):42–8.
97. Stasi MF, Amati D, Costa C, et al. Pet-therapy: a trial for institutionalized frail elderly patients. Arch Gerontol Geriatr Suppl. 2004;9:407–12.
98. Cole KM, Gawlinski A, Steers N, Kotlerman J. Animal-assisted therapy in patients hospitalized with heart failure. Am J Crit Care. 2007;16(6):575–85; quiz 586; discussion 587-578.
99. Braun C, Stangler T, Narveson J, Pettingell S. Animal-assisted therapy as a pain relief intervention for children. Complement Ther Clin Pract. 2009;15(2):105–9.
100. Caprilli S, Messeri A. Animal-assisted activity at A. Meyer Children's Hospital: a pilot study. Evid Based Complement Alternat Med. 2006;3(3):379–83.
101. Bouchard F, Landry M, Belles-Isles M, Gagnon J. A magical dream: a pilot project in animal-assisted therapy in pediatric oncology. Can Oncol Nurs J. 2004;14(1):14–7.
102. Lefebvre SL, Waltner-Toews D, Peregrine AS, et al. Prevalence of zoonotic agents in dogs visiting hospitalized people in Ontario: implications for infection control. J Hosp Infect. 2006;62(4):458–66.
103. Snider R, Landers S, Levy ML. The ringworm riddle: an outbreak of Microsporum canis in the nursery. Pediatr Infect Dis J. 1993;12(2):145–8.
104. Mossovitch M, Mossovitch B, Alkan M. Nosocomial dermatophytosis caused by Microsporum canis in a newborn department. Infect Control. 1986;7(12):593–5.
105. Richet HM, Craven PC, Brown JM, et al. A cluster of Rhodococcus (Gordona) Bronchialis sternal-wound infections after coronary-artery bypass surgery. N Engl J Med. 1991;324(2):104–9.
106. Lyons RW, Samples CL, DeSilva HN, Ross KA, Julian EM, Checko PJ. An epidemic of resistant Salmonella in a nursery. Animal-to-human spread. JAMA. 1980;243(6):546–7.
107. Chang HJ, Miller HL, Watkins N, et al. An epidemic of Malassezia pachydermatis in an intensive care nursery associated with colonization of health care workers' pet dogs. N Engl J Med. 1998;338(11):706–11.

108. Scott GM, Thomson R, Malone-Lee J, Ridgway GL. Cross-infection between animals and man: possible feline transmission of Staphylococcus aureus infection in humans? J Hosp Infect. 1988;12(1):29–34.

109. Bert F, Gualano MR, Camussi E, Pieve G, Voglino G, Siliquini R. Animal assisted intervention: a systematic review of benefits and risks. Eur J Integr Med. 2016;8(5):695–706.

110. Murthy R, Bearman G, Brown S, et al. Animals in healthcare facilities: recommendations to minimize potential risks. Infect Control Hosp Epidemiol. 2015;36(5):495–516.

111. US Department of Health and Human Services, Centers for Disease Control and Prevention. Guidelines for environmental infection control in health-care facilities. Atlanta: CDC (Centers for Disease Control). 2018. https://www.cdc.gov/infectioncontrol/pdf/guidelines/environmental-guidelines.pdf. Accessed 28 Sept 2018.

112. Committee on Infectious Diseases, American Academy of Pediatrics, Kimberlin D, Brady M, Jackson M, Long S. Recommendations for care of children in special circumstances. In: Kimberlin DW, Brady MT, Jackson MA, Long SS, editors. Red book. 30th ed. Elk Grove Village: American Academy of Pediatrics; 2015. p. 174–5.

113. Ivany A, LeBlanc C, Grisdale M, Maxwell B, Langley JM. Reducing infection transmission in the playroom: balancing patient safety and family-centered care. Am J Infect Control. 2016;44(1):61–5.

114. da Silva JR, Pizzoli LM, Amorim AR, et al. Using therapeutic toys to facilitate venipuncture procedure in preschool children. Pediatr Nurs. 2016;42(2):61–8.

115. Dales RE, Cakmak S, Brand K, Judek S. Respiratory illness in children attending daycare. Pediatr Pulmonol. 2004;38(1):64–9.

116. Nafstad P, Hagen JA, Oie L, Magnus P, Jaakkola JJ. Day care centers and respiratory health. Pediatrics. 1999;103(4 Pt 1):753–8.

117. Barros AJ. Child-care attendance and common morbidity: evidence of association in the literature and questions of design. Rev Saude Publica. 1999;33(1):98–106.

118. Cote SM, Petitclerc A, Raynault MF, et al. Short- and long-term risk of infections as a function of group child care attendance: an 8-year population-based study. Arch Pediatr Adolesc Med. 2010;164(12):1132–7.

119. Fraser A, Wohlgenant K, Cates S, et al. An observational study of frequency of provider hand contacts in child care facilities in North Carolina and South Carolina. Am J Infect Control. 2015;43(2):107–11.

120. Mahl MC, Sadler C. Virus survival on inanimate surfaces. Can J Microbiol. 1975;21(6):819–23.

121. Hughes WT, Williams B, Williams B, Pearson T. The nosocomial colonization of T. Bear. Infect Control. 1986;7(10):495–500.

122. Buttery JP, Alabaster SJ, Heine RG, et al. Multiresistant Pseudomonas aeruginosa outbreak in a pediatric oncology ward related to bath toys. Pediatr Infect Dis J. 1998;17(6):509–13.

123. Rogers M, Weinstock DM, Eagan J, Kiehn T, Armstrong D, Sepkowitz KA. Rotavirus outbreak on a pediatric oncology floor: possible association with toys. Am J Infect Control. 2000;28(5):378–80.

124. Avila-Aguero ML, German G, Paris MM, Herrera JF, Safe Toys Study G. Toys in a pediatric hospital: are they a bacterial source? Am J Infect Control. 2004;32(5):287–90.

125. Boretti VS, Correa RN, dos Santos SS, Leao MV, Goncalves e Silva CR. Sensitivity profile of Staphylococcus spp. and Streptococcus spp. isolated from toys used in a teaching hospital playroom. Rev Paul Pediatr. 2014;32(3):151–6.

126. Ruiz R, Quijandria J, Rojas-Vilca JL, Loyola S. High number of toys contaminated with Staphylococcus aureus in a pediatric hospitalization service. Rev Peru Med Exp Salud Publica. 2016;33(4):830–2.

127. Carducci A, Verani M, Lombardi R, Casini B, Privitera G. Environmental survey to assess viral contamination of air and surfaces in hospital settings. J Hosp Infect. 2011;77(3):242–7.

128. Siani H, Maillard JY. Best practice in healthcare environment decontamination. Eur J Clin Microbiol Infect Dis. 2015;34(1):1–11.

129. Evans HL, Shaffer MM, Hughes MG, et al. Contact isolation in surgical patients: a barrier to care? Surgery. 2003;134(2):180–8.

130. Saint S, Higgins LA, Nallamothu BK, Chenoweth C. Do physicians examine patients in contact isolation less frequently? A brief report. Am J Infect Control. 2003;31(6):354–6.
131. Kirkland KB, Weinstein JM. Adverse effects of contact isolation. Lancet. 1999;354(9185):1177–8.
132. Stelfox HT, Bates DW, Redelmeier DA. Safety of patients isolated for infection control. JAMA. 2003;290(14):1899–905.
133. Klein BS, Perloff WH, Maki DG. Reduction of nosocomial infection during pediatric intensive care by protective isolation. N Engl J Med. 1989;320(26):1714–21.
134. Cohen E, Austin J, Weinstein M, Matlow A, Redelmeier DA. Care of children isolated for infection control: a prospective observational cohort study. Pediatrics. 2008;122(2):e411–5.
135. Abad C, Fearday A, Safdar N. Adverse effects of isolation in hospitalised patients: a systematic review. J Hosp Infect. 2010;76(2):97–102.
136. Wassenberg MW, Severs D, Bonten MJ. Psychological impact of short-term isolation measures in hospitalised patients. J Hosp Infect. 2010;75(2):124–7.
137. Day HR, Perencevich EN, Harris AD, et al. Depression, anxiety, and moods of hospitalized patients under contact precautions. Infect Control Hosp Epidemiol. 2013;34(3):251–8.
138. Findik UY, Ozbas A, Cavdar I, Erkan T, Topcu SY. Effects of the contact isolation application on anxiety and depression levels of the patients. Int J Nurs Pract. 2012;18(4):340–6.
139. Austin D, Prieto J, Rushforth H. The child's experience of single room isolation: a literature review. Nurs Child Young People. 2013;25(3):18–24.
140. Koller DF, Nicholas DB, Goldie RS, Gearing R, Selkirk EK. When family-centered care is challenged by infectious disease: pediatric health care delivery during the SARS outbreaks. Qual Health Res. 2006;16(1):47–60.
141. Chan SS, Leung D, Chui H, et al. Parental response to child's isolation during the SARS outbreak. Ambul Pediatr. 2007;7(5):401–4.
142. Forsner M, Jansson L, Soderberg A. Afraid of medical care school-aged children's narratives about medical fear. J Pediatr Nurs. 2009;24(6):519–28.
143. Rees J, Davies HR, Birchall C, Price J. Psychological effects of source isolation nursing (2): patient satisfaction. Nurs Stand. 2000;14(29):32–6.

Part II

Major Healthcare-Associated Infection Syndromes

Fever in the Hospitalized or Critically Ill Child

5

J. Chase McNeil

Introduction

There is little rigorous data on the incidence or management of different infections specifically in hospitalized children with fever. Thus, recommendations must be gleaned from available studies of individual infections. Furthermore, most available studies on these subjects are highly weighted toward critically ill children. There are evidence-based guideliens for the assessment of fever in adult intensive care unit patients [1], however. In select cases, it may be reasonable to extrapolate such recommendations for adults to the pediatric population.

In general, temperature instability in any hospitalized child warrants a physical examination and careful evaluation for source. The value of a careful physical exam cannot be overemphasized in determining the source of fever and guiding diagnostic evaluation. Furthermore, in patients with ongoing illness, clinical assessment is an iterative and continuous process with the potential for new clues as to etiology to arise over time. It is valuable to consider individual patient risk factors for infection, particularly regarding medical foreign bodies/devices, underlying conditions, recent invasive procedures or surgeries, and medications. Finally, it is also of import to consider history of recent infections and their treatment as well as the appropriateness of previous diagnoses/therapy in order to guide management. Given the complexity of many patients in the pediatric and neonatal ICUs (PICU and NICU, respectively), specific guidelines are difficult to formulate which would apply to all patients, and in general care must be individualized. This chapter will provide a brief overview of the general considerations in the evaluation of the hospitalized child with fever (Fig. 5.1). A number of the topics discussed below are given a

J. C. McNeil
Department of Pediatrics, Section of Infectious Diseases, Baylor College of Medicine
and Texas Children's Hospital, Houston, TX, USA
e-mail: jm140109@bcm.edu

© Springer Nature Switzerland AG 2019
J. C. McNeil et al. (eds.), *Healthcare-Associated Infections in Children*,
https://doi.org/10.1007/978-3-319-98122-2_5

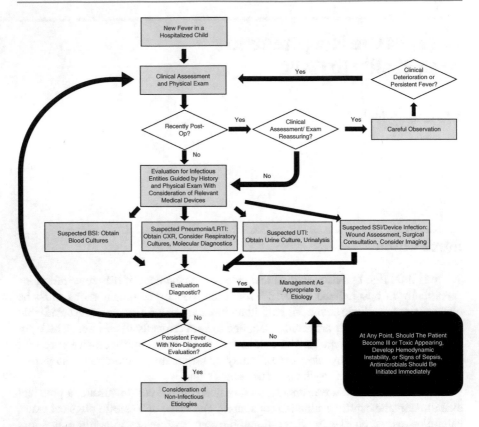

Fig. 5.1 Framework for the evaluation of the hospitalized child with fever. Abbreviations: Post-op, postoperative; BSI, bloodstream infection; LRTI, lower respiratory tract infection; UTI, urinary tract infection; SSI, surgical site infection. Disclaimer: This is to serve as a teaching tool regarding potential etiologies and the need for iterative evaluations of complex febrile children. This is not intended to serve as substitute for sound clinical judgment. The loop nature of this suggested algorithm is meant to emphasize the iterative nature of clinical assessment/diagnostic evaluation. Furthermore, the value of history (of events both prior to and during the hospitalization) and careful physical examination cannot be understated.

meticulous treatment in other dedicated chapters in this text; the interested reader is referred to these other chapters for greater detail.

Bloodstream Infection

Consideration must always be given to the possibility of a bacteremic infection in hospitalized children with fever, particularly when patients are immunocompromised or have central venous catheters in situ. Data from the Centers for Disease Control and Prevention (CDC) National Healthcare Safety Network has shown a steady decline in the incidence of nosocomial central line-associated bloodstream infection (CLABSI) developing in children in the United States [2]. Despite these strides, CLABSI still contributes substantially to morbidity in children along with increased hospital costs and length of stay [3]. A thorough discussion of CLABSI is provided in Chap. 6. Current Infectious Diseases Society of America (IDSA) and American College of Critical Care Medicine guidelines recommend obtaining blood cultures within 24 h of a new fever in adult ICU patients and preferably prior to the initiation of systemic antimicrobials [1]. For patients with a central venous line, at least one blood culture should be obtained from the catheter and one from a peripheral venipuncture; such measures help to distinguish true CLABSI from bacteremia secondary to another focus and may also help adjudicate whether or not a low-virulence pathogen represents true infection. Apart from identifying CLABSI, in the case of secondary bacteremia, blood culture results may also alert clinicians as to the potential for an occult focus of infection and its microbial etiology.

Blood cultures should be obtained judiciously, however, in order to maximize yield and minimize unnecessary diagnostic testing. In literature from the late 1990s, approximately 30% of adult ICU patients received at least one blood culture during the course of their ICU stay with approximately 10% of these yielding a microorganism [4]. Notably, of those positive blood cultures, nearly half were ultimately considered contaminants (e.g., *Micrococcus* spp., diphtheroids, etc.) [4]. Thus, it is important to consider the likely yield of blood culture and the potential consequences of false-positive results including unnecessary antibiotic exposure, additional diagnostic evaluation, and increased medical costs [5].

Studies of PICU patients have shown that institutional efforts to judiciously utilize blood cultures can be performed safely and effectively. As part of a quality improvement project, Johns Hopkins Bloomberg Children's Center utilized a checklist and algorithm approach to assist clinicians in determining the likely yield of blood culture. This intervention was associated with an almost 50% reduction in the rate of blood culture drawn per 100 patient days with no change in mortality, hospital/PICU readmission, or the rate of blood culture obtainment in patients with known/suspected sepsis [6].

Questions often arise as to the need for repeated blood cultures in hospitalized children with persistent fever of unknown origin. IDSA guidelines for adult ICU patients only recommend repeat cultures if there is clinical suspicion of ongoing bacteremia/fungemia, for test of cure after starting therapy for a positive culture or with other significant clinical changes [1]. Even among immunocompromised patients with persistent fever, the yield of repeat blood cultures in the setting of an initially negative culture is low in the absence of hemodynamic alterations or other clinical deteriorations. Current IDSA guidelines for the management of febrile neutropenia in adults and children recommend against additional blood cultures beyond day 3 of fever in the absence of clinical change or previous positive blood cultures [7]. In a study of pediatric febrile neutropenia at Comer Children's Hospital, of 294 febrile patients without bacteremia on day 1, 6 developed a positive blood culture beyond day 3, and only 1 of these was a true pathogen that occurred in the absence of hemodynamic instability (0.34%) [8]. Thus, while all hospitalized, febrile children are worthy of examination and careful consideration (especially if immunocompromised), the yield of repeat blood cultures in the face of previously negative studies and in the absence of other clinical changes is quite low.

Respiratory Infection and ICU-Acquired Pneumonia

Respiratory infections are quite common in the PICU or NICU setting with ventilator-associated pneumonia (VAP) having a reported incidence of 1–2/1000 ventilator days [2]. Principal clues toward VAP or other hospital-acquired respiratory infections include an increase in tracheal secretions, respiratory distress/increased work of breathing, need for increased ventilator support, and a new radiographic infiltrate. In general, a chest radiograph should be performed in febrile children with suspected hospital-acquired lower respiratory infection. Obtaining a lower respiratory specimen (e.g., sputum, tracheal aspirate, non-bronchoscopic bronchoalveolar lavage ["mini-BAL"], etc.) for Gram stain and culture can be helpful in determining the microbial etiology of respiratory infection; however, the results must be interpreted in the full clinical context. The upper airway is not sterile, and specimens for culture may be easily contaminated. Endotracheal tubes are colonized very rapidly after placement, and thus utilization of tracheal aspirates can lead to false-positive results [9]. Furthermore, quantitative cultures correlate very poorly with CDC criteria for VAP [9]. Thus, the results of respiratory cultures are very nonspecific in the diagnosis of lower respiratory infection and should not be interpreted in isolation but in the full clinical context along with other supportive diagnostic studies (e.g., new abnormal radiographic findings or leukocytosis). In general, however, when clinical examination reveals a high suspicion for a lower respiratory tract infection in an ICU patient, especially in the presence of radiographic infiltrate (and thus a high pretest probability), efforts should be made to obtain specimens for culture. Further discussion of this subject is provided in Chap. 7, Hospital-Acquired Pneumonia.

Urinary Tract Infection

The vast majority of urinary tract infections (UTI) occurring in the ICU setting are catheter-associated urinary tract infection (CAUTI), and conversely >80% of pediatric CAUTI occur in the ICU setting [10]. Catheter-associated urinary tract infections are very common in critically ill children, occurring with an incidence of 3–5.4/1000 catheter days [2, 11, 12]. Notably, while urinary catheters commonly become colonized with microorganisms, such colonization or bacteriuria is rarely symptomatic [13, 14]. Evaluation is further complicated by the fact that, based on data in adult ICU patients with true CAUTI, the typical signs/symptoms of UTI (e.g., dysuria) are often absent or subtle. Signs and symptoms attributed to CAUTI may be more systemic in nature and related to the critical illness of the ICU patient and include altered mental status, irritability, or hemodynamic instability. Thus a high index of suspicion must exist for this entity in hospitalized children.

In critically ill children without indwelling bladder catheters, urinary tract infection should be suspected when patients experience dysuria, frequency, urgency, suprapubic or costovertebral angle tenderness, and fever or have bacteremia secondary to an organism referable to the urinary tract (such as *Enterobacteriaceae* or *Enterococcus* spp.). The IDSA has published guidelines for the diagnosis, management, and prevention of CAUTI in adult patients [15]. According to these guidelines, CAUTI can be considered in patients with signs/symptoms compatible with a UTI along with $\geq 10^3$ organisms isolated from a catheter urine specimen or a midstream urine specimen in a patient whose catheter has been removed for at least 48 h. Given the high rate of asymptomatic bacteriuria in catheterized patients, however, efforts should be made to rule out other causes of fever prior to establishing the diagnosis of CAUTI. Similarly, urine cultures should be obtained judiciously in the catheterized patient. Specimens for culture should not be obtained from the collection bag as such vessels are often contaminated by high levels of microorganisms [16].

In general, urinary catheters should be removed promptly in the patients with known or suspected CAUTI. Adherence to infection prevention bundles as well as daily assessment for need of catheters has been shown to decrease CAUTI rates in children [12]. A thorough discussion of this topic is provided in Chap. 13, Healthcare-Associated Urinary Tract Infections.

Fever in the Post-surgical Pediatric Patient

The development of fever following surgery is extremely common in children, occurring in >30% of postoperative pediatric patients [17] and may be much higher in select populations [18]. While infection should always be considered in febrile patients, numerous studies have revealed that the vast majority of febrile episodes occurring within 48 h of surgery are noninfectious in nature and resolve without intervention [19]. Thus, while clinician assessment is imperative for every hospitalized child with new or persistent fever and while infection can present in the early postoperative period, diagnostic studies are not routinely recommended for patients with fever in the first 48 h after surgery. Diagnostic evaluations for children with fever early after surgery should only be guided by physical examination and the clinical appearance of the child. In limited pediatric studies, children in the ICU with early postoperative fever experienced a similar yield from diagnostic studies as postoperative fever patients outside the ICU [17]; thus even among the critically ill, most early postoperative fever is noninfectious in origin. Atelectasis is often attributed as a cause of early postoperative fever although it is difficult to attribute direct and sole causality of fever to this entity; atelectasis was noted in 46% of children with neuromuscular disorders who experienced postoperative fever in one series [18].

By contrast, fevers developing or lasting beyond 96 h postoperatively are likely to represent infection. Respiratory infections may develop postoperatively as a consequence of perioperative aspiration and/or mechanical ventilation or from community-acquired pathogens that were present and incubating in the host prior to surgery.

UTI postoperatively is typically a result of the use of urinary catheters with the risk of UTI associated with length of catheterization.

Infection involving the surgical site (SSI) should always be considered in the febrile postoperative child. Rates of SSI in pediatrics are typically reported as <2–3% of cases but vary depending on type of surgery/surgical indications, wound status (i.e., clean vs. contaminated vs. dirty), and medical comorbidities of the child [20–22]. While the signs and symptoms of SSI may manifest at any time in the postoperative course, presentation of SSI has classically been described to manifest at postoperative days 4–7 [19]. Importantly, high-virulence pathogens (such as group A *Streptococcus*) may manifest earlier after surgery. Thus, it is imperative that surgical wounds be examined in patients with persistent fever, drainage from wounds, or severe pain. If there is suspicion for SSI, prompt consultation with a surgeon for wound exploration is recommended along with institution of antimicrobials targeting the most likely pathogens. Finally, the presence of persistent fever in the absence of an alternative source and/or signs of local inflammation in patients with surgically implanted medical devices or hardware (e.g., ventriculoperitoneal shunts, spinal instrumentation, etc.) should raise suspicion for infection of such foreign bodies which may in turn necessitate removal. An extensive discussion of various pediatric SSIs is provided in Chaps. 8, 9, 10, and 11.

Soft Tissue Infections

During the course of examination, it is crucial to examine the patient fully as much as possible to evaluate for sources of infection, including fully disrobing the patient or rolling them over to examine the back and buttocks. Skin and soft tissue infections (SSTI) are frequently acquired in the hospital; in one series of pediatric nosocomial staphylococcal infections, SSTIs accounted for >25% of cases [23]. Patients may develop cellulitis, abscesses or phlebitis at sites of previous disruption to skin such as old venipuncture or intravenous line sites. In addition, very disabled patients or those who have required neuromuscular blockade may develop pressure wounds which can in turn become secondarily infected. Such potential diagnoses underscore the importance of careful physical examination in the diagnostic assessment.

Common Pediatric Illnesses Presenting in the Hospital Setting

Familiar clinical pearls shared in medical schools are the expressions "common things are common" and "when you hear hoof beats, think horses and not zebras." In the context of the above discussion, these adages refer to the fact that hospitalized children, particularly those newly hospitalized, can acquire many of the same common infections as children in the community. In hospitalized children with fever and upper respiratory symptoms, consideration should be given to respiratory viral infection [24]. Respiratory viral infections occuring in the hospital may be a consequence of nosocomial acquisition of infection or community-acquired viruses that were incubacting in the host prior to admission. Outbreaks of nosocomial respiratory viral infections (such as influenza and respiratory syncytial virus) have been described in hospitalized infants and children [25]. Additionally, upper respiratory symptoms raise the possibility of common bacterial infections such as otitis media and sinusitis. Among outpatients <6 years old, otitis media is the most common diagnoses associated with antibiotic prescription [26]. While precise incidence data are not available, anecdotally, otitis media may occur in hospitalized children; thus an otoscopic exam is warranted in children with unexplained fever and otherwise unrevealing physical exam. Similarly, gastrointestinal symptoms should alert the clinician to the possibility of routine viral gastroenteritis [27]. A more rigorous exploration of these topics is provided in Chap. 12, Healthcare-Associated Diarrhea, and Chap. 14, Healthcare-Associated Viral Infections.

Drug Fever and Drug Reaction with Eosinophilia and Systemic Symptoms (DRESS)

When infectious etiologies of fever have been reasonably excluded, consideration must be given to noninfectious causes of fever. A number of noninfectious entities have been described to cause fever including atelectasis, thyrotoxicosis, venous thrombosis, intracranial hemorrhage, and cerebrovascular accidents, and, most prominently, fever can exist as an adverse reaction to medications. While the entity of drug fever is well described, few studies exist which have sought to define its incidence. The majority of knowledge regarding drug fever is derived from case reports and limited case series with substantial potential for reporting bias. Nevertheless, it is critical for the clinician to be cognizant of this entity in order to spare patients unnecessary diagnostic tests and/or prolonged hospitalization. The mechanistic causes of drug fever are varied and may occur through altered thermoregulation, as a consequence of administration of drug (e.g., amphotericin), as a result of the pharmacologic activity of the drug, as a hypersensitivity reaction, or fever may develop in an idiosyncratic fashion [28].

A number of agents have been described to cause drug fever (Table 5.1) including anticonvulsants, furosemide, antineoplastics, anti-inflammatories, and antibiotics

Table 5.1 Commonly used drugs in pediatrics implicated in drug fever and/or DRESS syndrome

Drug fever		
Commonly implicated	Less commonly implicated	DRESS syndrome
Amphotericin B	Cimetidine	β-Lactams
Asparaginase	Furosemide	Carbamazepine
Barbiturates	Imipenem	Lamotrigine
β-Lactams	Isoniazid	Minocycline
Carbamazepine	Nifedipine	Nevirapine
Salicylates	NSAIDs	Oxcarbamazepine
Sulfonamides	Rifampin	Phenytoin
Tetracyclines		Sulfonamides
Vancomycin		Vancomycin

[29]. While fever may occur as a side effect of any antibiotic, this reaction is most commonly reported with β-lactam agents. Febrile illnesses secondary to piperacillin-tazobactam are frequently encountered due to the frequency of the use of this agent in many centers. Among children with cystic fibrosis, >18% receiving piperacillin-tazobactam developed a febrile adverse drug reaction [30]. In addition to fever, such drug reactions may produce other clinical findings including rash, hepatitis, and cytopenias, often spurring additional medical evaluation. Patel reported that among children who developed an adverse drug reaction with piperacillin-tazobactam, 7.5% developed fever, hematologic abnormalities, and rash at a median of 14.5 days of therapy [31]. Fever resolved in a mean of 1.5 days after discontinuing the offending antibiotic. Drug fever typically resolves in <48–72 h after discontinuing the causative agent; however, this response is variable and dependent on the clearance time of the individual medication. Importantly, no consistent lag time from the initiation of the drug to the time of onset of fever has been reported, and it is possible for patients who have been managed on a particular medication for a prolonged period (even years) to develop a febrile reaction to the drug (such as with anticonvulsants or diuretics) [32]. Tetracyclines, in particular minocycline taken for acne, are well-described causes of late-onset drug fever in adults and children [33, 34].

Although adverse reactions to drugs may manifest primarily with fever or with fever in isolation, some patients may develop a potentially life-threatening reaction characterized by eosinophilia and multi-organ dysfunction referred to as the drug reaction with eosinophilia and systemic symptoms (DRESS) syndrome. DRESS typically manifests with a combination of fever, cutaneous reactions, facial edema, leukocytosis with eosinophilia (typically >700/mm^3) and atypical lymphocytosis, transaminase elevation, and internal organ involvement including hepatitis, pancreatitis, pneumonitis, and interstitial nephritis. DRESS is associated with a long lag time from starting the offending medication to onset of symptoms, typically in the range of 2–6 weeks in duration [35]. Unlike the above described drug reactions, DRESS may be associated with a relapsing-remitting course and/or persistence of symptoms for months after drug discontinuation [36]. Recognition of this entity is critical as an appreciable (albeit variable) mortality of 1–10% has been reported in adults secondary to multi-organ failure or hemophagocytosis [35, 37, 38]. Both anticonvulsants and antimicrobials have been commonly reported as causes of DRESS syndrome in children (Table 5.1).

Hematologic Causes of Fever

Deep venous thrombosis is a well-described cause of postoperative fever and/or fever developing in the ICU setting in adult patients but is uncommon in pediatrics, even in very disabled patients [18]. Nevertheless, venous thrombosis should be considered in children, and especially adolescents, with unexplained fever and/or localized extremity edema or pain. Transfusions are common both in the ICU and in patients undergoing large surgical procedures. Hemolytic or nonhemolytic reactions to blood products may serve as a contributing factor in postoperative fever. Febrile nonhemo-lytic transfusion reactions account for >33% of adverse reactions with red cell trans-fusions [39]. Additionally, albeit rarely, blood products may serve as the source of pathogen transmission, and this should be considered in such patients when other etiologies of fever have been excluded (see Chap. 14 for more information).

Extracorporeal Membrane Oxygenation and Infection

The utilization of extracorporeal membrane oxygenation (ECMO) has allowed for survival of a number of children with medical conditions that were previously not considered consistent with life such as severe congenital anomalies or severe sepsis. Patients treated with ECMO, however, experience a very high rate of nosocomial infection during their hospitalization ranging from 26 to 30% [40, 41]; notably, the reported incidence of infection while on the ECMO circuit is much lower, ranging from 8 to 25% [40, 42]. Over 60% of infections reported while on ECMO are blood-stream infections which may be due to skin flora or more virulent hospital-acquired pathogens [40, 43]. One of the challenges in managing patients on ECMO is the difficulty of diagnosing infection early given that such patients may not be able to mount a fever or other inflammatory responses or develop leukocytosis. Furthermore, chest radiographs are often very difficult to interpret in this population. Close atten-tion to hemodynamics, oxygenation, and the need for increased support along with laboratory evidence of poor perfusion such as acidosis or rising lactate can serve as early clues to a new infection. There is some evidence from studies including largely adults that monitoring of procalcitonin along with C-reactive protein may serve as a useful adjunct in diagnosis for these complex patients [42].

Antimicrobial Management in Pediatric ICU Fever

In general, as discussed above, new fever in any critically ill child warrants an evalu-ation for infectious etiologies. Any patient with high suspicion for infection should be initiated on systemic antimicrobial therapy with specific choice individualized to the clinical condition of the child, underlying diagnoses, history of past infections and their treatment course, and local epidemiology/microbiology. Efforts should be made to obtain relevant cultures prior to the initiation of antimicrobials. In order to avoid selective pressure for drug-resistant pathogens in the individual patient and the hospital environment, therapy should be de-escalated as soon as feasible. As a gen-eral rule, once a specific infectious etiology is identified, therapy should be modified to target the specific organism of interest using the least broad spectrum agent pos-sible; using a bactericidal agent is recommended in the setting of severe infection. In the event that a specific organism is not identified, and reasonable efforts have been made to exclude infection, strong consideration should be given to the evaluation of noninfectious etiologies of ICU fever and discontinuation of antimicrobials.

Literature Cited

1. O'Grady NP, Barie PS, Bartlett JG, et al. Guidelines for evaluation of new fever in critically ill adult patients: 2008 update from the American College of Critical Care Medicine and the Infectious Diseases Society of America. Crit Care Med. 2008;36(4):1330–49.
2. Patrick SW, Kawai AT, Kleinman K, et al. Health care-associated infections among critically ill children in the US, 2007-2012. Pediatrics. 2014;134(4):705–12.
3. Goudie A, Dynan L, Brady PW, Rettiganti M. Attributable cost and length of stay for central line-associated bloodstream infections. Pediatrics. 2014;133(6):e1525–32.
4. Darby JM, Linden P, Pasculle W, Saul M. Utilization and diagnostic yield of blood cultures in a surgical intensive care unit. Crit Care Med. 1997;25(6):989–94.
5. Alahmadi YM, Aldeyab MA, McElnay JC, et al. Clinical and economic impact of contaminated blood cultures within the hospital setting. J Hosp Infect. 2011;77(3):233–6.
6. Fackler JC. The syndrome has been a good friend; now say goodbye-quickly. Pediatr Crit Care Med. 2017;18(1):83–5.
7. Freifeld AG, Bow EJ, Sepkowitz KA, et al. Clinical practice guideline for the use of antimicrobial agents in neutropenic patients with cancer: 2010 update by the Infectious Diseases Society of America. Clin Infect Dis Off Publ Infect Dis Soc Am. 2011;52(4):e56–93.
8. Petty LA, Sokol EA, Bartlett AH, McNeer JL, Alexander KA, Pisano J. Repeated blood cultures in pediatric febrile neutropenia: would following the guidelines alter the outcome? Pediatr Blood Cancer. 2016;63(7):1244–9.
9. Willson DF, Conaway M, Kelly R, Hendley JO. The lack of specificity of tracheal aspirates in the diagnosis of pulmonary infection in intubated children. Pediatr Crit Care Med. 2014;15(4):299–305.
10. Sen AI, Balzer K, Mangino D, et al. Electronic surveillance for catheter-associated urinary tract infections at a university-affiliated children's hospital. Am J Infect Control. 2016;44(5):599–601.
11. Stover BH, Shulman ST, Bratcher DF, et al. Nosocomial infection rates in US children's hospitals' neonatal and pediatric intensive care units. Am J Infect Control. 2001;29(3):152–7.
12. Davis KF, Colebaugh AM, Eithun BL, et al. Reducing catheter-associated urinary tract infections: a quality-improvement initiative. Pediatrics. 2014;134(3):e857–64.
13. Tambyah PA, Maki DG. Catheter-associated urinary tract infection is rarely symptomatic: a prospective study of 1,497 catheterized patients. Arch Intern Med. 2000;160(5):678–82.
14. Tambyah PA, Maki DG. The relationship between pyuria and infection in patients with indwelling urinary catheters: a prospective study of 761 patients. Arch Intern Med. 2000;160(5):673–7.
15. Hooton TM, Bradley SF, Cardenas DD, et al. Diagnosis, prevention, and treatment of catheter-associated urinary tract infection in adults: 2009 international clinical practice guidelines from the Infectious Diseases Society of America. Clin Infect Dis Off Publ Infect Dis Soc Am. 2010;50(5):625–63.
16. Shah PS, Cannon JP, Sullivan CL, Nemchausky B, Pachucki CT. Controlling antimicrobial use and decreasing microbiological laboratory tests for urinary tract infections in spinal-cord-injury patients with chronic indwelling catheters. Am J Health Syst Pharm. 2005;62(1):74–7.
17. Corkum KS, Hunter CJ, Grabowski JE, Lautz TB. Early postoperative fever workup in children: utilization and utility. J Pediatr Surg. 2017;53(7):1295–300.
18. Yousef MAA, Dranginis D, Rosenfeld S. Incidence and diagnostic evaluation of postoperative fever in pediatric patients with neuromuscular disorders. J Pediatr Orthop. 2017;8(2):e104–10.
19. Garibaldi RA, Brodine S, Matsumiya S, Coleman M. Evidence for the non-infectious etiology of early postoperative fever. Infect Control. 1985;6(7):273–7.
20. Ryan SL, Sen A, Staggers K, Luerssen TG, Jea A, Texas Children's Hospital Spine Study G. A standardized protocol to reduce pediatric spine surgery infection: a quality improvement initiative. J Neurosurg Pediatr. 2014;14(3):259–65.
21. Woodward C, Taylor R, Son M, et al. Multicenter quality improvement project to prevent sternal wound infections in pediatric cardiac surgery patients. World J Pediatr Congenit Heart Surg. 2017;8(4):453–9.

22. Serres SK, Cameron DB, Glass CC, et al. Time to appendectomy and risk of complicated appendicitis and adverse outcomes in children. JAMA Pediatr. 2017;171(8):740–6.
23. McNeil JC, Kok EY, Vallejo JG, et al. Clinical and molecular features of decreased chlorhexidine susceptibility among nosocomial Staphylococcus aureus isolates at Texas Children's Hospital. Antimicrob Agents Chemother. 2015;60(2):1121–8.
24. Sidler JA, Haberthur C, Dumoulin A, Hirsch HH, Heininger U. A retrospective analysis of nosocomial viral gastrointestinal and respiratory tract infections. Pediatr Infect Dis J. 2012;31(12):1233–8.
25. Zinna S, Lakshmanan A, Tan S, et al. Outcomes of nosocomial viral respiratory infections in high-risk neonates. Pediatrics. 2016; 138(5):pii: e20161675.
26. Vaz LE, Kleinman KP, Raebel MA, et al. Recent trends in outpatient antibiotic use in children. Pediatrics. 2014;133(3):375–85.
27. Tran A, Talmud D, Lejeune B, et al. Prevalence of rotavirus, adenovirus, norovirus, and astrovirus infections and coinfections among hospitalized children in northern France. J Clin Microbiol. 2010;48(5):1943–6.
28. Johnson DH, Cunha BA. Drug fever. Infect Dis Clin N Am. 1996;10(1):85–91.
29. Clegg HW, Riopel DA. Furosemide-associated fever. J Pediatr. 1995;126(5 Pt 1):817–8.
30. Reichardt P, Handrick W, Linke A, Schille R, Kiess W. Leukocytopenia, thrombocytopenia and fever related to piperacillin/tazobactam treatment – a retrospective analysis in 38 children with cystic fibrosis. Infection. 1999;27(6):355–6.
31. Patel A, Mao KR, McNeil JC, Kaplan SL, Vallejo JG. Fever and reversible laboratory abnormalities associated with prolonged use of piperacillin-tazobactam in children. Pediatr Infect Dis J. 2015;34(8):849–50.
32. Mackowiak PA, LeMaistre CF. Drug fever: a critical appraisal of conventional concepts. An analysis of 51 episodes in two Dallas hospitals and 97 episodes reported in the English literature. Ann Intern Med. 1987;106(5):728–33.
33. Gorard DA. Late-onset drug fever associated with minocycline. Postgrad Med J. 1990;66(775):404–5.
34. MacNeil M, Haase DA, Tremaine R, Marrie TJ. Fever, lymphadenopathy, eosinophilia, lymphocytosis, hepatitis, and dermatitis: a severe adverse reaction to minocycline. J Am Acad Dermatol. 1997;36(2 Pt 2):347–50.
35. Kardaun SH, Sekula P, Valeyrie-Allanore L, et al. Drug reaction with eosinophilia and systemic symptoms (DRESS): an original multisystem adverse drug reaction. Results from the prospective RegiSCAR study. Br J Dermatol. 2013;169(5):1071–80.
36. Husain Z, Reddy BY, Schwartz RA. DRESS syndrome: part I. Clinical perspectives. J Am Acad Dermatol. 2013;68(5):693. e1–14; quiz 706-8.
37. Chen YC, Chiu HC, Chu CY. Drug reaction with eosinophilia and systemic symptoms: a retrospective study of 60 cases. Arch Dermatol. 2010;146(12):1373–9.
38. Cacoub P, Musette P, Descamps V, et al. The DRESS syndrome: a literature review. Am J Med. 2011;124(7):588–97.
39. Kato H, Uruma M, Okuyama Y, et al. Incidence of transfusion-related adverse reactions per patient reflects the potential risk of transfusion therapy in Japan. Am J Clin Pathol. 2013;140(2):219–24.
40. Coffin SE, Bell LM, Manning M, Polin R. Nosocomial infections in neonates receiving extracorporeal membrane oxygenation. Infect Control Hosp Epidemiol. 1997;18(2):93–6.
41. O'Neill JM, Schutze GE, Heulitt MJ, Simpson PM, Taylor BJ. Nosocomial infections during extracorporeal membrane oxygenation. Intensive Care Med. 2001;27(8):1247–53.
42. Pieri M, Greco T, De Bonis M, et al. Diagnosis of infection in patients undergoing extracorporeal membrane oxygenation: a case-control study. J Thorac Cardiovasc Surg. 2012;143(6):1411–6.
43. Steiner CK, Stewart DL, Bond SJ, Hornung CA, McKay VJ. Predictors of acquiring a nosocomial bloodstream infection on extracorporeal membrane oxygenation. J Pediatr Surg. 2001;36(3):487–92.

Central Line-Associated Bloodstream Infection (CLABSI)

Galit Holzmann-Pazgal

Epidemiology

Pediatric central line-associated bloodstream infections (CLABSIs) represent a source of morbidity, mortality, and increased healthcare costs. Skin colonization, intraluminal contamination of central lines, hematogenous seeding, and infusate contamination are all potential sources of infection [1, 2].

Most data demonstrate that gram-positive cocci, predominantly coagulase-negative staphylococci, cause the majority of pediatric CLABSIs, followed by gram-negative bacilli, and fungal organisms [3, 4]. However, some studies demonstrate gram-negative organisms predominate among pediatric intensive care unit (PICU) patients with CLABSI [5].

CLABSIs place substantial burdens on the healthcare system. Attributable cost of pediatric CLABSI ranges from $39,000 to $46,000 per event in studies performed in Pediatric Intensive Care Units (PICUs) over 10 years ago, to nearly $70,000 in a more recent study of CLABSI costs in hematology/oncology patients [6–8]. Attributable length of stay is 21 days per more recent data [8].

Concerted efforts to decrease the incidence of CLABSI in adults and children have resulted in improvement over time in CLABSI rates. Data published by the National Healthcare Safety Network (NHSN) demonstrate a decrease in median CLABSI rates in pediatric medical/surgical intensive care units from 2.1 infections per 1000 catheter days in 2006 to 0.7 in 2013. Neonatal intensive care unit (NICU) CLABSI rates have declined from a high of 2.4 infections per 1000 catheter days in 2006 to 1.0 in 2013 [9, 10].

G. Holzmann-Pazgal
Department of Pediatrics, Section of Infectious Diseases, Baylor College of Medicine, Houston, TX, USA
e-mail: holzmann@bcm.edu

© Springer Nature Switzerland AG 2019
J. C. McNeil et al. (eds.), *Healthcare-Associated Infections in Children*,
https://doi.org/10.1007/978-3-319-98122-2_6

Risk Factors for CLABSI

Duration of catheterization, colonization of insertion site and catheter hubs, insertion site location, receipt of parenteral nutrition, and catheter care are all identified risk factors for development of CLABSI in adult patients [1]. Additional underlying risk factors for CLABSI in the pediatric population include presence of genetic and congenital abnormalities, extracorporeal membrane oxygenation (ECMO), prematurity, gastrointestinal (GI) disease, neutropenia/immune deficiency, and oncologic conditions [1]. For example, in one cohort study, CLABSI risk was 2.7 times higher in patients with GI disease and 2.6 times higher in patients with oncologic disease [3].

Several studies have demonstrated an increased risk of CLABSI within the first 30–60 days of catheter insertion in pediatric patients [4, 13]. A cohort study of CLABSI in the PICU population found a CLABSI risk of 0.27% per day after the 7th day of catheterization [3]. The subclavian insertion site was associated with an increased risk of infection in at least one study, while patients with a jugular vein insertion site had a significantly lower risk of CLABSI (RR 0.43) [3, 4]. While the femoral insertion site is associated with higher infection risk in adult patients, and likely in older pediatric patients, this association has not been demonstrated for short-term central venous catheters (CVCs) in the pediatric literature. In fact this site may have fewer insertion complications in children and can be used for short-term central vascular access in pediatric patients [14]. Additional risk factors for CLABSI include NICU admission, higher central line lumen count (2 versus 1), and using a non-transparent dressing [4]. In addition, blood product transfusions have been shown to be a risk factor in pediatric oncology patients [13, 15].

Risk factors for CLABSI in patients with a PICC line outside of the intensive care unit have also been studied. Younger age, underlying malignancy, underlying metabolic condition, having a lower extremity PICC line, and history of prior PICC-associated CLABSI are all identified risk factors [5].

Diagnosis

Standardized CLABSI surveillance definitions per NHSN are routinely utilized for identification of CLABSI [11]. CLABSIs are laboratory-confirmed bloodstream infections (LCBI) occurring in the presence of a central line. LCBIs are primary bloodstream infections that are not secondary to an infection at another site. According to NHSN definitions, intravascular central lines must terminate at or near the heart or in one of the great vessels to be considered in the CLABSI definition. Specific LCBI definitions are complex and vary with regard to organism type, patient age, and the duration the central line has been in place. The most current, up-to-date definitions are found on the NHSN website [11]. A subset of LCBI, termed mucosal barrier injury laboratory-confirmed bloodstream infections (MBI-LCBI), was recently defined. This category applies to allogeneic hematopoietic stem cell transplant recipients or neutropenic patients, who are at particularly high risk of infection from translocation of gastrointestinal or oral mucous membrane organisms [11].

Clinical definitions of catheter-related bloodstream infections (CRBSI) differ from surveillance definitions and should not be used interchangeably. The clinical definition relies on quantitative blood cultures drawn from both the catheter hub and a peripheral vein. Identifying CRBSI requires organism quantitation in blood drawn from the catheter hub to be ≥3-fold higher then the organism quantitation from a concurrent peripheral blood culture. Most clinical laboratories do not perform quantitative blood cultures. Alternately, differential time to positivity can be used to identify a CRBSI, which requires the organism from the catheter hub culture to grow at least 2 h prior to growth of the same organism from a peripheral blood culture obtained at same time. In the clinical setting, identifying whether a bloodstream infection originates from a central line is important in determining subsequent management [12].

Management of CRBSI

Management of CRBSI varies depending on the organism causing infection, the type of CVC, and the patient's clinical status.

The key decision from a patient care perspective is whether to remove or salvage the CVC. This decision should be based on type of central line (short term versus long term), the necessity of the central line to patient care, the patient's clinical status, and the infecting pathogen. Patients with known or suspected CRBSI who are exhibiting signs of sepsis/septic shock should have the line removed as soon as is clinically feasible. Current guidelines available from the Infectious Diseases Society of America (IDSA) recommend removal of CVCs when infected by high-virulence pathogens (such as *S. aureus*, or *Pseudomonas aeruginosa*). In addition, catheter removal is recommended when infection is caused by organisms with a high potential to form biofilm and relapse following discontinuation of therapy. In general, treatment of infections due to *Pseudomonas*, *S. aureus*, mycobacteria, and fungi requires catheter removal for successful outcomes. Finally, in cases where CRBSI is complicated by suppurative thrombophlebitis, endocarditis, metastatic infection (e.g., osteomyelitis), or, in the case of ports, tunnel infection or port abscess, prompt removal of CVCs is imperative. In cases where long-term catheters are necessary for survival and catheter access is limited, treatment through the line can be attempted, depending on the infecting pathogen, using both antibiotic lock therapy and systemic intravenous therapy. However, even when salvage is attempted, a low threshold for line removal is recommended with clinical deterioration. A major challenge in the management of CRBSI in the pediatric population, as acknowledged in the guidelines, is the limited alternative venous access in many medically complex children, particularly those with intestinal failure requiring long-term parenteral nutrition. Thus the need to ensure eradication of infection and minimization of recurrence (through CVC removal) must be balanced with the need to provide fluids, other medications, and nutrition (through ensuring venous access) to these fragile patients.

Duration of therapy for catheter-associated infections varies based on the organism and whether the catheter is removed or salvaged. For example, coagulase-negative staphylococci (CoNS) CRBSI can be treated with 5–7 days of systemic antibiotics after short term CVC removal, whereas uncomplicated *S. aureus* CRBSI requires at least 14 days of systemic therapy after removal. In contrast, a longer duration of therapy (10–14 days) is recommended for CoNS CRBSI when the catheter is retained. CRBSI secondary to gram-negative bacilli are recommended to be managed with 7–14 days of targeted antimicrobial therapy if the CVC is removed. Specific therapeutic recommendations can be found in the guidelines from the IDSA, "Diagnosis and Management of Intravascular Catheter-Related Infections." [12]

Prevention

There are multiple well-established recommendations designed to reduce the risk of CLABSI. Data supporting these recommendations are predominantly derived from studies focused on adult patients, but increasingly data from pediatric patients are available to support key practices with some modifications in certain instances.

Key prevention efforts focus on education of staff, insertion and maintenance of central lines, and patient hygiene. As central lines for pediatric patients in the outpatient setting are increasingly utilized, CLABSI prevention outside of the ICU setting has gained more attention as well.

Education/Staffing

CLABSI prevention begins with an adequately staffed infection prevention program that conducts timely, accurate surveillance for infections. Prevention efforts must also include education and training of healthcare providers inserting central lines and caring for patients with central lines. Providers should be educated regarding appropriate indications for central line placement, central line necessity and removal, and proper techniques for insertion and maintenance [1]. Designating competently trained staff to be responsible for line insertion and maintenance is also recommended [2]. The use of dedicated teams for central line insertion and/or maintenance has successfully decreased CLABSI rates in the NICU setting in several studies [16–18]. Periodic assessments of providers' knowledge of and adherence to recommended practices are essential to ensure ongoing compliance.

Maintaining proper nurse staffing levels has been shown to impact CLABSI rates, and guidelines from the Centers for Disease Control and Prevention (CDC) and Society for Healthcare Epidemiology of America (SHEA) recommend maintaining appropriate nurse staffing in the ICU setting [1, 2]. Several studies in pediatric and neonatal patients have found an increased risk of nosocomial infections when there is inadequate staffing of nurses in pediatric units [19–22]. Finally, providing feedback to providers regarding the incidence of CLABSI in their units in a timely fashion is a key component of prevention efforts.

Central Line Insertion

Central line placement in pediatric patients can be particularly challenging. Utilizing ultrasound guidance for line placement is recommended [2]. As pediatric patients often have smaller veins and limited venous access, this is particularly important in order to minimize the number of attempts needed for successful line insertion. Central lines with the minimal number of ports necessary should be selected [4]. Additionally, catheters inserted emergently should be replaced as soon as possible.

Central line insertion should be performed utilizing full barrier precautions including cap, mask, sterile gown, sterile gloves, and a sterile full-body drape. CDC and SHEA guidelines recommend that skin preparation agents should include an alcohol-based chlorhexidine preparation in patients >2 months of age [1, 2]. For patients under 2 months of age, product guidelines state that chlorhexidine should be used with caution due to concerns for systemic absorption and skin toxicity. It is noteworthy that surveys of pediatric centers reveal that more than 50% of pediatric centers utilize chlorhexidine-based products in patients less than 2 months of age with varying restrictions [23, 24] (see Chap. 15 for further discussion on CLABSI prevention in the NICU).

Central Line Maintenance

The proper maintenance and care of central lines is also a key component of prevention efforts. Maintenance efforts address central line dressing changes, accessing hubs of central lines, replacing central line tubing, and patient hygiene. Supplemental strategies include antimicrobial and ethanol locks as well as antimicrobial-coated central venous catheters.

Central line dressing changes should be performed with clean or sterile gloves [2]. Similar to catheter insertion recommendations, a chlorhexidine-alcohol-based product should be utilized to clean the site, and the site should then be covered with a transparent dressing so it can be easily visualized. Transparent dressings should be changed every 7 days or earlier if soiled or non-adherent [1, 2]. Gauze dressings may be utilized for oozing sites but should be changed at least every 48 h. In pediatrics, central lines are often not sutured, particularly in the neonatal/NICU population, in which case dressing changes may be performed as needed only when non-occlusive or soiled, in order to avoid the risk of catheter dislodgement [1, 2].

Utilization of a chlorhexidine-impregnated sponge over the catheter insertion site may be incorporated into an institution's CLABSI prevention program [1, 2].

Data demonstrate that these dressings decrease the incidence of CVC colonization in pediatric patients as well as in adults [25]. Pediatric data demonstrate an increased risk of contact dermatitis with the chlorhexidine patch in neonates with birth weight under 1000 g [25]. Two studies found a 5% incidence of mild erythema at the CVC insertion site using the chlorhexidine patch in neonatal patients [24, 26]. While chlorhexidine-impregnated sponges should generally be reserved for infants >2 months of age, some institutions have utilized them in neonates as young as 28 weeks gestational age with birth weight >1000 g in quality improvement efforts to decrease CLABSI [15].

Daily patient cleansing with 2% chlorhexidine wipes has been shown to decrease the incidence of CLABSI and is recommended for patients ≥2 months of age in guidelines [1]. This intervention has been demonstrated to decrease CLABSI in patients by at least 34% [27]. In a study of daily chlorhexidine bathing in pediatric patients, no trend of chlorhexidine accumulation in blood was noted in patients >2 months of age [28]. Daily bathing has also been studied in infants <2 months of age. CLABSI rates significantly decreased in NICU studies of daily chlorhexidine bathing in infants >28 days old and >1000 g birth weight with no adverse events noted [28, 29].

Central line administration set tubing should be changed at intervals no longer than every 96 h [1]. Needle-less systems should be changed at least as frequently as administration sets. Tubing used to administer blood products, lipids, or propofol should be changed more frequently according to accepted national guidelines [1, 2].

When accessing a central line, access ports should be scrubbed with an alcohol-based chlorhexidine product or 70% alcohol [1]. There are data demonstrating that the alcohol-based chlorhexidine product may be superior in decontaminating the hub as compared to alcohol alone [30, 31]. According to SHEA guidelines, the duration of the scrub should be at least 5 seconds(s) to decrease catheter hub colonization [1]. However, one study suggested a 15-s scrub with either alcohol-based chlorhexidine product or 70% alcohol is necessary to provide adequate disinfection [32]. A 15-s scrub has also been utilized in various studies of interventions to decrease CLABSI in pediatrics [16, 33, 34]. Alcohol-based disinfecting caps, which serve to passively disinfect catheter hubs, have also been demonstrated to decrease CLABSI incidence in several studies [35–37].

Central Line Bundles

Accepted practice encourages use of central line insertion and maintenance bundles to decrease the incidence of CLABSI. Insertion bundles can include checklists of necessary steps, empowering providers to stop and correct breaches in sterile technique or suboptimal practices (Fig. 6.1). Utilizing pre-assembled insertion kits or carts with all necessary supplies may facilitate bundle compliance.

Maintenance bundles, including a daily review and documentation of line necessity by providers and prompt removal of unnecessary lines, are an essential

Instructions: Audit practices related to insertion technique for central vascular lines, dialysis access ports, and central lines

Did the Provider/Staff Attending:	Please circle answer		Comments
Wash hands using soap or hand sanitizer prior to start? (ask if unsure)	Yes	No	
Prep the insertion site with Chlorhexidine for 30 seconds on a dry site or 2 minutes on a moist site?	Yes	No	
Wear a head cover, mask, sterile gown & sterile gloves during entire procedure?	Yes	No	
Drape the patient from head to toe?	Yes	No	
Was sterile field maintained during the procedure?	Yes	No	
Was Chlorhexidine patch placed at the insertion site?	Yes	No	
Was dressing labeled with insertion date and dressing date?	Yes	No	
Did the assisting physician/nurse:			
Wash hands using soap or hand sanitizer prior to start? (ask if unsure)	Yes	No	
Wear a head cover, mask, gown & gloves?	Yes	No	

Fig. 6.1 Central line insertion checklist – example

component of CLABSI prevention. Bundles can include documentation of dressing changes, tubing changes, scrub-the-hub compliance, daily chlorhexidine bathing, and use of disinfecting caps (Fig. 6.2).

There are increasing data that use of bundles is effective in decreasing CLABSI in neonatal, pediatric, and even outpatient settings [16, 33, 34, 38–40]. A survey of SHEA members involved in pediatrics demonstrated that 93% utilized some form of maintenance bundle as part of CLABSI prevention efforts [24].

Increasing attention has been given to pediatric patients with long-term CVCs, particularly oncology patients, outside the ICU, and in the outpatient setting. Studies have demonstrated that implementation and compliance with maintenance bundles effectively reduce the incidence of CLABSI in this growing population [41, 42].

Antibiotic and Ethanol Locks

Lock prophylaxis, particularly with ethanol, is an effective practice to decrease CLABSI in certain high-risk populations with long-term central access including dialysis and oncology patients and those with gastrointestinal (GI) disorders receiving parenteral nutrition. Studies in pediatric oncology and intestinal failure patients requiring long-term venous access have demonstrated significant decrease in

Physician "Necessity" Documented?		Is the central line dressing occlusive & intact?		Is CVC insertion site healthy without redness or drainage?		Date & time of last dressing change <7 days for transparent or <48 hrs for gauze dressing		All the CVC tubings are labeled with date & time ?		All CVC tubing dates adhere to policy (<96 hrs for IV fluid/meds; <24 hrs for lipids)?		If stopcock present, is covering/cap present over unused port?	
Yes	No	Yes	No	Yes	No	Yes	No	Yes	No	Yes	No	Yes	No

Fig. 6.2 Central line maintenance checklist – example

CLABSI rates with use of ethanol locks as compared to those not receiving locks [43, 44]. One trial in patients with intestinal failure demonstrated an 81% reduction in CLABSI when ethanol lock prophylaxis was added to maintenance interventions. Adverse events were rare [45]. Locking catheters with taurolidine decreased CLABSI incidence in oncology and GI patients, though this agent is not available in the United States [46, 47].

Antibiotic lock prophylaxis has been studied in pediatric patients as a preventative measure. Data predominantly using vancomycin lock therapy prophylactically demonstrate a reduction in CLABSI in neonates [48]. Use of vancomycin flush in pediatric oncology patients demonstrated mixed results in decreasing the incidence of CLABSI [49, 50]. Unlike a lock solution, an antibiotic flush may not necessarily dwell within the catheter lumen for a prolonged period of time. To minimize the emergence of antimicrobial resistance, CDC and SHEA guidelines recommend that antibiotic lock prophylaxis be considered in targeted patients with long-term CVC and a history of recurrent CLABSI or long-term hemodialysis [1, 2].

Antibiotic-Coated Catheters

Antibiotic-impregnated catheters can be effective in decreasing or delaying CLABSI in the pediatric population, and these can be considered if other recommended measures are not effective or sufficient in decreasing the incidence of CLABSI [51–53]. There are scarce data in neonates regarding efficacy of antimicrobial (silver zeolite)-coated umbilical catheters in decreasing CLABSI incidence in the NICU [54].

Implementation Strategies

All prevention processes require effective implementation in order to be successful. Suboptimal compliance with recommended processes is associated with higher hospital-acquired infections, including CLABSI rates [55]. Compliance with processes proven to prevent CLABSIs and other nosocomial infections must be a priority for healthcare organizations [55]. Resources, including adequate personnel, education, and equipment, must be provided and supported by organizational leadership. Frontline staff as well as senior leadership must be engaged, educated, and held accountable for patient safety [1]. Families and patients should also be educated regarding infection prevention and encouraged to participate in their care [56]. A culture of safety should be promoted, incorporating a team approach to implementation and compliance with infection prevention processes.

Conclusion

Successful CLABSI reduction, incorporating proven insertion and maintenance interventions, requires both employee and executive level hospital support. Bundle compliance must be monitored and barriers to best practice addressed. Feedback to providers and key stakeholders regarding CLABSI rates and performance metrics, as well as close scrutiny of all CLABSIs, are necessary components of successful infection prevention. Creating such a culture of safety and accountability is essential for successful quality improvement efforts.

References

1. Marschall J, Mermel LA, Fakih M, Hadaway L, Kallen A, O'Grady N, et al. Strategies to prevent central line associated bloodstream infections in acute care hospitals: 2014 update. Infect Control Hosp Epidemiol. 2014;35:753–71.
2. O'Grady NP, Alexander M, Burns LA, Dellinger P, Garland J, Heard SO, et al. Guidelines for prevention of intravascular catheter-related infections. Am J Infect Control. 2011;39:S1–34.
3. Niedner MF, Huskins WC, Colantuoni E, Muschelli J, Harris JM, Rice TB, et al. Epidemiology of central line-associated bloodstream infections in the pediatric intensive care unit. Infect Control Hosp Epidemiol. 2011;32:1200–8.
4. Carter JH, Langley JM, Kuhle S, Kirkland S. Risk factors for central venous catheter-associated bloodstream infection in pediatric patients: a cohort study. Infect Control Hosp Epidemiol. 2016;37:939–45.
5. Advani S, Reich NG, Sengupta A, Gosey L, Milstone AM. Central line-associated bloodstream infection in hospitalized children with peripherally inserted central venous catheters: extending risk analyses outside the intensive care unit. Clin Infect Dis. 2011;52:1108–15.
6. Slonim AD, Kurtines HC, Sprague BM, Singh N. The costs associated with nosocomial bloodstream infections in the pediatric intensive care unit. Pediatric Crit Care Med. 2001;2:170–4.
7. Elward AM, Hollenbeak CS, Warren DK, Fraser VJ. Attributable cost of nosocomial primary bloodstream infection in pediatric intensive care unit patients. Pediatrics. 2005;115:868–72.

8. Wilson MZ, Rafferty C, Deeter D, Comito MA, Hollenbeak CS. Attributable costs of central line-associated bloodstream infections in a pediatric hematology/oncology population. Am J Infect Control. 2014;42:1157–60.
9. Dudeck MA, Edwards JR, Allen-Bridson K, Gross C, Malpiedi PJ, Peterson KD, et al. National healthcare safety network report, data summary for 2013, device-associated module. Am J Infect Control. 2015;43:206–21.
10. Edwards JR, Peterson KD, Andrus ML, Dudeck MA, Pollock DA, Horan TC, et al. National healthcare safety network (NHSN) report, data summary for 2006 through 2007, issued November 2008. Am J Infect Control. 2008;36:609–26.
11. National Healthcare Safety Network, Centers for Disease Control and Prevention. The National Healthcare Safety Network (NHSN) manual: patient safety component protocol. 2018. Accessed 22 Feb 2018. http://www.cdc.gov/nhsn/PDFs/pscManual/4PSC_CLABScurrent.pdf.
12. Mermel LA, Allon M, Bouza E, Craven DE, Flynn P, O'Grady NP, et al. Clinical practice guidelines for the diagnosis and management of intravascular catheter-related infection: 2009 update by the infectious diseases society of America. Clin Infect Dis. 2009;49:1–45.
13. Kelly M, Conway M, Wirth K, Potter-Bynoe G, Billett AL, Sandora TJ. Moving CLABSI prevention beyond the ICU: risk factors in pediatric oncology patients. Infect Control Hosp Epidemiol. 2011;32:1079–85.
14. de Jonge RC, Polderman KH, Gemke RJ. Central venous catheter use in the pediatric patient: mechanical and infectious complications. Pediatr Crit Care Med. 2005;6:329–39.
15. Rogers AE, Eisenman KM, Dolan SA, Belderson KM, Zauche JR, Tong S, et al. Risk factors for bacteremia and central line-associated blood stream infections in children with acute myelogenous leukemia: a single institution report. Pediatr Blood Cancer. 2017;64:e26254.
16. Shepherd EG, Kelly TJ, Vinsel JA, Cunningham DJ, Keels E, Beauseau W, et al. Significant reduction of central-line associated bloodstream infections in a network of diverse neonatal nurseries. J Pediatr. 2015;167:41–6.
17. Holzmann-Pazgal G, Kubanda A, Davis K, Khan AM, Brumley K, Denson SE. Utilizing a line maintenance team to reduce central-line-associated bloodstream infections in a neonatal intensive care unit. J Perinatol. 2012;32:281–6.
18. Golombek SG, Rohan AJ, Parvez B, Salice AL, LaGamma EF. "Proactive" management of percutaneously inserted central catheters results in decreased incidence of infection in the ELBW population. J Perinatol. 2002;22:209–13.
19. Stratton KM. Pediatric nurse staffing and quality of care in the hospital setting. J Nurs Care Qual. 2008;23:105–14.
20. Archibald LK, Manning ML, Bell LM, Banerjee S, Jarvis WR. Patient density, nurse to patient ratio and nosocomial infection risk in a pediatric cardiac intensive care unit. Pediatr Infect Dis J. 1997;16:1045–8.
21. Haley RW, Bregman DA. The role of understaffing and overcrowding in recurrent outbreaks of staphylococcal infection in a neonatal special care unit. J Infect Dis. 1982;145:875–85.
22. Harbarth S, Sudre P, Dharan S, Cadenas M, Pittet D. Outbreak of Enterobacter cloacae related to understaffing, overcrowding and poor hygiene practices. Infect Control Hosp Epidemiol. 1999;20:598–603.
23. Tamma PD, Aucott SW, Milstone AM. Chlorhexidine use in the neonatal intensive care unit: results from a national survey. Infect Control Hosp Epidemiol. 2010;31:846–9.
24. Bryant KA, Zerr DM, Huskins WC, Milstone AM. The past, present, and future of healthcare-associated infection prevention in pediatrics: catheter-associated bloodstream infections. Infect Control Hosp Epidemiol. 2010;31:S27–31.
25. Levy I, Katz J, Solter E, Samra Z, Vidne B, Birk E, et al. Chlorhexidine-impregnated dressing for prevention of colonization of central venous catheters in infants and children a randomized controlled study. Pediatr Infect Dis J. 2005;24:676–9.
26. Garland JS, Alex CP, Mueller CD, Otten D, Shivpuri C, Harris MC, et al. A randomized trial comparing povidone iodine to a chlorhexidine gluconate impregnated dressing for prevention of central venous catheter infections in neonates. Pediatrics. 2001;107:1431–6.

27. Milstone AM, Elward A, Song X, Zerr DM, Orscheln R, Speck K, et al. Daily chlorhexidine bathing to reduce bacteremia in critically ill children: a multicenter, cluster-randomized, crossover trial. Lancet. 2013;381:1099–106.

28. Lee A, Harlan R, Breaud AR, Speck K, Perl TM, Clarke W, et al. Blood concentrations of chlorhexidine in hospitalized children undergoing daily chlorhexidine bathing. Infect Control Hosp Epidemiol. 2011;32:395–7.

29. Quach C, Milstone AM, Perpete C, Bonenfant M, Moore DL, Perreault T. Chlorhexidine bathing in a tertiary care neonatal intensive care unit: impact on central line-associated bloodstream infections. Infect Control Hosp Epidemiol. 2014;35:158–63.

30. Casey AL, Worthington T, Lambert PA, Quinn D, Faroqui MH, Elliott TS. A randomized prospective clinical trial to assess the potential infection risk associated with the Posiflow needleless connector. J Hosp Infect. 2003;54:288–93.

31. Soothill JS, Barvery K, Ho A, Macqueen S, Collins J, Lock P. A fall in bloodstream infections followed a change to 2% chlorhexidine in 70% isopropanol for catheter connection antisepsis: a pediatric single center before/after study on a hematopoietic stem cell transplant ward. Am J Infect Control. 2009;37:626–30.

32. Kaler W, Chinn R. Successful disinfection of needleless access ports: a matter of time and friction. JAVA. 2007;12:140–2.

33. Piazza AJ, Brozanski B, Provost L, Grover TR, Chuo J, Smith JR, et al. SLUG bug: quality improvement with orchestrated testing leads to NICU CLABSI reduction. Pediatrics. 2016;137:e20143642.

34. Erdei C, McAvoy LL, Gupta M, Pereira S, McGowan EC. Is zero central line-associated bloodstream infection rate sustainable? A 5 year perspective. Pediatrics. 2015;135:e1485.

35. Menyhay SZ, Maki DG. Preventing central venous catheter-associated bloodstream infections: development of an antiseptic barrier cap for needleless connectors. Am J Infect Control. 2008;36:S174e1–5e5.

36. Sweet MA, Cumpston A, Briggs F, Craig M, Hamadani M. Impact of alcohol-impregnated port protectors and needleless neutral pressure connectors on central line-associated bloodstream infections and contamination of blood cultures in an inpatient oncology unit. Am J Infect Control. 2012;40:931–4.

37. Wright MO, Tropp J, Schora DM, Dillon-Grant M, Peterson K, Boehm S, et al. Continuous passive disinfection of catheter hubs prevents contamination and bloodstream infection. Am J Infect Control. 2013;41:33–8.

38. Edwards JD, Herzig C, Liu H, Pogorzelska-Maziarz M, Zachariah P, Dick AW, et al. Central line-associated blood stream infections in pediatric ICU's: longitudinal trends and compliance with bundle strategies. Am J Infect Control. 2015;43:489–93.

39. Miller MR, Griswold M, Harris JM, Yenokyan G, Huskins WC, Moss M, et al. Decreasing PICU catheter-associated bloodstream infections: NACHRI's quality transformation efforts. Pediatrics. 2010;125:206–13.

40. Jeffries HE, Mason W, Brewer M, Oakes KL, Munoz EI, Gornick W, et al. Prevention of central venous catheter associated bloodstream infections in pediatric intensive care units: a performance improvement collaborative. Infect Control Hosp Epidemiol. 2009;30:645–51.

41. Rinke ML, Bundy DG, Chen AR, Milstone AM, Colantuoni E, Pehar M, et al. Central line maintenance bundles and CLABSIs in ambulatory oncology patients. Pediatrics. 2013;132:31403–e1412.

42. Bundy DG, Gaur AH, Billett AL, He B, Colantuoni EA, Miller MR. Preventing CLABSIs among pediatric hematology/oncology inpatients: National Collaborative Results. Pediatrics. 2014;134:e1678–85.

43. Schoot RA, van Ommen CH, Stijnen T, Tissing W, Michiels E, Abbink F, et al. Prevention of central venous catheter-associated bloodstream infections in pediatric oncology patients using 70% ethanol locks: a randomized controlled multi centre trial. Eur J Cancer. 2015;51:2031–8.

44. Ardura MI, Lewis J, Tansmore JL, Harp PL, Dienhart MC, Balint JP. Central catheter-associated bloodstream infection reduction with ethanol lock prophylaxis in pediatric intestinal failure. JAMA Pediatr. 2015;169:324–31.

45. Oliveira C, Nasr A, Brindle M, Wales PW. Ethanol locks to prevent catheter-related bloodstream infections in parenteral nutrition: a meta analysis. Pediatrics. 2012;129:318–29.
46. Handrup MM, Moller JK, Schroder H. Central venous catheters and catheter locks in children with cancer: a prospective randomized trial of taurolidine versus heparin. Pediatr Blood Cancer. 2013;60:1292–8.
47. Chu HP, Brind J, Tomar R, Hill S. Significant reduction in central venous catheter related bloodstream infections in children on HPN after starting treatment with Taurolidine line lock. JPGN. 2012;55:403–7.
48. Garland JS, Alex CP, Henrickson KJ, McAuliffe TL, Maki DG. A vancomycin-heparin lock solution for prevention of nosocomial bloodstream infection in critically ill neonates with peripherally inserted central venous catheters: a prospective, randomized trial. Pediatrics. 2005;116:e198–205.
49. Rackoff WR, Weiman M, Jakobowski D, Hirschl R, Stallings V, Bilodeau J, et al. A randomized controlled trial of the efficacy of a heparin and vancomycin solution in preventing central venous catheter infections in children. J Pediatr. 1995;127:147–51.
50. Henrickson KJ, Axtell RA, Hoover SM, Kuhn SM, Pritchett J, Kehl SC, et al. Prevention of central venous catheter related infections and thrombotic events in immunocompromised children by the use of vancomycin/ciprofloxacin/heparin flush solution: a randomized, multicenter, double blind trial. J Clin Oncol. 2000;18:1269–78.
51. Chelliah A, Heydon KH, Zaoutis TE, Rettig SL, Dominguez TE, Lin R, et al. Observational trial of antibiotic coated central venous catheters in critically ill pediatric patients. Pediatr Infect Dis J. 2007;26:816–20.
52. Bhutta A, Gilliam C, Honeycutt M, et al. Reductions of bloodstream infections associated with catheters in paediatric intensive care unit: stepwise approach. BMJ. 2007;334:362–5.
53. Weber JM, Sheridan RL, Fagan S, Ryan CM, Pasternack MS, Tompkins RG. Incidene of catheter associated bloodstream infection after introduction of minocycline and rifampin antimicrobial coated catheters in a pediatric burn population. J Burn Care Res. 2012;33:539–43.
54. Bertini G, Elia S, Ceciarini F, Dani C. Reduction of catheter related bloodstream infections in preterm infants by the use of catheters with AgION antimicrobial system. Early Hum Dev. 2013;89:21–5.
55. Zachariah P, Furuya EY, Edwards J, Dick A, Liu H, Herzig C, et al. Compliance with prevention practices and their association with central line-associated bloodstream infections in neonatal intensive care units. Am J Infect Control. 2014;42:847–51.
56. Suresh GK, Edwards WH. Central line-associated bloodstream infections in neonatal intensive care: changing the mental model from inevitability to preventability. Am J Perinatol. 2012;29:57–64.

Ventilator-Associated Pneumonias

7

Amy S. Arrington

Introduction

Despite providing quality care for hospitalized children, nosocomial infections remain a challenge, particularly in critical care settings. Among these infections, hospital-acquired pneumonias, and specifically ventilator-associated pneumonias (VAP), are the most common complication in the course of intubated patients. VAPs are the leading cause of death in critical care settings worldwide, in addition to being the first cause of antibiotic prescription in intensive care units (ICUs). Recent surveys using the National Healthcare Safety Network (NHSN) criteria indicate that in the adult population in 2011, an approximated 157,000 healthcare-associated pneumonias occurred in US hospitals and an estimated 39% of these were VAPs [1]. Additionally, the suspicion of VAPs in pediatric ICU (PICU) patients increases the overall exposure rate to antibiotics by over twofold, and the high rate of prescribed antibiotics for presumed VAP supersedes even that for suspected bloodstream infections [2–4], increasing overall PICU length of stay significantly in some studies. Patients with confirmed VAPs experience an increased length of mechanical ventilation by more than 11 days, and a recent multicenter study of pediatric VAP showed a three-fold increase in severity-adjusted PICU mortality [5] as well as additional direct cost of more than $50,000 [6, 7]. Healthcare systems are now required to report VAPs, among other healthcare-associated infections (HAIs) through the Centers for Disease Control and Prevention (CDC) NHSN, focused on quality, infection tracking, and prevention nationwide, as well as for Medicaid and Medicare reimbursement [8].

In the past, there has been great variability in both the surveillance and reporting of VAPs in both the adult and pediatric population, leading to a redefining of VAPs

A. S. Arrington
Pediatric Critical Care Medicine, Global Biologic Preparedness, Baylor College of Medicine/Texas Children's Hospital, Houston, TX, USA
e-mail: aa691762@bcm.edu

© Springer Nature Switzerland AG 2019
J. C. McNeil et al. (eds.), *Healthcare-Associated Infections in Children*,
https://doi.org/10.1007/978-3-319-98122-2_7

by the CDC in 2012. The new paradigm provided more objective documentation and recognized ventilator-associated complications other than infection. It also redefined the language to describe and classify VAP. In this chapter, these definitions and the newly revised criteria, as well as the pathogenesis, diagnosis, and treatment strategies for VAPs, will be discussed.

VAPs: Defined

Hospital-acquired pneumonias are considered any nosocomial pneumonia, while ventilator-associated pneumonias (VAP) are specific to patients who are mechanically ventilated and are of great consequence to quality patient care in critical care settings. National surveillance for VAP has long been a challenge because of the lack of objective, reliable definitions. The incidence of VAPs is also used as a quality benchmark indicator, though data shows that there is great variability in the accuracy of reporting VAPs due to a lack of objective, reliable definitions [8–10]. The standardization of clinical criteria for VAPs was first developed in 2002 by the CDC and National Nosocomial Infections Surveillance (NNIS) to promote consistent diagnosis and reporting. These criteria consisted of radiographic, clinical, and laboratory evidence supporting the diagnosis. However, after several years of data collection, analyses revealed that application of these criteria resulted in poor outcomes with inconsistent and imprecise reporting due to these initial criteria being poorly defined, time-consuming, and subjective in this complicated patient cohort [11–15].

To address these issues, the National Healthcare Safety Network (NHSN) *replaced* surveillance for VAPs in adult inpatient locations with surveillance for ventilator-associated events (VAE) in January of 2013 [1]. In this updated criterion, patients on mechanical ventilation must meet a minimum threshold of worsening oxygenation as evidenced by increased positive end-expiratory pressure (PEEP) or fraction of inspired oxygen (FiO_2), must have evidence for infection (fever or abnormal serum leukocyte count), and must be treated with a new antibiotic for 4 or more days. To date, these new criteria have yet to be validated in pediatric populations.

In attempts to include more objective and inclusive guidelines, several new definitions were added to the 2013 NHSN criteria, comprising different "levels" of ventilator-associated events (Fig. 7.1) (https://www.cdc.gov/nhsn/pdfs/pscmanual/10-vae_final.pdf):

1. *Ventilator-associated conditions (VACs)*: occurs on or after 3 days of mechanical ventilation and within 2 days before or after the onset of worsening oxygenation, where the patient has (a) temperature >38 °C or <36 °C or (b) has a white blood cell count ≥12,000 cell/mm³ or ≤4000/mm³ and (c) a new antimicrobial agent(s) added to the patient's treatment regimen
2. *Infection-related VACs (IVACs)*: which aim to identify the subset of VAC cases potentially caused by infection through culture or other forms of laboratory identification of infectious organisms
3. *Possible VAP (PVAP)*: which aims to identify the subset of IVAC cases caused by pneumonia

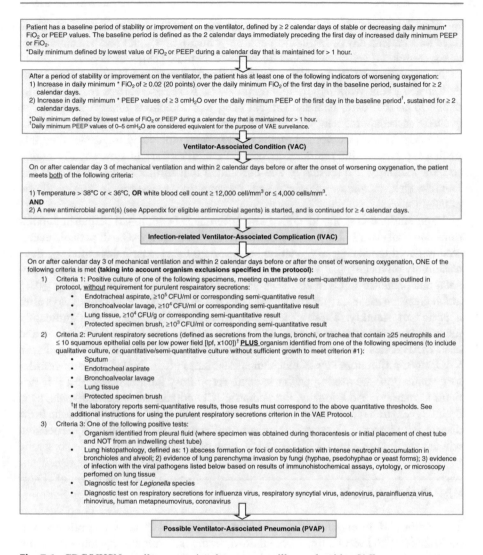

Patient has a baseline period of stability or improvement on the ventilator, defined by ≥ 2 calendar days of stable or decreasing daily minimum* FiO$_2$ or PEEP values. The baseline period is defined as the 2 calendar days immediately preceding the first day of increased daily minimum PEEP or FiO$_2$.
*Daily minimum defined by lowest value of FiO$_2$ or PEEP during a calendar day that is maintained for > 1 hour.

After a period of stability or improvement on the ventilator, the patient has at least one of the following indicators of worsening oxygenation:
1) Increase in daily minimum * FiO$_2$ of ≥ 0.02 (20 points) over the daily minimum FiO$_2$ of the first day in the baseline period, sustained for ≥ 2 calendar days.
2) Increase in daily minimum * PEEP values of ≥ 3 cmH$_2$O over the daily minimum PEEP of the first day in the baseline period†, sustained for ≥ 2 calendar days.

*Daily minimum defined by lowest value of FiO$_2$ or PEEP during a calendar day that is maintained for > 1 hour.
†Daily minimum PEEP values of 0–5 cmH$_2$O are considered equivalent for the purpose of VAE surveillance.

Ventilator-Associated Condition (VAC)

On or after calendar day 3 of mechanical ventilation and within 2 calendar days before or after the onset of worsening oxygenation, the patient meets both of the following criteria:

1) Temperature > 38°C or < 36°C, **OR** white blood cell count ≥ 12,000 cell/mm^3 or ≤ 4,000 cells/mm^3.
AND
2) A new antimicrobial agent(s) (see Appendix for eligible antimicrobial agents) is started, and is continued for ≥ 4 calendar days.

Infection-related Ventilator-Associated Complication (IVAC)

On or after calendar day 3 of mechanical ventilation and within 2 calendar days before or after the onset of worsening oxygenation, ONE of the following criteria is met **(taking into account organism exclusions specified in the protocol):**
1) Criteria 1: Positive culture of one of the following specimens, meeting quantitative or semi-quantitative thresholds as outlined in protocol, without requirement for purulent respiratory secretions:
   • Endotracheal aspirate, ≥10^5 CFU/ml or corresponding semi-quantitative result
   • Bronchoalveolar lavage, ≥10^4 CFU/ml or corresponding semi-quantitative result
   • Lung tissue, ≥10^4 CFU/g or corresponding semi-quantitative result
   • Protected specimen brush, ≥10^3 CFU/ml or corresponding semi-quantitative result
2) Criteria 2: Purulent respiratory secretions (defined as secretions from the lungs, bronchi, or trachea that contain ≥25 neutrophils and ≤ 10 squamous epithelial cells per low power field [lpf, x100])† **PLUS** organism identified from one of the following specimens (to include qualitative culture, or quantitative/semi-quantitative culture without sufficient growth to meet criterion #1):
   • Sputum
   • Endotracheal aspirate
   • Bronchoalveolar lavage
   • Lung tissue
   • Protected specimen brush
   †If the laboratory reports semi-quantitative results, those results must correspond to the above quantitative thresholds. See additional instructions for using the purulent respiratory secretions criterion in the VAE Protocol.
3) Criteria 3: One of the following positive tests:
   • Organism identified from pleural fluid (where specimen was obtained during thoracentesis or initial placement of chest tube and NOT from an indwelling chest tube)
   • Lung histopathology, defined as: 1) abscess formation or foci of consolidation with intense neutrophil accumulation in bronchioles and alveoli; 2) evidence of lung parenchyma invasion by fungi (hyphae, psedohyphae or yeast forms); 3) evidence of infection with the viral pathogens listed below based on results of immunohistochemical assays, cytology, or microscopy perfomed on lung tissue
   • Diagnostic test for *Legionella* species
   • Diagnostic test on respiratory secretions for influenza virus, respiratory syncytial virus, adenovirus, parainfluenza virus, rhinovirus, human metapneumovirus, coronavirus

Possible Ventilator-Associated Pneumonia (PVAP)

Fig. 7.1 CDC/NHSN ventilator-associated events surveillance algorithm [16]

The current NHSN definition for adults specifically identifies a VAC when, after a period of stability or improvement on the ventilator, a patient has one or both of the following indicators of worsening oxygenation: (1) the minimum daily fraction of inspired oxygen (Fio$_2$) increases at least 0.20 over the daily minimum Fio$_2$ in the preceding two calendar days and the increase is sustained for at least 2 days or (2) the minimum daily positive end-expiratory pressure (PEEP) values increase at least 3 cm H$_2$O over the daily minimum PEEP in the preceding two calendar days and the increase is sustained for at least 2 days [17, 18] (https://www.cdc.gov/nhsn/pdfs/pscmanual/6pscvapcurrent.pdf). Defining VAP and its prevalence in the pediatric population is challenging. VAP surveillance using the criteria found in the CDC/NHSN 2014 guidelines excludes neonates and is only available in pediatric inpatient locations where denominator data can be collected (consisting of device days and patient days), including pediatric critical care units and specialty care areas, step-down units, wards, and long-term care units [18].

In September 2012, the CDC convened the Pediatric and Neonatal Ventilator-Associated Event Working Group, comprised of 20 representatives from pediatric, pediatric critical care, neonatal critical care, and infectious disease societies, to evaluate and adapt the new VAE surveillance methods for use in pediatric and neonatal ICUs. While this work is ongoing, the group elucidated important data that pediatric patients with ventilator-associated conditions are at substantially higher risk for mortality and morbidity and concluded that further studies are needed to identify risk factors, etiologies, and preventative measures in the pediatric population.

Importantly, this group identified key differences in adult and pediatric populations and considered 12 alternative definitions for pediatric VAC. All patients evaluated required worsening oxygenation be sustained for at least 2 days after ≥ 2 days of stability on mechanical ventilation. Two criteria were found to best capture neonatal and pediatric VACs in all ICUs: an increase in minimum daily Fio_2 by ≥ 0.25 and increase in mean airway pressure (MAP) by ≥ 4 cm H_2O for 2 or more days after a period of stability. These criteria helped to identify patients at significantly increased risk for adverse outcomes. The authors modified the adult definition and used MAP instead of positive end-expiratory pressure (PEEP) to define pediatric VAC, since different modes of mechanical ventilation (e.g., high-frequency oscillatory ventilation) are used in pediatric acute respiratory failure, where PEEP is difficult to measure. Additionally, the pediatric ICU population is quite diverse, as is their oxygenation requirements: patients may range from infants with cyanotic heart disease with lower SpO_2 goals, to neonates with persistent pulmonary hypertension which may require a higher FIO_2 or MAP than other patients [19].

VAP Pathogenesis

The etiology of nosocomial pneumonias in ICU patients is likely complicated and multifactorial and results from a breakdown in the host immune system on several levels in the mechanically ventilated patient. Traditionally, it was assumed that these infections were likely caused by the direct inoculation of bacteria into a sterile lung via the endotracheal tube or the bloodstream in critically ill patients. It is well accepted that the aspiration of colonized oropharyngeal secretions across the endotracheal tube (ETT) cuff plays a significant role in the pathogenesis of VAP. The ETT and its placement and care are also independent factors contributing to VAP; the ETT is a direct conduit for bacteria to reach the airways and acts as a substrate that allows the adherence of various microorganisms (biofilm).

As VAP infrequently occurs as a direct consequence of bacteremia, the majority of these infections appear to result from aspiration of potential pathogens that have colonized the mucosal surfaces of the oropharyngeal airways. Introduction of a foreign body into the airway of a critically ill patient compromises the natural barrier between the oropharynx and trachea and may facilitate the entry of bacteria into the lung by pooling and leakage of contaminated secretions around the endotracheal tube cuff. Additionally, the longer a patient has been hospitalized, the more risk they are at for colonization of the upper airway with pathogens including gram-negative bacteria and *Staphylococcus aureus* [20]. Also, according to the gastro-pulmonary hypothesis of colonization, pathogens may translocate from the stomach into the oropharynx, especially in patients in the supine, fully horizontal position or in patients who have aspirated [21].

Newer research suggests that the host lung and airway possess an incredibly complex microbiome, which is altered in mechanically ventilated critically and chronically ill patients. Endogenous airway bacteria maintain a balance between host immune activation and suppression, but shifts in the airway environment likely contribute to VAP. Factors including bacteria, viruses, and critical illness itself may cause this imbalance, leading to a suppression of host immune responses and infectious consequences [22].

Host Risk Factors

Second only to bloodstream infections, VAPs are among the most frequently occurring healthcare-associated infection in PICUs and account for up to 20% of infections in this patient population, increasing length of stay and cost, as well as morbidity and mortality [23, 24].

In a recent case-control study of 600 pediatric ICU patients, Guess et al. found an association between VAEs and several new risk factors in critically ill children. This study found that in univariate analysis acute kidney injury (AKI) (defined as a greater than 50% change in creatinine clearance per pediatric RIFLE {acronym for risk for renal dysfunction, injury to the kidney, failure of kidney function, loss of kidney function, and end-stage renal disease} guidelines), increased peak cumulative fluid overload, mean peak inspiratory pressure (PIP), mean airway pressure, using neuromuscular blockade (NMB), and steroids were associated with VAC. Subsequently, following multivariable analyses, the authors concluded that AKI and mean PIP were independent risk factors for VAC and that AKI and NMB infusion were independent risk factors for IVAC [25].

In a separate pediatric retrospective cohort study, researchers identified children with pediatric VACs and matched them to children without VACs ($n = 192$). This cohort of children was taken from pediatric, cardiac, and neonatal ICUs of six different US hospitals. Similar to other studies, several possible risk factors were identified for pediatric patients, including neuromuscular blockade (odds ratio, 2.29; 95% CI, 1.08–4.87), positive fluid balance (highest quartile compared with the lowest, odds ratio, 7.76; 95% CI, 2.10–28.6), and blood product use (odds ratio, 1.52; 95% CI, 0.70–3.28). Additionally, potential protective factors were identified, including reduced sedation or interruption of sedation (odds ratio, 0.44; 95% CI, 0.18–1.11). In neonatal patients, risk factors included blood product use (odds ratio, 2.99; 95% CI, 1.02–8.78), neuromuscular blockade (odds ratio, 3.96; 95% CI,

0.93–16.9), and recent surgical procedures (odds ratio, 2.19; 95% CI, 0.77–6.28). Weaning or interrupting sedation was also found to be potentially protective (odds ratio, 0.07; 95% CI, 0.01–0.79) in neonates [26]. Additionally, in premature infants, a birth weight less than 750 g has been shown to be an independent risk factor for the development of VAP. Patients with VACs had longer length of stays and incurred higher hospital costs as well [27].

A recent study in PICU patients using the framework for VAEs adapted for critically ill pediatric patients by Cocoros et al. specifically utilized an escalation in mean airway pressure (MAP, ≥ 4 cm H_2O) and a larger increase in inspired oxygen as criteria to identify "ventilator-associated conditions" [17, 28, 29]. Patients were further diagnosed with a pediatric VAP (PVAP) if they had a positive respiratory culture. Two hundred seventy-seven children representing a diverse group of PICU patients who had been initially diagnosed with VAPs were included in the study. This study revealed that few children with a ventilator-associated pneumonia diagnosis met the proposed PVAP criteria (16%, $n = 45$), with only 18% ($n = 49$) having any ventilator-associated condition using the proposed revised pediatric guidelines. Failure to fulfill new definitions was based largely on inadequate increase in mean airway pressure in 90% or Fio_2 in 92%, suggesting that additional study is needed before new definitions for VAP are introduced for children.

In adults, the incidence of VAP in mechanically ventilated trauma patients has been reported to be as high as 29%, and a subset of these patients (13%) develop bacteremia as well. Perhaps the most significant risk factor for bloodstream infections in this subset of patients has been found to be transfusion with packed red blood cells (pRBCs). Bochicchio et al. demonstrated that blood product transfusion is an independent risk factor for the development of VAP in trauma patients and that this risk increased as more units were transfused [30]. Moreover, all blood products were shown to have an increase in VAPs, including pRBCs, fresh frozen plasma, and platelets.

VAPs have also been associated with inappropriate empiric antimicrobial therapy. In the study done by Kunac et al., 32% of patients with VAP treated with ineffective therapy became bacteremic compared with only 11% of those treated with appropriate initial antimicrobial agents ($p < 0.05$) [31]. Additional studies in adult ICU patients have demonstrated more than twice the mortality rate in patients who received inappropriate early antibiotic coverage compared to those who received appropriate empiric coverage [32].

Prolonged mechanical ventilation for more than 48 h is perhaps the most important risk factor associated with healthcare-associated pneumonia. However, VAP may occur within the first 48 h after intubation. It is also important to consider the timing of the infection, as "early-onset VAP," occurring within the first 4 days of ventilation, is typically less severe as compared to "late-onset VAP" and often has different causative agents [33, 34].

VAP is thought to be a common complication in critically ill patients with acute respiratory distress syndrome (ARDS), though the diagnosis of pulmonary infections in patients with ARDS can be difficult, and studies vary on the incidence of VAP in ARDS patients, ranging from 15% to 60% [33, 35–38]. A common risk factor associated with both ARDS and VAP is hyperoxemia, which is common in critically ill mechanically ventilated patients. Hyperoxemia leads to acute lung injury, inhibition of surfactant production, reduced bacterial clearance in the lung by impairing mucociliary clearance, and the impaired antimicrobial action capacity of macrophages and immune cells, increasing the risk for VAPs [39].

Lastly, additional studies have also evaluated various other risk factors for mechanically ventilated patients, such as patient positioning, endotracheal tube material, and open versus closed suction systems for ventilated patients. A 2016 Cochrane review evaluating semi-recumbent positioning versus supine positioning in mechanically ventilated patients found that a semi-recumbent position of $\geq 30°$ may reduce clinically suspected VAP compared to a $0°–10°$ supine position [40]. Additional risk factors which should be considered in the diagnosis and treatment of VAP include admission from long-term care facilities, patients on dialysis, immunosuppression, gastric acid suppression, recent hospital admissions, and patients with greater severities of illness [41–44].

Diagnosis

Following CDC/NHSN guidelines, there is a tiered approach to diagnosing patients with ventilator-associated conditions, ranging from VAC to IVAC, to possible ventilator-associated pneumonias (PVAP) (see section "VAPs: Defined"). To differentiate these conditions and accurately diagnose VAPs in mechanically ventilated patients, specific criteria must be met. These diagnostic criteria are detailed in Fig. 7.1.

Next-generation diagnostic tools are up and coming and offer promising advances in both the rapid and specific identification of VAPs. Several studies have also looked at the use of biomarkers in the diagnosis and management of VAPs. The BioVAP study (biomarkers in the diagnosis and management of ventilator-associated pneumonia) is a prospective, multicenter, observational study evaluating the kinetics of procalcitonin (PCT) and C-reactive protein (CRP) in patients with VAP following initiation of antibiotic therapy in order to recognize patients with poor outcome early in their clinical course as well as to identify the individual patterns of CRP and PCT kinetics following antibiotics. This study found that CRP rate of decline significantly differed between survivors and non-survivors ($p = 0.026$ and $p = 0.005$, respectively). On day 4 of antibiotic therapy, CRP of survivors was 47% of the initial value, while it was 96% in non-survivors. These data suggest that perhaps C-reactive protein kinetics can be used to identify VAP patients with poor outcome as soon as 4 days after the initiation of treatment [45]. Additionally, multiplex PCR allows for not only pathogen identification (bacterial and non-bacterial) but can also reveal the presence of the most frequently encountered drug-resistance genes. As such, this modality may serve as a useful adjunct in the rapid identification of VAP pathogens. Lastly, exhalome analysis is an up and coming, noninvasive methodology of diagnosing respiratory infections in patients, based on the detection of ethanol in exhaled breath using mass spectrometry, and has shown promising results in diagnosing patients with VAPs [46].

Microbiology

In a study describing pathogen distribution and antimicrobial resistance patterns for healthcare-associated infections (HAIs) reported to the NHSN from pediatric locations during 2011–2014, a total of 1366 VAP pathogens were reported. Among these, 63% were reported from NICUs and 37% from PICUs. *S. aureus*, *Pseudomonas aeruginosa*, *Klebsiella* spp., and *Enterobacter* spp. were the four most common pathogens in both location types. *Streptococcus pneumoniae* ranked fifth in PICUs, and *E. coli* ranked fifth in NICUs [47]. Interestingly, in previous reporting from 2006 to 2008, the most common pathogen was *P. aeruginosa* (16.1% of 830 reported pathogens) followed closely by *S. aureus* (15.8%). Additional data from the 2011 to 2014 cohort showed that for pediatric patients with VAPs due to *K. pneumoniae/K. oxytoca* and *P. aeruginosa*, resistance was higher overall in PICUs than in NICUs. In PICUs, >10% of *K. pneumoniae/K. oxytoca* and *P. aeruginosa* were resistant to carbapenems [47].

In adult populations, *Acinetobacter baumannii*, *P. aeruginosa*, and methicillin-resistant *S. aureus* (MRSA) were the most common causative microorganisms for VAP. Information on the causative organisms of VAP at one's own institution and their antibiotic susceptibility profiles, along with the regular monitoring of resistance patterns, is important to make effective empiric antibiotic choices. Thus, every hospital should monitor its own microbial flora and rates of resistance to antibiotics [34]. While resistant bacteria may be present even in early-onset VAP, taking length of stay (LOS) into consideration may improve estimates of the presence of resistant bacteria. One study reported that patients admitted for longer than 48 h are more likely to be colonized with *Pseudomonas* spp. and MRSA [48]. Conversely, Karakuzu et al. found *A. baumannii*, *P. aeruginosa*, *K. pneumoniae*, and MRSA to be the most common bacteria seen in early-onset VAP. Important factors associated with these organisms were patients who had been in the hospital for longer than 48 h *before* admission to the ICU (and prior to mechanical ventilation) and those having received prior antimicrobial therapy [34]. Chastre et al. also demonstrated that LOS and prior antibiotic treatment were the major risk factors for resistant bacteria in VAP [33]. A summary of the most common bacteria found in VAPs is shown in Table 7.1. Lastly, viral pathogens, including influenza, RSV, adenovirus, human metapneumovirus, and parainfluenza must be considered as common causes of VAP in the pediatric population.

Table 7.1 Common bacteria in ventilator-associated pneumonias (VAP) [49]

Gram-positive pathogens
Methicillin-resistant *Staphylococcus aureus* (MRSA)
Methicillin-sensitive *Staphylococcus aureus* (MSSA)
Streptococcus pneumoniae
Gram-negative pathogens
Haemophilus influenzae
Lactose fermenting gram-negative bacilli
Enterobacteriaceae
Enterobacter spp.
Escherichia coli
Klebsiella pneumonia
Proteus spp.
Serratia spp.
Non-lactose fermenting gram-negative bacilli
Pseudomonas aeruginosa
Acinetobacter baumannii
Burkholderia spp.

Management

An important determinant of the morbidity and mortality of VAP is the timing of appropriate antibiotic therapy administered for its treatment. Delay in the initiation of empiric antibiotic therapy until culture results are available is associated with negative clinical outcomes [50, 51]. With the increasing development of multidrug-resistant (MDR), extensively drug-resistant (XDR), and pandrug-resistant (PDR) organisms, it is crucial that each organization is aware of their own microbial ecology, antibiotic resistance profiles, and frequency of specific pathogens causing VAP in their ICU patient populations to help tailor empiric antibiotic coverage. Additionally, in choosing empiric antibiotics, it is important to consider certain features present on admission, such as severe hypoxemia, bilateral infiltrates, and presence of pleural effusion, as these factors could point toward a more virulent or resistant pathogen [52].

A recent prospective, observational cohort study conducted in 47 PICUs in the United States, Canada, and Australia evaluated the clinical variables associated with continuing antibiotics after initial evaluation for suspected ventilator-associated infection to determine whether clinical variables or antibiotic treatment influenced outcomes. Positive respiratory cultures were the primary determinant of continued antibiotic treatment in children with suspected VAPs. Positive cultures were, however, not associated with worse outcomes regardless of antibiotic therapy [53].

Antibiotic Therapy and Antimicrobial Resistance

In adults, published guidelines for the diagnosis and management of hospital- and ventilator-acquired pneumonias are available and well delineated by the Infectious

Diseases Society of America and the American Thoracic Society [54]. These guidelines include the following recommendations and can be adapted to pediatric patients:

- All hospitals should regularly summarize and report a local antibiogram, and empiric therapy regimen should be guided by local distribution of pathogens associated with VAP and their antimicrobial susceptibilities.
- Early, appropriate, broad-spectrum, antibiotic therapy should be prescribed with adequate doses to optimize antimicrobial efficacy.
- Combination empiric therapy (two antipseudomonal antibiotics from different classes) may be considered in instances of suspected *P. aeruginosa* pneumonia, in patients in septic shock, those at risk for resistant isolates or until susceptibility data are available.
- Linezolid is an alternative to vancomycin, and unconfirmed, preliminary data suggest it may have an advantage for proven VAP due to MRSA.
- Colistin should be considered as therapy for patients with VAP due to a carbapenem-resistant *Acinetobacter* species.
- Aerosolized antibiotics may have value as adjunctive therapy in patients with VAP due to some MDR pathogens. For organisms only susceptible to aminoglycosides or colistin, both inhaled and systemic antimicrobials should be considered.
- Antibiotic therapy should be de-escalated once susceptibility data are available based on the results of lower respiratory tract cultures and the patient's clincial response.
- A shorter duration of antibiotic therapy (7 days) is recommended for patients with uncomplicated VAP who have received initially appropriate therapy with good clinical response.

Of note, in the largest meta-analysis to date, a Cochrane review in 2016 found no difference in outcome between monotherapy and combination therapy for the treatment of adult patients with VAP [55].

In choosing appropriate antibiotic coverage in the pediatric ICU, the value of understanding common bacterial infections and resistance patterns cannot be overstated. Typically for ICU patients, *S. aureus* coverage along with a third-generation cephalosporin, and possibly *Pseudomonas* coverage, is necessary depending upon the patient population. Risk factors for multidrug resistance in VAP include prior intravenous antibiotic use within 90 days, septic shock at the time of VAP, ARDS preceding the diagnosis of VAP, 5 or more days of hospitalization prior to the occurrence of VAP, and acute renal replacement therapy prior to VAP onset [54]. These factors should be considered in the choice of antimicrobial therapies for critically ill patients.

Duration of Treatment

Meta-analyses demonstrate comparable patient outcomes in those receiving 7 days of antimicrobial therapy versus 10–14 days. Therefore, 7 days of therapy is recommended for most VAP patients, with the caveat that longer course may be necessary for patients who respond slowly. Prior recommendations have suggested longer treatment in patients with VAP secondary to non-lactose fermenting gram-negative bacteria, including *Pseudomonas* spp. and *Acinetobacter* spp., because of a perception that there is a higher rate of recurrent VAP if such patients are treated with 7–8 days of therapy [54], which was supported by a 2015 Cochrane review [56]. However, additional meta-analyses evaluating short versus long courses in patients with VAP due to these organisms showed no differences in mortality, recovery, disease recurrence, and duration of mechanical ventilation. Therefore, 7 days of therapy are recommended as the standard for most patients with VAP though, depending upon unique patient responses, longer courses may be appropriate, and clinical judgment is indicated [57].

New Agents

New antibiotics with activity against MRSA such as tedizolid, ceftaroline, and eravacycline represent promising options for the treatment of VAP in patients with risk factors for this organism. Tedizolid, a new oxazolidinone approved by Food and Drug Administration for the treatment of acute bacterial skin and soft tissue infections in adults, demonstrated potent in vitro activity against MRSA and vancomycin-resistant *enterococci* (VRE), including some linezolid-resistant strains. While still in phase III trials for patients with VAPs, this drug has advantages to linezolid with an improved side effect profile [58]. Ceftaroline is a cephalosporin with activity against MRSA and drug-resistant pneumococci and has been approved to treat community-acquired pneumonia and skin and soft tissue infection in children >2 years and could conceivably have a place in the treatment of MRSA VAP. Additionally, new antimicrobials such as ceftolozane-tazobactam and ceftazidime-avibactam with broad-spectrum activity against MDR gram-negative bacteria will enhance the available armamentarium for VAP. Notably, however a limited number of new compounds have shown activity against MDR *Acinetobacter baumannii* [59].

Nebulized antibiotics are also advantageous in the treatment of VAPs, with the key advantage of being able to deliver high concentrations of drug directly to the site of infection without the systemic side effects [60]. New inhaled antibiotic options are currently under development for the treatment of VAP including inhaled ciprofloxacin, arbekacin, murepavadin, and amikacin [61–63]. As many of these drugs are still in phase II and III trials, it is unclear if/when they will be available for use in the pediatric population.

Prevention

Many evidence-based clinical practice guidelines exist for preventing VAP, although data show only an estimated 50% of patients receive such evidence-based recommended care in hospital settings [64, 65].

VAP bundles In an effort to reduce the number of VAPs in intensive care units, ventilator "bundles" were developed by the Institute for Healthcare Improvement (IHI). These bundles are defined as a set of evidence-based practices that when each element is executed individually, it improves the patient recovery process and outcomes; when all of the practices are executed together, however, they provide better outcomes than when implemented individually [66]. The ventilator care bundle consists of five interventions: head of bed elevation, daily sedative holidays and assessment of readiness to extubate, peptic ulcer prophylaxis, deep vein thrombosis prophylaxis, and daily oral care with chlorhexidine. Additionally, some institutions have added additional evidence-based interventions to the IHI VAP bundle, creating customized VAP bundles for decreasing VAP rates, and data have shown that the implementation of these tailored VAP bundles results in improved patient outcomes [67, 68]. Additional interventions added to VAP bundles commonly include hand hygiene and endotracheal tube cuff pressure monitoring.

Probiotics Several published studies have demonstrated that probiotics are safe for patients in the ICU setting and much interest exists in the utilization of probiotics for the prevention of HAIs. Some studies suggest that the use of probiotics is associated with a reduction in the incidence of VAP; however, the quality of the evidence is low. Furthermore, the available evidence is not clear regarding any decrease in ICU or in hospital mortality associated with probiotic use [69].

Respiratory Infections in the Chronically Ventilated Child

When considering the pediatric population most at risk for ventilator-associated conditions, one must also include patients with tracheostomies who are ventilator-dependent due to chronic respiratory failure. This unique population of children is at risk for increased hospital admissions, morbidity, and mortality. In a 2008 study examining 70 hospitalized patients who received tracheostomies at a large tertiary pediatric hospital, 81% of children were discharged home; 63% of these children were readmitted within 6 months, with 11% of those patients requiring four or more admissions [70]. It is estimated that hospitalizations in pediatric patients with pre-existing tracheostomy resulted in an estimated $1.4 billion in hospital charges in 2012 alone [71]. A majority of pediatric patients (up to 90%) with tracheostomies will have respiratory cultures positive for *P. aeruginosa* at some point in time, with limited oral treatment options, resulting in repeated and often frequent hospitalizations. Likewise, over 70% of chronically ventilated pediatric patients hospitalized with respiratory tract infections receive empiric antibiotics that target *P. aeruginosa*.

In a study describing the respiratory pathogens in a cohort of pediatric patients with tracheostomies, McCaleb et al. found the most common organism isolated to be *P. aeruginosa* (90.3%), with gram-negative organisms as a whole predominating. However, 55.9% of the study population also had isolation of MRSA from a respiratory culture, underscoring the often polymicrobial nature of such infections. The organism found to be isolated earliest after tracheostomy placement was methicillin-sensitive *S. aureus* (MSSA) [72].

Furthermore, it is important to differentiate between ventilator-associated tracheobronchitis (VAT) and ventilator-associated pneumonia (VAP). Key differences include a new and persistent infiltrate on chest radiograph as well as at least moderate bacterial growth in cultures from bronchoscopic bronchoalveolar lavage in VAPs as opposed to VATs [73]. Findings of recent study of VAT by Nseir et al. and a systematic review by Agrafiotis et al. of randomized controlled trials demonstrated that patients treated for VAT were less likely to progress to VAP [74, 75], emphasizing that it is critical to adequately and properly treat identified VATs in tracheostomized children to prevent the progression to worsening disease. Simpson et al. reported 3.4% VAT incidence in pediatric ventilated patients and a significant association between VAT and tracheostomy and between VAT and chronic ventilator dependence. In addition, patients with VAT experienced significantly more ventilator days and a longer ICU length of stay [76].

Conclusions

The definition, pathogenesis, and treatment of VAP in pediatric patients are complex, and VAP remains the most common healthcare-associated infection in critically ill, mechanically ventilated patients. A continued need for improved methods of diagnosis and treatment remains, and surveillance definitions for ventilator-associated pneumonia in children are currently in the process of being updated. A critical piece in the quality of care of these patients includes recognizing those children most at risk and diagnosing these patients early by utilizing the CDC guidelines provided in this chapter. Additionally, the adherence to evidence-based ventilator bundles has been proven to significantly improve outcomes in this patient population, particularly when combined with tailoring appropriate antimicrobial therapy based on cultures and regional antimicrobial resistance profiles. With these interventions and preventative steps, the rate of VAPs can be reduced, and long-term outcomes can be optimized in pediatric patients.

References

1. Magill SS, Edwards JR, Bamberg W, et al. Multistate point-prevalence survey of health care-associated infections, 2011. N Engl J Med. 2014;370:1198–208.
2. Fischer JE, Ramser M, Fanconi S. Use of antibiotics in pediatric intensive care and potential savings. Intensive Care Med. 2000;26(7):959–66.
3. Fayon MJ, Tucci M, Lacroix J, Farrell CA, Gauthier M, Lafleur L, et al. Nosocomial pneumonia and tracheitis in a pediatric intensive care unit: a prospective study. Am J Respir Crit Care Med. 1997;155:162–9.
4. Fagon JY, Chastre J, Vuagnat A, Trouillet JL, Novara A, Gibert C. Nosocomial pneumonia and mortality among patients in intensive care units. JAMA. 1996;275(11):866–9.

5. Gupta S, Boville BM, Blanton R, et al. A multicentered prospective analysis of diagnosis, risk factors, and outcomes associated with pediatric ventilator- associated pneumonia. Pediatr Crit Care Med. 2015;16(3):e65–73.
6. Bigham MT, Amato R, Bondurrant P, et al. Ventilator-associated pneumonia in the pediatric intensive care unit: Characterizing the problem and implementing a sustainable solution. J Pediatr. 2009;154:582–587.e2.
7. Brilli RJ, Sparling KW, Lake MR, et al. The business case for preventing ventilator-associated pneumonia in pediatric intensive care unit patients. Jt Comm J Qual Patient Saf. 2008;34:629–38.
8. Klompas M. Interobserver variability in ventilator-associated pneumonia surveillance. Am J Infect Control. 2010;38:237–9.
9. Dudeck MA, et al. National Healthcare Safety Network (NHSN) report, data summary for 2012, Device-associated module. Am J Infect Control. 2013;41:1148–66.
10. Klompas M, et al. Risk of misleading ventilator-associated pneumonia rates with use of standard clinical and microbiological criteria. Clin Infect Dis. 2008;46:1443–6.
11. Beyersmann J, Gastmeier P, Grundmann H, et al. Use of multistate models to assess prolongation of intensive care unit stay due to nosocomial infection. Infect Control Hosp Epidemiol. 2006;27(5):493–9.
12. Safdar N, Dezfulian C, Collard HR, et al. Clinical and economic consequences of ventilator-associated pneumonia: a systematic review. Crit Care Med. 2005;33(10):2184–93.
13. Suka M, Yoshida K, Uno H, et al. Incidence and outcomes of ventilator- associated pneumonia in Japanese intensive care units: the Japanese nosocomial infection surveillance system. Infect Control Hosp Epidemiol. 2007;28(3):307–13.
14. Cordero L, Ayers LW, Miller RR, et al. Surveillance of ventilator-associated pneumonia in very-low-birth-weight infants. Am J Infect Control. 2002;30(1):32–9.
15. Emori TG, Edwards JR, Culver DH, et al. Accuracy of reporting nosocomial infections in intensive-care-unit patients to the National Nosocomial Infections Surveillance system: a pilot study. Infect Control Hosp Epidemiol. 1998;19(5):308–16.
16. https://www.cdc.gov/nhsn/pdfs/pscmanual/10-vae_final.pdf. Accessed 17 Apr 2018.
17. Cocoros NM, et al. Ventilator-associated events in neonates and children – a new paradigm. Crit Care Med. 2016;44(1):14–22.
18. https://www.cdc.gov/nhsn/pdfs/pscmanual/6pscvapcurrent.pdf. Accessed 17 Apr 2018.
19. Mhanna MJ. Ventilator-associated events in neonates and children: a single definition for a heterogeneous population. Crit Care Med. 2016;44(1):233–4.
20. American Thoracic Society. Hospital-acquired pneumonia in adults: diagnosis, assessment of severity, initial antimicrobial therapy, and preventive strategies. A consensus statement, American Thoracic Society, November 1995. Am J Respir Crit Care Med. 1996;153:1711–25.
21. Pinciroli R, et al. Respiratory therapy device modifications to prevent ventilator-associated pneumonia. Curr Opin Infect Dis. 2013;26:175–83.
22. Mourani PM, Sontag MK. Ventilator-associated pneumonia in critically ill children: a new paradigm. Pediatr Clin N Am. 2017;64:1039–56.
23. Foglia E, Meier MD, Elward A. Ventilator-associated pneumonia in neonatal and pediatric intensive care unit patients. Clin Microbiol Rev. 2007;20(3):409–25.
24. Elward AM. Pediatric ventilator-associated pneumonia. Pediatr Infect Dis J. 2003;22(5):445–6.
25. Guess R, et al. Risk factors for ventilator-associated events in a PICU. Pediatr Crit Care Med. 2018;19:e7–e13.
26. Cocoros NM. Factors associated with pediatric ventilator-associated conditions in 6 US hospitals: a nested case-control study. Pediatr Crit Care Med. 2017;18(11):e536–45.
27. Thatrimontrichai A, et al. Outcomes and risk factors of ventilator-associated pneumonia in neonates. World J Pediatr. 2017;13(4):328–34.
28. Cocoros NM, Priebe GP, Logan LK, et al. A pediatric approach to ventilator-associated events surveillance. Infect Control Hosp Epidemiol. 2017;38:327–33.
29. Gionfriddo A, et al. Retrospective application of new pediatric ventilator-associated pneumonia criteria identifies a high-risk population. Pediatr Crit Care Med. 2018;19:507. https://doi.org/10.1097/PCC.0000000000001522.

30. Bochicchio GV, Napolitano L, Joshi M, et al. Blood product transfusion and ventilator-associated pneumonia in trauma patients. Surg Infect. 2008;9:415–22.
31. Kunac A, Sifri ZC, Mohr AM, Horng H, Lavery RF, Livingston DH. Bacteremia and ventilator-associated pneumonia: a marker for contemporaneous extra-pulmonic infection. Surg Infect. 2014;15(2):77–83.
32. Luna CM, et al. Blood cultures have limited value in predicting severity of illness and as a diagnostic tool in ventilator-associated pneumonia. Chest. 1999;116:1075–84.
33. Chastre J, Fagon JY. Ventilator-associated pneumonia. Am J Respir Crit Care Med. 2002;165(7):867–903.
34. Karakuzu Z, et al. Prognostic risk factors in ventilator-associated pneumonia. Med Sci Monit. 2018;24:1321–8.
35. Sutherland KR, Steinberg KP, Maunder RJ, Milberg JA, Allen DL, Hudson LD. Pulmonary infection during the acute respiratory distress syndrome. Am J Respir Crit Care Med. 1995;152:550–6.
36. Chastre J, Trouillet JL, Vuagnat A, Joly-Guillou ML, Clavier H, Dombret MC, Gibert C. Nosocomial pneumonia in patients with acute respiratory distress syndrome. Am J Respir Crit Care Med. 1998;157:1165–72.
37. Delclaux C, Roupie E, Blot F, Brochard L, Lemaire F, Brun-Buisson C. Lower respiratory tract colonization and infection during severe acute respiratory distress syndrome: incidence and diagnosis. Am J Respir Crit Care Med. 1997;156:1092–8.
38. Markowitz P, Wolff M, Djedaini K, Cohen Y, Chastre J, Delclaux C, Merrer J, Herman B, Veber B, Fontaine A, et al. Multicenter prospective study of ventilator-associated pneumonia during acute respiratory distress syndrome. Incidence, prognosis, and risk factors. ARDS Study Group. Am J Respir Crit Care Med. 2000;161:1942–8.
39. Six S, et al. Hyperoxemia as a risk factor for ventilator-associated pneumonia. Crit Care. 2016;20:195.
40. Wang L, et al. Semi-recumbent position versus supine position for the prevention of ventilator-associated pneumonia in adults requiring mechanical ventilation. Cochrane Database Syst Rev. 2016;(1):CD009946.
41. Shorr AF, Zilberberg MD, Micek ST, Kollef MH. Prediction of infection due to antibiotic-resistant bacteria by select risk factors for healthcare-associated pneumonia. Arch Intern Med. 2008;168:2205–10.
42. Aliberti S, Di Pasquale M, Zanaboni AM, et al. Stratifying risk factors for multidrug-resistant pathogens in hospitalized patients coming from the community with pneumonia. Clin Infect Dis Off Publ Infect Dis Soc Am. 2012;54:470–8.
43. Shindo Y, Ito R, Kobayashi D, et al. Risk factors for drug-resistant pathogens in community-acquired and healthcare-associated pneumonia. Am J Respir Crit Care Med. 2013;188: 985–95.
44. Maruyama T, Fujisawa T, Okuno M, et al. A new strategy for healthcare- associated pneumonia: a 2-year prospective multicenter cohort study using risk factors for multidrug-resistant pathogens to select initial empiric therapy. Clin Infect Dis Off Publ Infect Dis Soc Am. 2013;57:1373–83.
45. Povoa P, et al. Biomarkers kinetics in the assessment of ventilator-associated pneumonia response to antibiotics – results from the BioVAP study. J Crit Care. 2017;41:91–7.
46. Bos LD, Martin-Loeches I, Kastelijn JB, et al. The volatile metabolic fingerprint of ventilator-associated pneumonia. Intensive Care Med. 2014;40:761–2.
47. Lake JG, et al. Pathogen distribution and antimicrobial resistance among pediatric healthcare-associated infections reported to the National Healthcare Safety Network, 2011-2014. Infect Control Hosp Epidemiol. 2018;39:1–11.
48. Olsen B, Weinstein RA, Nathan C, et al. Epidemiology of endemic *Pseudomonas aeruginosa*: why infection control efforts have failed. J Infect Dis. 1984;150:808–16.
49. Oliveira J, et al. Prevention of ventilator-associated pneumonias. Rev Port Pneumol. 2014;20(3):152–61.
50. Baker AM, Meredith JW, Chang M, et al. Bronchoscopically guided management of ventilator-associated pneumonia in trauma patients. J Bronchology. 2003;10:7–16.

51. Muscedere JC, et al. The adequacy of timely empiric antibiotic therapy for ventilator-associated pneumonia: an important determinant of outcome. J Crit Care. 2012;27:322.e7–322.e14.
52. Falcone M, Russo A, Giannella M, et al. Individualizing risk of multidrug- && resistant pathogens in community-onset pneumonia. PLoS One. 2015;10:e0119528.
53. Wilson DF, et al. Pediatric ventilator-associated infections: the ventilator-associated infection study. Pediatr Crit Care Med. 2017;18:e24–34.
54. Kalil AC, Metersky ML, Klompas M, et al. Management of adults with hospital-acquired and ventilator-associated pneumonia: 2016 clinical practice guidelines by the infectious diseases Society of America and the American Thoracic Society. Clin Infect Dis. 2016;63(5):e61–111.
55. Arthur LE et al. Antibiotics for ventilator-associated pneumonia. Cochrane Database Syst Rev. 2016;(10):CD004267.
56. Pugh R1, Grant C, Cooke RP, Dempsey G. Short-course versus prolonged-course antibiotic therapy for hospitalacquired pneumonia in critically ill adults. Cochrane Database Syst Rev. 2015;8:1–43.
57. Metersky ML, Kalil AC. New guidelines for nosocomial pneumonia. Curr Opin Pulm Med. 2017;23(3):211–7.
58. Lodise TP, Drusano GL. Use of pharmacokinetic/pharmacodynamic systems analyses to inform dose selection of tedizolid phosphate. Clin Infect Dis. 2014;58(Suppl 1):S28–34.
59. Bassetti M, et al. New antibiotics for ventilator-associated pneumonia. Curr Opin Infect Dis. 2018;31:177–86.
60. Sole-Lleonart C, Rouby JJ, Blot S, et al. Nebulization of antiinfective agents in invasively mechanically ventilated adults: a systematic review and meta analysis. Anesthesiology. 2017;126:890–908.
61. Niederman MS, Chastre J, Corkery K, et al. BAY41-6551 achieves bactericidal tracheal aspirate amikacin concentrations in mechanically ventilated patients with Gram-negative pneumonia. Intensive Care Med. 2012;38:263–71.
62. Kaku N, Morinaga Y, Takeda K, et al. Efficacy and pharmacokinetics of ME1100, a novel optimized formulation of arbekacin for inhalation, com- pared with amikacin in a murine model of ventilator-associated pneumonia caused by Pseudomonas aeruginosa. J Antimicrob Chemother. 2017;72:1123–8.
63. Falco V, Burgos J, Papiol E, et al. Investigational drugs in phase I and phase II & clinical trials for the treatment of hospital-acquired pneumonia. Expert Opin Investig Drugs. 2016;25:653–65.
64. Cabana MD, Rand CS, Powe NR, Wu AW, Wilson MH, Abboud PC, et al. Why don't physicians follow clinical practice guidelines? A framework for improvement. JAMA. 1999;282:1458–65.
65. Marwick C, Davey P. Care bundles: the holy grail of infectious risk management in hospital? Curr Opin Infect Dis. 2009;22:364–9.
66. Institute for Healthcare Improvement. How to guide: prevent ventilator- associated pneumonia. Cambridge, MA. Available from: http://www.ihi.org.
67. Alcan AO, Korkmaz FD, Uyar M. Prevention of ventilator-associated pneumonia: Use of the care bundle approach. Am J Infect Control. 2016;44:e173–6.
68. Eom JS, et al. The impact of a ventilator bundle on preventing ventilator-associated pneumonia: a multicenter study. Am J Infect Control. 2014;42:34–7.
69. Bo L, et al. Probiotics for preventing ventilator-associated pneumonia. Cochrane Database Syst Rev. 2014;(10):CD009066.
70. Graf JM, Montagnino BA, Hueckel R. McPherson ML. Pediatric tracheostomies: a recent experience from one academic center. 2008;9:96–100.
71. AHRQ. Agency for healthcare research and quality. HCUP KID database 2012.
72. McCaleb R, et al. Description of respiratory microbiology of children with long-term tracheostomies. Respir Care. 2016;61(4):447–52.
73. Craven DE, Hudcova J, Rashid J. Antibiotic therapy for ventilator-associated tracheobronchitis: a standard of care to reduce pneumonia, morbidity and costs? Curr Opin Pulm Med. 2015;21(3):250–9.

74. Nseir S, Martin-Loeches I, Makris D, et al. Impact of appropriate antimicrobial treatment on transition from ventilator-associated tracheobronchitis to ventilator-associated pneumonia. Crit Care. 2014;18:R129.
75. Agrafiotis M, Siempos II, Falagas ME. Frequency, prevention, outcome and treatment of ventilator-associated tracheobronchitis: systematic review and meta-analysis. Respir Med. 2010;104:325–36.
76. Simpson VS, Bailey A, Higgerson RA, Christie LM. Ventilator-associated tracheobronchitis in a mixed medical/surgical pediatric ICU. Chest. 2013;144:32–8.

Infections Complicating Abdominal Surgery Procedures

8

Lucila Marquez

Epidemiology

Much of the data regarding the epidemiology of surgical site infections (SSI) in pediatric patients undergoing abdominal surgery in the United States comes from data reported to the National Surgical Quality Improvement Program for Pediatrics (NSQIP-P) [1]. The NSQIP-P maintains a database of prospective information from a sample of pediatric surgical cases from institutions participating in the program.

The most common abdominal condition that requires surgery in children is appendicitis. Cases of appendicitis are categorized into either simple or complicated appendicitis [2]. In the later, the appendix is found to be either gangrenous or perforated. Perforated appendicitis is more likely to occur in infants and young children than in adolescents. Categorizing cases of appendicitis is important with regard to patient management and subsequent risk for SSI.

In a multi-institution study that utilized NSQIP-P data, SSI occurred in 2.5% of all pediatric patients undergoing appendectomy [2]. This study demonstrated that the frequency of SSI differs greatly between patients with simple appendicitis (1.2%) compared to those with complicated appendicitis (5.7%). In the multivariate analysis, complicated appendicitis, longer symptom duration prior to the operation, and sepsis were significantly associated with SSI. Delay in time to surgery from presentation to the emergency department or from admission was not associated with an increased risk for SSI [3].

Other studies provide insight into the prevalence of SSI in other pediatric abdominal procedures. Using data reported to NSQIP-P between 2012 and 2013 from 50 hospitals, the frequency of SSIs in pediatric colorectal procedures was 5.9% (169/2872) [1]. In comparison, the frequency of SSIs in adult colorectal procedures has been reported to be as high as 45% [1]. For pediatric colorectal procedures, total

L. Marquez
Pediatric Infectious Diseases, Baylor College of Medicine, Houston, TX, USA
e-mail: lm043062@bcm.edu

© Springer Nature Switzerland AG 2019
J. C. McNeil et al. (eds.), *Healthcare-Associated Infections in Children*,
https://doi.org/10.1007/978-3-319-98122-2_8

abdominal colectomy was associated with a higher frequency of SSIs compared to partial colectomy, which in turn had a higher frequency than colostomy closure. The conditions most commonly associated with SSIs due to colorectal procedures included inflammatory bowel disease, Hirschsprung's disease, anorectal malformations, and necrotizing enterocolitis, in descending order.

NSQIP-P data have also been used to estimate overall rates of composite morbidity, SSI, and mortality for common pediatric surgical procedures. In the study by Saito et al. [4], composite morbidity included infectious complications as well as cardiac, pulmonary, renal, neurologic, and hematologic events. Review of 10,907 pediatric (non-neonatal) abdominal surgeries revealed that the proportion of cases that experienced composite morbidity, SSI, and mortality were 6.7%, 3.3%, and 0.3%, respectively. Outcomes were worse in the 1803 neonatal abdominal cases reviewed where morbidity occurred in 17.7%, SSI in 4.3%, and mortality in 2.7%.

There are numerous risk factors for SSIs in patients undergoing abdominal surgical procedures. In common with other surgical procedures, abdominal procedures that are long in duration or performed emergently have a higher rate of SSIs [5]. Additionally, open procedures in general have higher SSI rates than laparoscopic procedures. Of note, laparoscopic appendectomies have been associated with lower rates of superficial or deep SSIs but with higher rates of organ/space SSIs [5]. In gastroduodenal procedures, reduced gastric acidity and motility and reduced integrity of the mucosa (including bleeding and perforation) have been shown to increase the risk for an SSI [5, 6]. In biliary procedures, acute cholecystitis and bile spillage have been associated with developing an SSI [5, 7]. In colon procedures, rectal resection has a higher risk of infection than intraperitoneal colon resection [5].

Clinical Manifestations

The symptoms of postoperative abdominal infections vary by anatomic location. Infections of surgical incisions can manifest as warmth, erythema, induration, and/or pain. Purulent drainage and dehiscence of the wound can be observed. Manifestations of deep or organ space infections generally include fever and abdominal pain. Individuals with postoperative abdominal infections often experience nausea and emesis, intolerance of feeds, and abnormal bowel function. Physical examination can reveal abdominal distention, reduced bowel sounds, tenderness, and guarding; patients with infections of the biliary tract may have associated jaundice.

Diagnosis

The National Healthcare Safety Network of the Centers for Disease Control and Prevention provides surveillance definitions for SSI [8]. These include superficial incisional, deep incisional, and organ/space SSIs. Superficial incisional SSIs occur within 30 days of the procedure, involve only the skin and subcutaneous tissues, and must meet specific clinical criteria: either (1) purulent drainage; (2) recovery of organisms in culture; (3) symptoms of pain, swelling, erythema, or heat in the context of deliberate opening of the wound by a medical provider; or (4) diagnosis of a superficial SSI by a medical provider. Deep incisional SSIs occur within 90 days of the procedure, involve deep soft tissues (fascia and muscles), and must meet specific clinical criteria: either (1) purulent drainage, (2) presence of fever or pain and recovery of organisms in culture from a wound that dehisces or is deliberately opened by a medical provider, or (3) abscess or infection detected on gross anatomical or histopathologic exam or imaging. Organ/space SSIs occur within 90 days of the procedure, involve any body part deeper than the fascial/muscle layers, and must meet specific clinical criteria: (1) purulent drainage, (2) recovery of organisms in culture from the organ/space, or (3) abscess or infection detected on gross anatomical or histopathologic exam or imaging.

The Infectious Diseases Society of America Guidelines for the Diagnosis and Management of Complicated Intra-abdominal Infection in Adults and Children emphasize that routine history, physical examination, and laboratory studies should identify most patients with suspected intra-abdominal infection [9]. Imaging studies can confirm and localize an organ/space infection. For example, in the setting of complicated appendicitis, children who continue to have fever and/or are unable to tolerate a regular diet 7–10 days after surgery should undergo imaging studies with a goal toward identifying a postoperative infection (e.g., an intra-abdominal abscess) [10]. In adults, computed tomography (CT) is considered the imaging study of choice. Though CT is more sensitive in this setting, many pediatric institutions consider abdominal ultrasound as an initial imaging modality in order to avoid radiation associated with CT.

Microbiology

As is the case for all surgical procedures, superficial infections complicating abdominal procedures can occur as a result of wound contamination with skin flora, including *Staphylococcus aureus* and *Streptococcus pyogenes*. With regard to SSIs specifically complicating abdominal surgical procedures, enteric organisms are predominant etiologies of infection and the precise frequency of organisms contributing to SSI vary somewhat with the organ of interest. Organisms that typically colonize the stomach and duodenum include streptococci, lactobacilli, diphtheroids, and fungi, and these are usually found in small numbers [5]. The flora of the jejunum is very similar to that of the duodenum; by contrast, the biliary tract is usually sterile. The lower intestinal tract, including the ileum and colon, is heavy colonized with anaerobes (of which *Bacteroides fragilis* is the most common organism) and gram-negative organisms (of which *E. coli* is the predominant aerobe) [11]. In the colon, the concentration of anaerobes is 1,000–10,000-fold higher than the concentration of aerobes. In the setting of small bowel obstruction, the flora of the small intestine more closely resembles that of the colon. Other organisms can be present in the gastrointestinal tract of children and can play a role in postoperative infections. *Pseudomonas* has been found in up to 25–30% of intra-abdominal infections in children [9, 12]. Nearly one-fifth of patients with gastrointestinal perforations will have *Candida* species identified in culture, and *Candida* peritonitis can rarely occur as a complication of abdominal surgery.

Management

Given that appendectomy is the most common pediatric abdominal procedure, it is worth noting that national guidelines dictate postoperative antibiotic management for complicated appendicitis. A Cochrane Review published in 2011 found that the use of antibiotics for patients undergoing appendectomy was superior to placebo for preventing wound infection and intra-abdominal abscess [13]. Subsequent guidelines by the Surgical Infection Society and the American Pediatric Surgical Association recommend preoperative antibiotics for all pediatric patients with appendicitis and continuation of antibiotics postoperatively only for patients with complicated appendicitis [14, 15]. For children with perforated appendicitis, parenteral antibiotics should be continued until the patient is afebrile, has resolution of symptoms (resolution of pain, return of normal bowel function, tolerance of diet), and the white blood cell count normalizes [14]. The American Pediatric Surgical Association recommends that if parenteral antibiotics are administered for less than 5 days, then oral antibiotics should be given to complete a total course of 7 days [14]. However, there is mounting evidence that additional days of oral antibiotics do not affect outcomes for complicated appendicitis if the patient has met the aforementioned criteria for discontinuation of parenteral therapy [10].

Cellulitis of a surgical incision may be managed with empiric antibiotics orally or parenterally depending on severity of illness. Fluctuant surgical incisions should be explored, irrigated, and debrided. Purulent drainage should be cultured and results of this used to guide antimicrobial therapy. Empiric antibiotics should have activity against skin flora in addition to activity against the flora expected at the surgical site. Based on local epidemiology and patient risk factors, consideration should be given to including coverage for methicillin-resistant *S. aureus* (MRSA).

Management of complicated abdominal infections is detailed in the Infectious Diseases Society of America Guidelines for the Diagnosis and Management of Complicated Intra-abdominal Infection in Adults and Children [9]. Timely administration of antibiotics and source control are recommended. Source control requires urgent intervention and should not be delayed beyond 24 h. Abscesses or well-defined fluid collections should be drained. Percutaneous drainage is preferred over open surgical drainage as long as there is no other indication for laparotomy, such as hollow-organ perforation or acute peritonitis.

In general, antibiotic-resistant flora are more often expected in postoperative infections compared with community-acquired abdominal infections where they are not. Empiric antibiotic regimens should be guided by local epidemiology and influenced in particular by the frequency of extended spectrum beta-lactamase-producing *Enterobacteriaceae* and cephalosporin-resistant *Pseudomonas aeruginosa* at a given institution. Carbapenems and piperacillin-tazobactam can be used as single agents, instead of multidrug combination therapy, as they provide broad gram-negative and anaerobic coverage. The addition of an aminoglycoside should be considered in institutions that frequently encounter multidrug-resistant gram-negative infections. In settings with low prevalence of resistant organisms, ceftazidime or cefepime in combination with metronidazole can be used. Clindamycin is not recommended for anaerobic coverage given high rates of resistance to this antibiotic by *Bacteroides fragilis*. Studies suggest that only 48–80% of *B. fragilis* isolates are susceptible to clindamycin [16]. Of note, empiric coverage of *Enterococcus* species is recommended for healthcare-associated intra-abdominal infections. Antibiotics with activity against *Enterococcus* species include carbapenems, piperacillin-tazobactam, ampicillin and vancomycin. Of note, enterococci are intrinsically resistant to all cephalosporins. Anti-MRSA therapy should be considered for individuals colonized with MRSA or who are at risk for this infection such as those with a prior history of MRSA infection. Antifungal therapy is only recommended if *Candida* is recovered in culture and, in general, should not be administered empirically.

Prevention

There is a large body of evidence in adults that supports the use of antibiotic surgical prophylaxis for the prevention of SSIs. Recommendations for this are nicely summarized in the Clinical Practice Guidelines for Antimicrobial Prophylaxis in Surgery developed jointly by the American Society of Health-System Pharmacists, the Infectious Diseases Society of America, and the Society for Healthcare Epidemiology of America [5]. The guidelines address the surgical procedures for which antimicrobial prophylaxis is indicated and the antimicrobial agents, doses, and interval for redosing for each indicated procedure (Table 8.1). The first dose of antibiotic prophylaxis should be administered beginning within 60 min of surgical incision, unless the antibiotic is vancomycin or a fluoroquinolone in which case it should be administered beginning within 120 min of surgical incision. Redosing should occur if the duration of the procedure exceeds two half-lives of the antibiotic. There are studies that also support antibiotic surgical prophylaxis in children. In a prospective cohort study that reviewed compliance with antibiotic prophylaxis in over five thousand pediatric cases, compliance was associated with a 30% decreased risk of SSI [17].

With regard to abdominal surgeries, the following anatomic sites and/or procedures have distinct recommendations: gastroduodenal, biliary tract, appendectomy, small intestine, and colorectal [5]. The distinction is necessary as different portions of the gastrointestinal tract have distinct compositions of microbial flora, as discussed previously, which dictates the need for varying antimicrobial agents. Antimicrobial prophylaxis is recommended for gastroduodenal procedures in which the lumen of the intestinal tract is entered, biliary tract procedures for which the patient is at high risk of infection (including open procedures), all cases of

Table 8.1 Antimicrobial prophylaxis for abdominal procedures [4]

Procedure	Antimicrobial agent	Dose (children)[b]
Gastroduodenal	Cefazolin	30 mg/kg
Biliary tract, *open and high risk*[a]	Cefazolin	30 mg/kg
Appendectomy, *simple*	Cefazolin + metronidazole OR Cefoxitin OR Cefotetan	30 mg/kg + 15 mg/kg 40 mg/kg 40 mg/kg

Small intestine
  Unobstructed
  Obstructed
	
	Cefazolin
	Cefazolin + metronidazole OR
	Cefoxitin OR
	Cefotetan
		
		30 mg/kg
		30 mg/kg + 15 mg/kg
		40 mg/kg
		40 mg/kg

Colorectal	Cefazolin + metronidazole OR Cefoxitin OR Cefotetan	30 mg/kg + 15 mg/kg 40 mg/kg 40 mg/kg

[a]High risk of infectious complications in adults includes emergency procedures, diabetes, long procedure duration, intraoperative gallbladder rupture, age >70 years, ASA class 3 or greater, episode of colic within 30 days before the procedure, re-intervention in less than 1 month, acute cholecystitis, bile spillage, jaundice, pregnancy, non-functioning gallbladder, immunosuppression, and insertion of prosthetic device
[b]Excludes neonates

suspected appendicitis, small bowel surgery that includes incision or resection of the small intestine, and colon procedures. Surgical antibiotic prophylaxis should be discontinued after the surgical incision is closed, even in the presence of a drain, for clean and clean-contaminated procedures [18]. Clean wounds include uninfected operative wounds and procedures where the alimentary tract is not entered. Clean-contaminated wounds include procedures where the alimentary tract is entered but under controlled conditions and without unusual contamination [8].

The American Pediatric Surgical Association does not recommend mechanical bowel preparation for colorectal procedures in children, as data suggest this does not offer any advantage for SSI prevention over what is offered by parenteral antibiotic prophylaxis [19]. Due to limited pediatric data, the guidelines make no recommendation on the use of enteral antibiotics combined with mechanical bowel preparation for pediatric colorectal procedures, though there is strong evidence for this in adults.

The reader is referred to the 2017 Centers for Disease Control and Prevention Guidelines for other general measures recommended for SSI prevention [18]. A thorough discussion of other topics related to SSI prevention, including patient bathing, antiseptics, and sterilization, is provided in Chap. 2.

References

1. Feng C, Sighwa F, Cameron D, Glass C, Rangel S. Rates and burden of surgical site infections associated with pediatric colorectal surgery: insight from the national surgery quality improvement program. J Pediatr Surg. 2016;51:970–4.

2. Boomer LA, Cooper JN, Anandalwar S, et al. Delaying appendectomy does not lead to higher rates of surgical site infections: a multi-institutional analysis of children with appendicitis. Ann Surg. 2016;264(1):164–8.

3. Serres SK, Cameron DB, Glass CC, et al. Time to appendectomy and risk of complicated appendicitis and adverse outcomes in children. JAMA Pediatr. 2017;171(8):740–6.

4. Saito JM, Chen LE, Hall BL, et al. Risk-adjusted hospital outcomes for children's surgery. Pediatrics. 2013;132(3):e677–88.

5. Bratzler DW, Dellinger EP, Olsen KM, et al. Clinical practice guidelines for antimicrobial prophylaxis in surgery. Am J Health Syst Pharm. 2013;70(3):195–283.

6. Pessaux P, Msika S, Atalla D, Hay JM, Flamant Y. French Association for Surgical R. Risk factors for postoperative infectious complications in noncolorectal abdominal surgery: a multivariate analysis based on a prospective multicenter study of 4718 patients. Arch Surg. 2003;138(3):314–24.

7. den Hoed PT, Boelhouwer RU, Veen HF, Hop WC, Bruining HA. Infections and bacteriological data after laparoscopic and open gallbladder surgery. J Hosp Infect. 1998;39(1):27–37.

8. Center for Disease control and Prevention. Surgical Site Infection (SSI) event. In: National healthcare safety network patient safety component manual. Atlanta; 2018. www.cdc.gov/nhsn/pdfs/pscmanual/9pscssicurrent.pdf. Accessed 22 Jan 2018.

9. Solomkin JS, Mazuski JE, Bradley JS, et al. Diagnosis and management of complicated intra-abdominal infection in adults and children: guidelines by the surgical infection society and the Infectious Diseases Society of America. Clin Infect Dis. 2010;50(2):133–64.

10. Wesson D. Acute appendicitis in children: management. In: Singer J, editor. UpToDate. 2018. www.uptodate.com/contents/acute-appendicitis-in-children-management. Accessed 23 Jan 2018.

11. Stone HH. Bacterial flora of appendicitis in children. J Pediatr Surg. 1976;11(1):37–42.

12. Fallon SC, Hassan SF, Larimer EL, et al. Modification of an evidence-based protocol for advanced appendicitis in children. J Surg Res. 2013;185(1):273–7.

13. Andersen BR, Kallehave FL, Andersen HK. Antibiotics versus placebo for prevention of postoperative infection after appendicectomy. Cochrane Database Syst Rev. 2005;(3):CD001439.

14. Lee SL, Islam S, Cassidy LD, et al. Antibiotics and appendicitis in the pediatric population: an American Pediatric Surgical Association Outcomes and Clinical Trials Committee systematic review. J Pediatr Surg. 2010;45(11):2181–5.

15. Nadler EP, Gaines BA, Therapeutic Agents Committee of the Surgical Infection Society. The surgical infection society guidelines on antimicrobial therapy for children with appendicitis. Surg Infect. 2008;9(1):75–83.

16. Foster C, Marquez L, Buckingham SC. Bacteroides, fusobacterium, prevotella and porphyromonas. In: Cherry JD, Demmler-Harison G, Kaplan S, Steinbach WJ, Hotez PJ, editors. Feigin and Cherry's textbook of pediatric infectious diseases, vol. 1. Philadelphia: Elsevier; 2018. p. 1316–23.

17. Khoshbin A, So JP, Aleem IS, et al. Antibiotic prophylaxis to prevent surgical site infections in children: a prospective cohort study. Ann Surg. 2015;262(2):397–402.

18. Berrios-Torres SI, Umscheid CA, Bratzler DW, et al. Centers for disease control and prevention guideline for the prevention of surgical site infection, 2017. JAMA Surg. 2017;152(8):784–91.

19. Rangel SJ, Islam S, St Peter SD, et al. Prevention of infectious complications after elective colorectal surgery in children: an American Pediatric Surgical Association Outcomes and Clinical Trials Committee comprehensive review. J Pediatr Surg. 2015;50(1):192–200.

Infections Complicating Orthopedic Surgery and Implants

9

Zachary Stinson, Scott Rosenfeld, and J. Chase McNeil

Introduction

Orthopedic surgical procedures as a group are among the most common forms of surgery performed in the pediatric population. Based on administrative data from the Kids' Inpatient Database (KID) of the Agency for Healthcare Research and Quality (AHRQ), orthopedic conditions are the second most common indication for surgical admission in children, accounting for >20% of cases [1]. Surgical implants are commonly used in orthopedic surgery to stabilize fractures, correct deformity and/or support function and ensure optimal long-term growth in children. While infections complicate the minority of pediatric orthopedic surgeries (<2%) [2], they can contribute substantially to morbidity, given the potential consequences for growth and development. The management of such infections is often complicated by the presence of hardware and implants. This chapter will briefly review the available literature regarding the epidemiology, microbiology, and medical and surgical management of infection complicating spinal instrumentation and the fixation of fractures in children.

Z. Stinson · S. Rosenfeld
Department of Orthopedic Surgery, Division of Pediatric Orthopedic Surgery, Baylor College of Medicine, Houston, TX, USA

J. C. McNeil (✉)
Department of Pediatrics, Section of Infectious Diseases, Baylor College of Medicine and Texas Children's Hospital, Houston, TX, USA
e-mail: jm140109@bcm.edu

© Springer Nature Switzerland AG 2019
J. C. McNeil et al. (eds.), *Healthcare-Associated Infections in Children*,
https://doi.org/10.1007/978-3-319-98122-2_9

Infections Complicating Spinal Instrumentation

Epidemiology

There is a wide variation in the reported rates of infection complicating pediatric spine surgery, ranging from 0.9% to 5% for adolescent idiopathic scoliosis (AIS) and 4% to 20% for neuromuscular scoliosis [3–7]. Data collected from the Scoliosis Research Society (SRS) database identified postoperative infection rates of 5.7%, 5.5%, 2.2%, and 1.4% for post-traumatic, neuromuscular, congenital, and idiopathic causes of scoliosis, respectively, and an overall infection rate of 2.6% following pediatric scoliosis surgery [7].

Patients with neuromuscular scoliosis have multiple factors placing them at increased risk of postoperative infection including poor bowel/bladder control, longer surgical times, increased implant density, instrumentation that often extends to the pelvis, cognitive impairment, altered sensation, relative immuno-compromised state, impaired nutritional status, and history of previous spinal surgery and frequent urinary tract infections compared to otherwise healthy children. One study that evaluated risk factors specific to patients with cerebral palsy identified older age, increased magnitude of primary curve, presence of gastrostomy tube, increased preoperative serum white blood cell count, and increased operative time as significant risk factors for the development of infection [5]. Additional risk factors pertinent to all scoliosis patients include the inappropriate choice, dose, timing, or frequency of perioperative antibiotics, use of allograft bone, and increased implant density [4, 6, 8, 9]. Other studies suggest that revisions to growing constructs are associated with a high risk of infection with rates as high as 10.2% [10].

Clinical Features

An infection may occur early or late in the postoperative period. There is, however, not a standard time cutoff used in the literature to define early vs. late infection. The definition of early infection has ranged from less than 30 days up to 6 months and late infection defined as those occurring beyond this time period [11–15]. The presence of an infection may not be obvious, and a high index of suspicion should be used in any patient with pain, fever, malaise, or wound drainage. Back pain and wound drainage have been identified as two of the most common presenting symptoms of spinal implant infection [4]. A sinus tract or wound dehiscence may also be present. Laboratory studies such as erythrocyte sedimentation rate (ESR) and C-reactive protein (CRP) may be elevated, but not consistently. Imaging modalities, including plain radiographs and computed tomography may be useful to evaluate for successful fusion. Ultrasound and MRI may also be considered to evaluate for a fluid collection; however, in the early postoperative period, it may be difficult to distinguish between normal surgical hematoma and abscess, limiting the utility of such studies.

Diagnosis

If a superficial or deep infection is suspected, a wound aspiration under sterile conditions may be utilized. A superficial swab of the wound is unreliable and is likely to result in the isolation of skin flora. With regard to the aspiration procedure, a deep aspiration should be performed first. Proper needle location can be confirmed by placing it up against the implant prior to aspiration. This should then be followed by performing a separate superficial aspiration just below the skin. Both samples should then be analyzed separately. Diagnosis of infection is made unequivocal by a positive culture result. Diagnosis of deep infection requires surgical confirmation of communication of the infectious material with the instrumentation or fusion mass. The presence of a hematoma or seroma without a positive culture result does not rule out the presence of infection. Any patient with clinical features of an infection along with a draining spinal wound or postoperative seroma or hematoma should be treated with a high index of suspicion and further managed with surgical irrigation and debridement at a minimum.

Microbiology

Specific data regarding the contemporary microbiology of spinal instrumentation infections is largely limited to single-center retrospective case series. It is apparent, however, from the available research that the relative frequency of causative pathogens is influenced by both the indication for spinal instrumentation as well as the time since initial surgery (Table 9.1). When deep operative cultures are obtained, a pathogen can be identified in approximately 70–92% of cases. Much lower culture yield is reported in studies that included superficial wound swabs [10, 16, 17]. As a whole, gram-positive pathogens predominate in spinal instrumentation infection, accounting for up to 87% of culture-positive cases [18, 19]. Infections are reported to be polymicrobial in 30–42% of cases [18, 20].

Among children with idiopathic scoliosis, *Staphylococcus aureus* and coagulase-negative staphylococci (CoNS) are the predominant organisms isolated; together these organisms account for up to 81% of isolates [18]. The proportion of cases secondary to methicillin-resistant *S. aureus* (MRSA) has been relatively low in the reported literature (1.4–17.5%); however this would be anticipated to vary geographically with the relative prevalence of MRSA in the community and healthcare settings [18, 21]. Among those children who have spinal instrumentation performed for reasons other than idiopathic scoliosis (which can be referred to as non-idiopathic scoliosis), gram-negative bacilli are far more common in these infections accounting for up to 57% of cases [10, 18]. Maesani et al. [18], in a series of pediatric spinal instrumentation infections at a tertiary care hospital in Paris, reported a greater than threefold increased risk of gram-negative enteric spinal instrumentation infection among patients with neuromuscular disease compared to those with idiopathic scoliosis. Other identified risk factors associated with gram-negative etiologies include body weight <30 kg and fusion extending to

Table 9.1 Microbiology of infections complicating spinal instrumentation based on published literature

Etiology[a]	All cases	Idiopathic scoliosis	Non-idiopathic scoliosis	Early-onset infection	Late-onset infection
Staphylococcus aureus	33–50.8	76	10–37.5	15–43.9	8.3–22
Coagulase-negative staphylococci	13.4–21.1	4.8–15	37.5–45	10–35	18–50
Enterococcus spp.	2.7–15.7	3.3	25	25	40
Propionibacterium spp.	6.8	10–13.3	4.5	3–10.5	12–85
Enterobacteriaceae	14–39	0–14	57–60	13–40	2–60
Pseudomonas spp.	12–17.3	10–14	4–13.6	12.6	9.1–20
Anaerobic bacteria[b]	2–7.8	16.7	10.5–13	3	2
Atypical mycobacteria[c]	5.9–8.6	–	–	1.7	2
Candida[c]	1	–	–	1.5	0
Polymicrobial infection	14–34	34	25–52	23–40	24–60

References: [11, 12, 14, 17, 19, 21–23, 25, 29]
Values expressed are percentages of reported cases in literature
[a]Categories are not mutually exclusive
[b]Excluding *Propionibacterium* species
[c]Data are extremely limited regarding the frequency of *Candida* and mycobacteria in spinal instrumentation infections

the sacrum. In this series, gram-negative organisms were also more likely to exist as components of polymicrobial infections, whereas gram-positive infections were more often monomicrobial.

In addition to underlying conditions, the timing of onset of infection following surgery can also be used to predict the microbiologic etiology [11–13]. Overall, organisms of higher virulence, such as *S. aureus* and gram-negative enterics, are predominant in early-onset infections. Notably, nearly a third of early-onset infections are secondary to CoNS, an organism of fairly low intrinsic virulence. While *S. aureus* and *Enterobacteriaceae* may be found in late-onset infections, lower virulence organisms more often typify these infections, including CoNS, *Enterococcus* spp., and anaerobes. A number of authors have reported a high degree of medical therapy failure in late-onset spinal infections and recommend earlier implant removal in this scenario [11].

As stated above, anaerobic and facultative anaerobic bacteria have also been implicated in spinal instrumentation infection. The true prevalence of anaerobic bacteria in these infections is unclear as most of the literature does not discuss whether or not anaerobic cultures and/or molecular methods (such as 16s PCR) are utilized in the microbiologic diagnosis. This is complicated by the intrinsic difficulties of isolating and identifying anaerobic bacteria including challenges related to obtaining and handling specimens and limited resources of many clinical microbiology laboratories in this arena. Anaerobic species identified in spinal instrumentation infections have included organisms belonging to a wide range of genera including *Corynebacterium, Peptostreptococcus, Finegoldia, Bacteroides, Actinomyces,* and *Propionibacterium* [12, 18, 21–23]. Anaerobic organisms are typically isolated as components of polymicrobial infections, frequently in patients with neuromuscular scoliosis. One exception to this rule is organisms of the *Propionibacterium* genus. *Propionibacterium* species (notably *P. acnes*) are well-described causes of orthopedic implant infections in adults and children [11, 18, 24] and contribute substantially to late-onset spinal instrumentation infections, accounting for >50% of cases in some series [23, 25]. *P. acnes* was implicated in ~13% of infections following posterior fusion for idiopathic scoliosis in a 12-year single-center review [26]. Notably, the clinical presentation of infections caused by *P. acnes* is often subtle, frequently without systemic symptoms and often at a time point far removed from initial surgery (presentation beyond a year after implantation has been described) [23, 26]. Thus a high index of suspicion for this pathogen must exist [27]. Given the reported difficulty in eradicating this organism with implants in situ, some authors recommend implant removal when this organism is isolated (see sections "Surgical Management" and "Medical Management" below) [28]. Other rare causes of spinal instrumentation infection include fungi (most often *Candida* spp.) and non-tuberculous mycobacteria [23, 29]. Despite the limited data regarding fungal and mycobacterial instrumentation infection, it is generally believed that these organisms are inoculated into the surgical site at the time of implantation. While these infections typically present in a more subacute or chronic fashion than typical bacterial infections, rapidly growing mycobacteria (such as *M. abscessus*) have also been reported as causes of early-onset spinal instrumentation infection [23].

A pathogen is unable to be definitively identified in 3–12% of spinal instrumentation infections as a whole [10, 12, 17] but may be much higher in late-onset infections [11]. The utilization of molecular microbiology methods may serve as a useful adjunct for pathogen identification. In studies of adults with prosthetic joint infections undergoing implant removal, the use of 16s PCR sequencing was able to identify a pathogen in up to 90% of patients [30–32]. There is little data available however to assess the utility of molecular methods in spinal instrumentation infections or pediatric orthopedic infections in general. Despite these caveats, such laboratory testing may be useful in cases in which difficult-to-culture pathogens are suspected such as late-onset infections or among those with subtle symptoms.

Surgical Management

Initial management of a suspected or confirmed early or late infection should include surgical wound exploration with irrigation and debridement of devitalized tissue and involved implants. Careful exploration of the fusion mass should also be performed in order to confirm successful fusion. Additional considerations include implant removal vs. retention, wound management, and the need for additional debridements.

In the setting of infected implants, removal of the implant is optimal for the greatest opportunity for infection eradication. However, implant removal may not be the best option in the setting of an acute- or early-onset infection. The increased difficulty of eradicating an infection associated with implant retention must be weighed against the risks of implant removal including a lengthy surgery with potential for large blood loss, as well as increased risk of curve progression and pseudarthrosis associated with implant removal. Curve progression is likely to occur in patients with both early and late infection following implant removal [11, 14, 16, 33]. Larger main thoracic and kyphotic curves have been shown to be particularly prone to progression in this setting [33]. One study reported a significantly increased rate of Cobb angle progression with implant removal in both early and late infections and a 38% pseudarthrosis rate with implant removal vs. 0% with implant retention. In this study the majority of the pseudarthrosis cases (7 out of 8) occurred in patients with implants removed following late infection, indicating that it is very difficult to definitively confirm a spine fusion [14]. Additionally, it has been postulated that pseudarthrosis may be a predisposing factor for the development of a late infection [34, 35].

While retention of implants is desirable from the standpoint of preventing curve progression, it has been well documented that implant retention increases the likelihood of infection recurrence, with one recent study demonstrating a 47% rate of recurrence of infection and subsequent debridements associated with implant retention compared to 20% with implant removal [12]. An additional study demonstrated 100% success at eradicating infection with implant removal and also showed a significant increase in hospitalization time and financial burden associated with attempted implant retention [13]. Failed eradication of infection with implant retention is likely due to presence of the biofilm on retained metal implants [34]. Therefore, the option of implant exchange may serve as a successful alternative approach in removing biofilm while minimizing the risks associated with complete implant removal. In a small series of patients with late-onset infection, patients treated with either acute or delayed implant exchange had better outcomes with respect to final Cobb angle when compared to patients treated with complete implant removal [16]. Another study employing the use of implant exchange in acute infections was successful in ultimately eradicating the infection in 76% of cases. Even in those patients who experienced a recurrence of infection, they did so at an average follow-up of 18 months, which provided additional time for fusion to occur prior to ultimate implant removal [15]. Patients with stainless steel implants and older age were significantly more likely to have recurrence of infection. In both of these studies, it was recommended to exchange stainless steel implants with newer-generation low-profile titanium implants. The specific infecting organism is another factor to consider when deciding whether to remove implants, and this is discussed further in the section on medical management.

Following initial irrigation and debridement, with or without implant retention, wounds are typically closed primarily over drains. Vacuum-assisted closure (VAC) devices have been shown to be very useful, especially in the setting of treating infections associated with neuromuscular scoliosis [36, 37]. A closed suction-irrigation system is another option to consider and was shown to be effective in a retrospective review, with success demonstrated in two-thirds of patients with acute infections and implant retention. The remaining third of patients ultimately cleared the infection after an additional irrigation and debridement followed by a second round of closed suction-irrigation [38]. Finally, the use of antibiotic-loaded polymethylmethacrylate (PMMA) bone cement used in combination with implant retention can be considered. While this is a common technique used in the treatment of prosthetic joint infections (PJI), there is little information in the literature on its use for the treatment of instrumented spine infections. One case series in adult patients demonstrated the successful use of this technique when there was a recurrence of infection following initial management of instrumented spine infection with implant retention. Antibiotic-loaded cement tailored to the cultured specimen was placed around the retained implants, and all patients remained free of infection without the need for additional debridements [39]. The long-term local and systemic effects of retained antibiotic-loaded cement in the pediatric population have not been reported and would need further investigation prior to making specific recommendations on its use.

Medical Management

There is little published literature available to provide high-quality evidence-based guidance for the medical management of spinal instrumentation infections in children, and most recommendations are extrapolated from studies of PJI or spinal implant infections in adults. Some combination of surgical intervention along with effective antimicrobial agents is necessary for good clinical outcome and as such requires a multidisciplinary approach. While, in general, infections associated with orthopedic implants are treated most effectively with implant removal, situations may arise in which removal of implants may not be able to be performed safely (such as very early after placement) or may not be required for good outcome. Furthermore, as previously discussed, removal of spinal implants is associated with risks beyond that of the operation itself including a greater rate of pseudoarthrosis development and continued curve progression [14, 22]. The Infectious Diseases Society of America (IDSA) practice guideline for the management of PJI in adults outlines recommended criteria for when Debridement, Antibiotics and Implant Retention (DAIR) may be appropriate (Table 9.2) [40]. Additionally, the likelihood of success with DAIR may in part be dependent on the infecting

Table 9.2 Infectious Diseases
Society of America Proposed
Criteria for Debridement,
Antibiotics and Implant
Retention (DAIR) for Prosthetic
Joint Infections [40]

Duration of symptoms <3 weeks
<30 days since implant placed
Well-fixed prosthesis
Absence of a sinus tract
Organisms susceptible to oral agents

organism. In a retrospective series of children with infection following surgery for neuromuscular scoliosis, DAIR was more often successful in gram-positive rather than gram-negative infections [29].

Patients with spinal instrumentation infection are typically treated with 2–6 weeks of parenteral antimicrobial therapy [11, 21] which may be followed by prolonged oral suppression when instrumentation is retained (Fig. 9.1). Kowalski et al. examined outcomes among adults with spinal implant infections with particular attention to the impact of oral antimicrobial suppression, defined as ≥6 months of effective oral antimicrobials following at least 2 weeks of parenteral therapy [11]. These investigators found that patients with early-onset infection treated with DAIR receiving at least 6 months of suppressive antimicrobial therapy had substantially lower rates of treatment failure at 2-year follow-up than those who received a shorter duration of suppression (20% vs. 67%). In this study, the oral suppressive therapy was continued for a median of 468 days. This evidence supports the use of suppressive therapy for 6–12 months in spinal instrumentation infection following surgical irrigation and debridement with implant retention. It is worth noting however, that in a recent study of 89 primarily adult patients with orthopedic implant infections (including spinal instrumentation) while antimicrobial suppression was associated with a better outcome, there was no benefit to 6 months of suppression over 3 months [41]. Thus the exact duration of suppression necessary is unclear, with some experts favoring indefinite suppression in the case of PJI in adults [40]. Among adults undergoing PJI treatment with DAIR, an increased risk of treatment failure and relapse was observed following discontinuation of antibiotics regardless of how long suppression had been utilized [42]. Messina et al. in a series of children with spinal implant infections who were treated successfully with DAIR reported a wide range of total antibiotic duration ranging from 42 to 597 days with resolution of symptoms and normalization of inflammatory markers (ESR and CRP) being in part used to gauge when to discontinue antimicrobials [21]. Furthermore, while a period of parenteral antimicrobial therapy is typically prescribed in these infections prior to transitioning to oral therapy, it is conceivable that utilization of an antibiotic regimen with high oral bioavailability may be just as efficacious [40]. It is important to note, however, that even with optimal medical therapy, there is still a substantial risk of treatment failure with implant retention ranging from 18% to 53% [11, 21, 41].

Final antibiotic choice should be based on the results of culture and antimicrobial susceptibility testing. While it is a common dogma in infectious diseases practice that bactericidal cell-wall active agents (such as β-lactams) should be utilized whenever possible, concern exists for the activity of these agents against organisms living in the relatively metabolic inert state of biofilm that often exists in orthopedic device

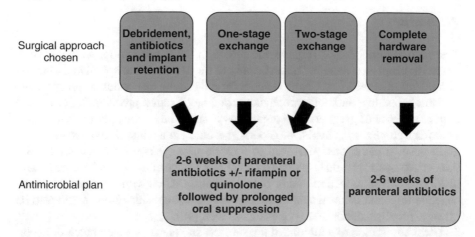

Fig. 9.1 Medical and surgical approaches to spinal instrumentation infections

infections. In particular, rifampin and fluoroquinolones are known to have good activity against bacteria living in biofilm. Ex vivo and animal models of *S. aureus* orthopedic implant-associated osteomyelitis have demonstrated the synergistic activity of vancomycin and rifampin in reducing bacterial burden [43]. Among adults with staphylococcal orthopedic implant infection treated with retention, the use of rifampin along with vancomycin or flucloxacillin was associated with improved eradication [44]. While data is limited regarding its use in spinal instrumentation infection, the IDSA PJI guidelines recommend 2–6 weeks of directed parenteral antimicrobial therapy in combination with rifampin followed by 3–6 months of rifampin in combination with another orally active agent (preferably a fluoroquinolone) for staphylococcal PJI treated with DAIR or one-stage exchange [40]. Recent studies would also suggest a potential benefit to rifampin combination therapy even in streptococcal PJI [45], suggesting that this agent may have a benefit for other gram-positive orthopedic hardware infections. Similarly in two studies of gram-negative orthopedic hardware infections, the use of fluoroquinolone-containing regimens was associated with higher rates of treatment success [46, 47].

Prognosis

Despite the need for additional surgical procedures and hospitalization, with appropriate management, patients with spinal instrumentation infection can ultimately have an outcome similar to patients who did not experience this complication. This is especially true for patients who were able to have implants retained, as their risk of curve progression greatly decreases, with one review showing a progression rate of 0.2 degrees per year in patients with retained implants compared to 5.8 degrees per year for those patients who had implants removed [14]. Despite this, aggressive treatment and close follow-up should be utilized in such patients to avoid further complications, such as sepsis and vertebral osteomyelitis.

Prevention

The general principles of surgical site infection (SSI) prevention, which are discussed in detail elsewhere in this text, apply to the prevention of spinal instrumentation infection as well (see Chaps. 2 and 8 for a thorough discussion of preoperative screening, bathing, antibiotic prophylaxis, and sterilization procedures). Given the high prevalence of gram-positive organisms in these infections, perioperative antimicrobial prophylaxis should, in general, be directed against *S. aureus* and other gram-positive pathogens. The need to provide prophylactic coverage for MRSA (i.e., vancomycin) should be guided by local prevalence of this organism and patient history of MRSA infection and/or colonization. In cases with high risk of gram-negative infection (such as neuromuscular scoliosis), consideration should also be given to prophylaxis for these organisms as well [48].

Local application of antibiotic at the surgical site (such as vancomycin or gentamicin powder) has been utilized by many surgeons in attempts to prevent infection at the surgical site. In studies of adults undergoing spinal instrumentation, results have been conflicting with regard to the utility of intraoperative vancomycin powder. In a systematic review (which largely included studies of adult patients) intra-site vancomycin powder appears to provide some reduction in incidence of SSI compared to historical controls [49]. Gans et al. described a series of 87 pediatric patients who received intra-site vancomycin powder for prevention of SSI; no patient experienced acute kidney injury or other systemic side effects leading the authors to conclude that vancomycin powder can be utilized safely in children [50]. Consensus guidelines created by pediatric spine surgeons and infectious disease specialists advocate the use of intraoperative vancomycin powder in children undergoing spine surgery [48]. Notably, one series reported a high rate of gram-negative and polymicrobial infection among spine surgery patients who received intraoperative vancomycin powder; such findings likely reflect the selection for organisms for which vancomycin would not be effective therapy [51]. Evidence is currently insufficient to support the use of topical/local gentamicin routinely for the prevention of SSI [52].

Some experts have advocated double gloving to prevent SSI in patients undergoing spinal instrumentation. In one study of 389 adults undergoing spinal instrumentation, removal of the outer pair of gloves by the surgeon prior to handling of implants was associated with an almost 80% reduction in SSI compared to when surgeons maintained the same pair of gloves throughout the operation [53]. Notably, however, this center reported a baseline SSI rate of 3.9% in the control group, higher than reported in many institutions, and this may have influenced the observed efficacy of double gloving.

In addition, there is some data suggesting that the material of which the implant is constructed may influence infection risk. Early-generation stainless steel spine implants were associated with a higher incidence of delayed infection compared to later-generation titanium implants [15, 26, 54]. Given temporal changes in design of implants as well as surgical practices, however, it is difficult to definitively assign risk to the material itself [52]. Based on such limited data, the preferential use of titanium implants is neither endorsed nor discouraged by consensus guidelines [48, 55].

There is not a consensus on the most effective type of irrigation method and solution to use prior to closure. Bulb irrigation is most commonly used, followed by pulse lavage, cysto tubing and directly pouring irrigation solution into the wound. Saline solution is used most routinely, followed by bacitracin. Adult spinal instrumentation studies have demonstrated the effective use of dilute povidone-iodine solution in the prevention of postoperative infection; these solutions are reportedly used 9% of the time in pediatric spinal surgery [52].

Infections Complicating Internal and External Fixation of Fractures and Pins/Pin Tracts

Epidemiology

Infection of buried or exposed metal implants used for the treatment of pediatric fractures or elective reconstructive surgery varies based on the type of implants and clinical history. Patients treated for open fractures are at higher risk of infection [56], with those rates decreased by timely administration of antibiotics [57]. When implants are used for closed fractures, there is no difference in the reported infection rates for fractures treated with exposed or buried implants. One study reported an infection rate of 3.5% for buried implants versus 2.3% for exposed implants in the treatment setting of forearm fractures [58].

Pinning of pediatric supracondylar humerus fractures, a very common indication for the use of exposed pins, has a relatively low infection rate, with reports ranging from 0.81% to 2.34% [59, 60]. Possible clinical factors associated with infection risk include patient compliance with cast care, timely removal of pins, and improper use of perioperative antibiotics [59]. Elastic stable intramedullary nailing (ESIN) used most commonly for forearm and femur fractures has a reported 2% rate of developing late osteomyelitis [61]. In addition, these cases are often associated with local skin irritation at the sites of insertion, with rates of 8% and 12% for forearm fractures and femur fractures, respectively [61]. The rates of infection associated with ESIN, however, vary across centers with a separate study identifying only one superficial infection and no deep infections out of 202 forearm fractures treated with ESIN [62]. Telescopic intramedullary Fassier-Duval rods, commonly used for the treatment of osteogenesis imperfecta, have a very low risk of infection, with one review reporting 0 cases out of 24 developing rod infection [63].

Infections associated with circular external fixators used for elective reconstructive surgery occur at a rate of 4.0% per pin site observation, with infections more commonly associated with periarticular pins than diaphyseal pins, at rates of 4.5% and 1.6%, respectively [64]. The vast majority of these infections are superficial; in one study of 46 patients and another with 27 patients, there were no occurrences of deep infections involving the bone [64, 65]. Since pin site infection is a well-known complication associated with external fixators, close clinical follow-up with vigilant observation of pin sites helps make deep infection a rare occurance [64].

Clinical Features

Increased pain at the surgical site is the most common symptom of a postoperative infection. The patient may also present with fever and have a history of a wet cast or missed follow-up appointments and late removal of pins [59, 66]. ESR and CRP may be elevated, but not consistently [66]. The timing of postoperative pin site infection is variable and may occur early on or several weeks postoperatively [59, 66]. One study noted that the majority of infections occurred more than 3 weeks postoperatively [66]. Once an infection of an exposed pin is identified, thorough inspection around the pin sites should be performed to determine if there is purulent drainage or an associated deep soft tissue abscess. Plain radiographs, or even advanced imaging, may be needed in the setting of suspected osteomyelitis. Infection of a buried implant is less obvious and requires a high index of suspicion.

External fixator smooth wires and half pins used for elective deformity correction have different clinical considerations due to the length of time they are left in place. Given that pin site infection is a common concern related to this treatment modality, these patients should be monitored frequently. All pins should be routinely checked for appropriate tension, and skin around pin sites must be completely free of tension. It has been noted that pain often precedes the clinical appearance by 2–3 days and thus index of suspicion must be high for the patient with unexpected pain even when other signs of infection are not present [64].

Diagnosis

An infection associated with a buried or exposed implant is most often a clinical diagnosis. Further diagnostic considerations should include if the infection is superficial or deep. The clinical appearance of pin site infections has been described using different grading systems. Paley divides abnormal pin site appearances into three grades that include soft tissue inflammation (grade 1), soft tissue infection (grade 2) and bone infection (grade 3) [65]. Alternatively, pin site appearances may also be graded by the system described by Dahl using a 0–5 scale (Table 9.3) [64]. A superficial infection may present as localized inflammation around a pin site or diffuse cellulitis. Deep infections can include a soft tissue abscess with or without a

Table 9.3 Comparison of Paley and Dahl scales for grading pin site infections

Scale	Paley [65]	Dahl [64]
0	–	Clean
1	Soft tissue inflammation	Pain or erythema, no drainage
2	Soft tissue infection	Pain, erythema, serous drainage
3	Osteomyelitis	Pain, erythema and purulent drainage
4	–	Pain, erythema and purulent drainage with osteolytic lesion
5	–	Ring sequestrum or osteomyelitis

draining sinus tract, osteomyelitis, or even septic arthritis [66]. A case of toxic shock syndrome following percutaneous pinning of a supracondylar humerus fracture has also been reported [66].

Infections involving ringed fixator pin sites may be described according to the grading systems noted above, with Paley grade 3 or Dahl grade 4 or 5 being the only categories that require surgery. It should also be noted if the infection is associated with a diaphyseal or periarticular pin or wire, with periarticular infections at risk for causing septic arthritis.

Microbiology

The most common microbial etiologies to contribute to infections of pins, wires and external fixators used to manage fractures in children are gram-positive bacteria. The two most frequently isolated organisms in published studies of these infections are *S. aureus* accounting for 17–33% of cases and CoNS accounting for 20–27% [67, 68]. Gram-negative enterics and *Pseudomonas* spp. have also been isolated from these infections in 5–12% of cases [66, 68]. Other typical commensal organisms of low virulence such as α-streptococci and diphtheroids have also been frequently isolated from these infections although their significance in infection is unclear [67, 69]. Mahan et al. [69] reported that of 214 pins removed from patients with and without signs of inflammation/infection, 74.8% of pin tips grew bacteria on culture; however only 42% grew virulent organisms (which they defined to include *S. aureus, S. haemolyticus, Pseudomonas, Proteus mirabilis*, and *E. coli*). Notably, the presence of virulent organisms was strongly associated with loose pins and grossly inflamed pin tracts, and this was far less often the case with low-virulence organisms. Thus it is likely that organisms of low virulence frequently colonize external fixation devices without causing true infection. By contrast, other organisms such as *S. aureus* more often contribute to actual clinical infections.

Surgical Management

If a deep infection of a buried or exposed implant is suspected, then surgical management with irrigation and debridement should be performed as soon as possible. Some difficult cases may require staging with serial debridements [66]. From a stability standpoint, implants should be left in place until bone healing is evident whenever possible [61]. Alternatively, exposed pins may be removed and replaced in a different location during surgical debridement, if needed [66]. In the setting of chronic osteomyelitis, the mainstay of treatment is thorough debridement of the necrotic bone. If a significant bone void is left behind, then additional procedures, such as bone transport or the use of autograft or allograft bone may be needed after the infection is cleared. A thorough evaluation of the adjacent joint should be performed for implants placed near a joint. If septic arthritis is suspected, irrigation and debridement of the joint through an arthrotomy should be performed.

For pin-tract infections associated with the use of external fixators, most superficial infections can be addressed with topical or oral antibiotics, but periarticular pins or pins with surrounding cellulitis should be removed. Paley grade 3 or Dahl grade 4 and 5 infections involving the bone should be treated with implant removal and debridement [65].

Medical Management

While orthopedic pin tract and pin site infections are quite common and often mild in nature, the need to be vigilant for the possibility of deeper infection cannot be overemphasized. That being stated, up to 17% of superficial pin tract infections were successfully treated with topical antimicrobials in one series [67]. Other investigators have reported that 10/18 pin tract infections developing after external fixation of humerus fractures were successfully treated with oral antibiotics [68].

While infection may be limited to the superficial skin and be amenable to oral or topical antimicrobial therapy [67, 70], a high degree of suspicion must exist for infection communicating with bone and producing an underlying osteomyelitis. Efforts should be made to distinguish between these but in the absence of clear evidence, providers should assume infection encompasses the bone. While there is very limited high-quality literature to guide medical management for infections complicating orthopedic fixation devices, the principles that pertain to spinal instrumentation infection or PJI are applicable. When at all possible, implants should be removed and patients treated for osteomyelitis with 4–6 weeks of effective therapy. When implants are unable to be removed whether due to instability or medical comorbidity, patients should be treated with a course of parenteral therapy followed by prolonged oral suppression as discussed above.

Prognosis

The clinical outcomes associated with these complications vary in significance, depending on the extent of the infection and the interventions utilized to eradicate the infection. The majority of patients will experience an outcome similar to patients who did not experience an infection. There is, however, the potential for permanent morbidity. A case of total elbow joint destruction following treatment of septic arthritis that occurred secondary to a pin site infection has been reported. In that same case series, two patients experienced marked arthrofibrosis and limited elbow range of motion following multiple debridements for the treatment of pin site infections [66].

Prevention

Prevention of pin site infection starts at the time of insertion. Avoidance of thermal injury when using drills intraoperatively and prevention of excessive tension on skin are generally regarded as means to reduce pin site infection by minimizing soft tissue injury [71]. Many different regimens have been prescribed for pin site care including the use of povidone-iodine, hydrogen peroxide, chlorhexidine and normal saline solutions as well as soap and water and sterile dressing changes. A Cochrane Systematic Review found no benefit to the use of any particular cleanser compared to no cleansing agents and thus the review concluded that evidence was insufficient to support the use of any particular agent [72, 73]. In a separate prospective cohort study, patients who underwent pin site care with chlorhexidine-containing solutions had lower rates of positive pin site cultures compared to those who received pin care with normal saline; there was no difference in clinically defined pin site infections, however. Thus chlorhexidine-containing solutions may have some benefit at decreasing microorganism colonization of fixation pins [74]; that being said, given the lack of benefit on incidence of true infection, the value of such practices is unclear. Similarly, evidence is limited to recommend any one particular frequency of pin site cleansing over another. Thus, data are insufficient to support any specific regimen for pin site care in the outpatient setting.

As discussed in previous chapters, the use of preoperative intravenous antibiotics is recommended for open procedures involving the use of metal implants. However, there is not a consensus regarding the use of preoperative antibiotics for the treatment of fractures with percutaneous pinning. While one study reported no advantage to the use of preoperative antibiotics for the prevention of infection [60], another study identified that 100% of patients who developed a postoperative infection were not treated with preoperative antibiotics [59]. Additionally, this study identified timely pin removal at 3–4 weeks and appropriate cast care as factors related to preventing infection. Such data emphasize the importance of timely orthopedic follow-up and basic fracture care in prevention and early identification/management of infection.

References

1. Tzong KY, Han S, Roh A, Ing C. Epidemiology of pediatric surgical admissions in US children: data from the HCUP kids inpatient database. J Neurosurg Anesthesiol. 2012;24(4):391–5.
2. Ciofi Degli Atti ML, Serino L, Piga S, Tozzi AE, Raponi M. Incidence of surgical site infections in children: active surveillance in an Italian academic children's hospital. Ann Ig. 2017;29(1):46–53.
3. Bachy M, Bouyer B, Vialle R. Infections after spinal correction and fusion for spinal deformities in childhood and adolescence. Int Orthop. 2012;36(2):465–9.
4. Aleissa S, Parsons D, Grant J, Harder J, Howard J. Deep wound infection following pediatric scoliosis surgery: incidence and analysis of risk factors. Can J Surg. 2011;54(4):263–9.
5. Sponseller PD, Jain A, Shah SA, Samdani A, Yaszay B, Newton PO, et al. Deep wound infections after spinal fusion in children with cerebral palsy: a prospective cohort study. Spine (Phila Pa 1976). 2013;38(23):2023–7.
6. Subramanyam R, Schaffzin J, Cudilo EM, Rao MB, Varughese AM. Systematic review of risk factors for surgical site infection in pediatric scoliosis surgery. Spine J. 2015;15(6):1422–31.
7. Smith JS, Shaffrey CI, Sansur CA, Berven SH, Fu KM, Broadstone PA, et al. Rates of infection after spine surgery based on 108,419 procedures: a report from the Scoliosis Research Society Morbidity and Mortality Committee. Spine (Phila Pa 1976). 2011;36(7):556–63.

8. Milstone AM, Maragakis LL, Townsend T, Speck K, Sponseller P, Song X, et al. Timing of preoperative antibiotic prophylaxis: a modifiable risk factor for deep surgical site infections after pediatric spinal fusion. Pediatr Infect Dis J. 2008;27(8):704–8.

9. Linam WM, Margolis PA, Staat MA, Britto MT, Hornung R, Cassedy A, et al. Risk factors associated with surgical site infection after pediatric posterior spinal fusion procedure. Infect Control Hosp Epidemiol. 2009;30(2):109–16.

10. Mackenzie WG, Matsumoto H, Williams BA, Corona J, Lee C, Cody SR, et al. Surgical site infection following spinal instrumentation for scoliosis: a multicenter analysis of rates, risk factors, and pathogens. J Bone Joint Surg Am. 2013;95(9):800–6. S801-802

11. Kowalski TJ, Berbari EF, Huddleston PM, Steckelberg JM, Mandrekar JN, Osmon DR. The management and outcome of spinal implant infections: contemporary retrospective cohort study. Clin Infect Dis. 2007;44(7):913–20.

12. Ho C, Skaggs DL, Weiss JM, Tolo VT. Management of infection after instrumented posterior spine fusion in pediatric scoliosis. Spine (Phila Pa 1976). 2007;32(24):2739–44.

13. Hedequist D, Haugen A, Hresko T, Emans J. Failure of attempted implant retention in spinal deformity delayed surgical site infections. Spine (Phila Pa 1976). 2009;34(1):60–4.

14. Khoshbin A, Lysenko M, Law P, Wright JG. Outcomes of infection following pediatric spinal fusion. Can J Surg. 2015;58(2):107–13.

15. Glotzbecker MP, Gomez JA, Miller PE, Troy MJ, Skaggs DL, Vitale MG, et al. Management of spinal implants in acute pediatric surgical site infections: a multicenter study. Spine Deform. 2016;4(4):277–82.

16. Muschik M, Luck W, Schlenzka D. Implant removal for late-developing infection after instrumented posterior spinal fusion for scoliosis: reinstrumentation reduces loss of correction. A retrospective analysis of 45 cases. Eur Spine J. 2004;13(7):645–51.

17. Clark CE, Shufflebarger HL. Late-developing infection in instrumented idiopathic scoliosis. Spine (Phila Pa 1976). 1999;24(18):1909–12.

18. Maesani M, Doit C, Lorrot M, Vitoux C, Hilly J, Michelet D, et al. Surgical site infections in pediatric spine surgery: comparative microbiology of patients with idiopathic and nonidiopathic etiologies of spine deformity. Pediatr Infect Dis J. 2016;35(1):66–70.

19. Master DL, Poe-Kochert C, Son-Hing J, Armstrong DG, Thompson GH. Wound infections after surgery for neuromuscular scoliosis: risk factors and treatment outcomes. Spine (Phila Pa 1976). 2011;36(3):E179–85.

20. Labbe AC, Demers AM, Rodrigues R, Arlet V, Tanguay K, Moore DL. Surgical-site infection following spinal fusion: a case-control study in a children's hospital. Infect Control Hosp Epidemiol. 2003;24(8):591–5.

21. Messina AF, Berman DM, Ghazarian SR, Patel R, Neustadt J, Hahn G, et al. The management and outcome of spinal implant-related infections in pediatric patients: a retrospective review. Pediatr Infect Dis J. 2014;33(7):720–3.

22. Cahill PJ, Warnick DE, Lee MJ, Gaughan J, Vogel LE, Hammerberg KW, et al. Infection after spinal fusion for pediatric spinal deformity: thirty years of experience at a single institution. Spine (Phila Pa 1976). 2010;35(12):1211–7.

23. LaGreca J, Hotchkiss M, Carry P, Messacar K, Nyquist AC, Erickson M, et al. Bacteriology and risk factors for development of late (greater than one year) deep infection following spinal fusion with instrumentation. Spine Deform. 2014;2(3):186–90.

24. Petrini B, Welin-Berger T, Nord CE. Anaerobic bacteria in late infections following orthopedic surgery. Med Microbiol Immunol. 1979;167(3):155–9.

25. Hahn F, Zbinden R, Min K. Late implant infections caused by Propionibacterium acnes in scoliosis surgery. Eur Spine J. 2005;14(8):783–8.

26. Di Silvestre M, Bakaloudis G, Lolli F, Giacomini S. Late-developing infection following posterior fusion for adolescent idiopathic scoliosis. Eur Spine J. 2011;20(Suppl 1):S121–7.

27. Rihn JA, Lee JY, Ward WT. Infection after the surgical treatment of adolescent idiopathic scoliosis: evaluation of the diagnosis, treatment, and impact on clinical outcomes. Spine (Phila Pa 1976). 2008;33(3):289–94.

28. Collins I, Wilson-MacDonald J, Chami G, Burgoyne W, Vineyakam P, Berendt T, et al. The diagnosis and management of infection following instrumented spinal fusion. Eur Spine J. 2008;17(3):445–50.
29. Sponseller PD, LaPorte DM, Hungerford MW, Eck K, Bridwell KH, Lenke LG. Deep wound infections after neuromuscular scoliosis surgery: a multicenter study of risk factors and treatment outcomes. Spine (Phila Pa 1976). 2000;25(19):2461–6.
30. Bereza P, Ekiel A, Augusciak-Duma A, Aptekorz M, Wilk I, Kusz D, et al. Comparison of cultures and 16S rRNA sequencing for identification of bacteria in two-stage revision arthroplasties: preliminary report. BMC Musculoskelet Disord. 2016;17:138.
31. Bereza PL, Ekiel A, Augusciak-Duma A, Aptekorz M, Wilk I, Kusz DJ, et al. Identification of silent prosthetic joint infection: preliminary report of a prospective controlled study. Int Orthop. 2013;37(10):2037–43.
32. Bjerkan G, Witso E, Nor A, Viset T, Loseth K, Lydersen S, et al. A comprehensive microbiological evaluation of fifty-four patients undergoing revision surgery due to prosthetic joint loosening. J Med Microbiol. 2012;61(Pt 4):572–81.
33. Rathjen K, Wood M, McClung A, Vest Z. Clinical and radiographic results after implant removal in idiopathic scoliosis. Spine (Phila Pa 1976). 2007;32(20):2184–8.
34. Richards BS. Delayed infections following posterior spinal instrumentation for the treatment of idiopathic scoliosis. J Bone Joint Surg Am. 1995;77(4):524–9.
35. Viola RW, King HA, Adler SM, Wilson CB. Delayed infection after elective spinal instrumentation and fusion. A retrospective analysis of eight cases. Spine (Phila Pa 1976). 1997;22(20):2444–50; discussion 2450–1
36. Canavese F, Marengo L, Corradin M, Mansour M, Samba A, Andreacchio A, et al. Deep postoperative spine infection treated by negative pressure therapy in patients with progressive spinal deformities. Arch Orthop Trauma Surg. 2018;138(4):463–9.
37. Kale M, Padalkar P, Mehta V. Vacuum-assisted closure in patients with post-operative infections after instrumented spine surgery: a series of 12 cases. J Orthop Case Rep. 2017;7(1):95–100.
38. Rohmiller MT, Akbarnia BA, Raiszadeh K, Raiszadeh K, Canale S. Closed suction irrigation for the treatment of postoperative wound infections following posterior spinal fusion and instrumentation. Spine (Phila Pa 1976). 2010;35(6):642–6.
39. Masuda S, Fujibayashi S, Otsuki B, Kimura H, Matsuda S. Efficacy of target drug delivery and dead space reduction using antibiotic-loaded bone cement for the treatment of complex spinal infection. Clin Spine Surg. 2017;30(9):E1246–50.
40. Osmon DR, Berbari EF, Berendt AR, Lew D, Zimmerli W, Steckelberg JM, et al. Diagnosis and management of prosthetic joint infection: clinical practice guidelines by the Infectious Diseases Society of America. Clin Infect Dis. 2013;56(1):e1–e25.
41. Keller SC, Cosgrove SE, Higgins Y, Piggott DA, Osgood G, Auwaerter PG. Role of suppressive oral antibiotics in orthopedic hardware infections for those not undergoing two-stage replacement surgery. Open Forum Infect Dis. 2016;3(4):ofw176.
42. Byren I, Bejon P, Atkins BL, Angus B, Masters S, McLardy-Smith P, et al. One hundred and twelve infected arthroplasties treated with 'DAIR' (debridement, antibiotics and implant retention): antibiotic duration and outcome. J Antimicrob Chemother. 2009;63(6):1264–71.
43. Jorgensen NP, Skovdal SM, Meyer RL, Dagnaes-Hansen F, Fuursted K, Petersen E. Rifampicin-containing combinations are superior to combinations of vancomycin, linezolid and daptomycin against Staphylococcus aureus biofilm infection in vivo and in vitro. Pathog Dis. 2016;74(4):ftw019.
44. Zimmerli W, Widmer AF, Blatter M, Frei R, Ochsner PE. Role of rifampin for treatment of orthopedic implant-related staphylococcal infections: a randomized controlled trial. Foreign-Body Infection (FBI) Study Group. JAMA. 1998;279(19):1537–41.
45. Lora-Tamayo J, Senneville E, Ribera A, Bernard L, Dupon M, Zeller V, et al. The not-so-good prognosis of streptococcal periprosthetic joint infection managed by implant retention: the results of a large multicenter study. Clin Infect Dis. 2017;64(12):1742–52.

46. Martinez-Pastor JC, Munoz-Mahamud E, Vilchez F, Garcia-Ramiro S, Bori G, Sierra J, et al. Outcome of acute prosthetic joint infections due to gram-negative bacilli treated with open debridement and retention of the prosthesis. Antimicrob Agents Chemother. 2009;53(11):4772–7.

47. Rodriguez-Pardo D, Pigrau C, Lora-Tamayo J, Soriano A, del Toro MD, Cobo J, et al. Gram-negative prosthetic joint infection: outcome of a debridement, antibiotics and implant retention approach. A large multicentre study. Clin Microbiol Infect. 2014;20(11):O911–9.

48. Vitale MG, Riedel MD, Glotzbecker MP, Matsumoto H, Roye DP, Akbarnia BA, et al. Building consensus: development of a Best Practice Guideline (BPG) for surgical site infection (SSI) prevention in high-risk pediatric spine surgery. J Pediatr Orthop. 2013;33(5):471–8.

49. Kang DG, Holekamp TF, Wagner SC, Lehman RA Jr. Intrasite vancomycin powder for the prevention of surgical site infection in spine surgery: a systematic literature review. Spine J. 2015;15(4):762–70.

50. Gans I, Dormans JP, Spiegel DA, Flynn JM, Sankar WN, Campbell RM, et al. Adjunctive vancomycin powder in pediatric spine surgery is safe. Spine (Phila Pa 1976). 2013;38(19):1703–7.

51. Ghobrial GM, Thakkar V, Andrews E, Lang M, Chitale A, Oppenlander ME, et al. Intraoperative vancomycin use in spinal surgery: single institution experience and microbial trends. Spine (Phila Pa 1976). 2014;39(7):550–5.

52. Glotzbecker MP, Riedel MD, Vitale MG, Matsumoto H, Roye DP, Erickson M, et al. What's the evidence? Systematic literature review of risk factors and preventive strategies for surgical site infection following pediatric spine surgery. J Pediatr Orthop. 2013;33(5):479–87.

53. Rehman A, Rehman AU, Rehman TU, Freeman C. Removing outer gloves as a method to reduce spinal surgery infection. J Spinal Disord Tech. 2015;28(6):E343–6.

54. Soultanis KC, Pyrovolou N, Zahos KA, Karaliotas GI, Lenti A, Liveris I, et al. Late postoperative infection following spinal instrumentation: stainless steel versus titanium implants. J Surg Orthop Adv. 2008;17(3):193–9.

55. Glotzbecker MP, St Hilaire TA, Pawelek JB, Thompson GH, Vitale MG, Children's Spine Study G, et al. Best practice guidelines for surgical site infection prevention with surgical treatment of early onset scoliosis. J Pediatr Orthop. 2017 [epub ahead of print].

56. Gustilo RB, Anderson JT. Prevention of infection in the treatment of one thousand and twenty-five open fractures of long bones: retrospective and prospective analyses. J Bone Joint Surg Am. 1976;58(4):453–8.

57. Patzakis MJ, Wilkins J. Factors influencing infection rate in open fracture wounds. Clin Orthop Relat Res. 1989;243:36–40.

58. Kelly BA, Shore BJ, Bae DS, Hedequist DJ, Glotzbecker MP. Pediatric forearm fractures with in situ intramedullary implants. J Child Orthop. 2016;10(4):321–7.

59. Combs K, Frick S, Kiebzak G. Multicenter study of pin site infections and skin complications following pinning of pediatric supracondylar Humerus fractures. Cureus. 2016;8(12):e911.

60. Bashyal RK, Chu JY, Schoenecker PL, Dobbs MB, Luhmann SJ, Gordon JE. Complications after pinning of supracondylar distal humerus fractures. J Pediatr Orthop. 2009;29(7):704–8.

61. Lascombes P, Haumont T, Journeau P. Use and abuse of flexible intramedullary nailing in children and adolescents. J Pediatr Orthop. 2006;26(6):827–34.

62. Kruppa C, Bunge P, Schildhauer TA, Dudda M. Low complication rate of elastic stable intramedullary nailing (ESIN) of pediatric forearm fractures: a retrospective study of 202 cases. Medicine (Baltimore). 2017;96(16):e6669.

63. Birke O, Davies N, Latimer M, Little DG, Bellemore M. Experience with the Fassier-Duval telescopic rod: first 24 consecutive cases with a minimum of 1-year follow-up. J Pediatr Orthop. 2011;31(4):458–64.

64. Gordon JE, Kelly-Hahn J, Carpenter CJ, Schoenecker PL. Pin site care during external fixation in children: results of a nihilistic approach. J Pediatr Orthop. 2000;20(2):163–5.

65. Paley D. Problems, obstacles, and complications of limb lengthening by the Ilizarov technique. Clin Orthop Relat Res. 1990;250:81–104.

66. Tosti R, Foroohar A, Pizzutillo PD, Herman MJ. Kirschner wire infections in pediatric orthopaedic surgery. J Pediatr Orthop. 2015;35(1):69–73.

67. Schalamon J, Petnehazy T, Ainoedhofer H, Zwick EB, Singer G, Hoellwarth ME. Pin tract infection with external fixation of pediatric fractures. J Pediatr Surg. 2007;42(9):1584–7.
68. Shabtai L, Dolkart O, Chechik O, Amar E, Steinberg E, Mozes G, et al. Incidence and severity of infections after closed reduction and external fixation of proximal humeral fractures. J Orthop Trauma. 2013;27(4):e81–6.
69. Mahan J, Seligson D, Henry SL, Hynes P, Dobbins J. Factors in pin tract infections. Orthopedics. 1991;14(3):305–8.
70. Desai A, Dramis A, Thompson N, Board T, Choudhary A. Discharging pin sites following K-wire fixation of distal radial fractures: a case for pin removal? Acta Orthop Belg. 2009;75(3):310–5.
71. Kazmers NH, Fragomen AT, Rozbruch SR. Prevention of pin site infection in external fixation: a review of the literature. Strategies Trauma Limb Reconstr. 2016;11(2):75–85.
72. Lethaby A, Temple J, Santy J. Pin site care for preventing infections associated with external bone fixators and pins. Cochrane Database Syst Rev. 2008;(4):CD004551.
73. Lethaby A, Temple J, Santy-Tomlinson J. Pin site care for preventing infections associated with external bone fixators and pins. Cochrane Database Syst Rev. 2013;(12):CD004551.
74. W-Dahl A, Toksvig-Larsen S. Pin site care in external fixation sodium chloride or chlorhexidine solution as a cleansing agent. Arch Orthop Trauma Surg. 2004;124(8):555–8.

Infections Complicating Neurosurgical Procedures/Devices

10

William Whitehead and J. Chase McNeil

Introduction

Modern neurological surgery has made significant advancements over the last 100 years. These advancements are largely due to improvements in anesthesia, localization techniques, neuroimaging, the operating microscope, and a multitude of intraoperative technological advancements [1]. Surgical wound infections and infections associated with the implantation of devices, however, continue to plague the field resulting in significant morbidity, mortality, and costs for patients and healthcare systems. In this chapter, the most common neurosurgical postoperative infections including those associated with neurosurgical implantable devices are reviewed.

Ventricular Shunt and External Ventricular Drain (EVD) Infections

Ventriculoperitoneal, Ventriculopleural, Ventriculoatrial Shunts

Cerebrospinal fluid (CSF) shunt placement and revision for hydrocephalus is the most common procedure performed by pediatric neurosurgeons. Shunts are composed of a proximal catheter with the hole-bearing tip within the ventricle, a valve with a fixed or adjustable opening pressure, and a distal catheter placed within a

W. Whitehead
Department of Neurosurgery, Division of Pediatric Neurosurgery, Baylor College of Medicine, Houston, TX, USA

J. C. McNeil (✉)
Department of Pediatrics, Section of Infectious Diseases, Baylor College of Medicine and Texas Children's Hospital, Houston, TX, USA
e-mail: jm140109@bcm.edu

© Springer Nature Switzerland AG 2019
J. C. McNeil et al. (eds.), *Healthcare-Associated Infections in Children*,
https://doi.org/10.1007/978-3-319-98122-2_10

Table 10.1 Common etiologies for pediatric hydrocephalus

Etiology	% of cases
Intraventricular hemorrhage of prematurity	21.8–31.4
Myelomeningocele	15.8–25.5
Posterior fossa tumor	10.5
Aqueductal stenosis	8.1
Tumor, other	8.0
Congenital communicating	7.7–10.2
Genetic syndrome	1–5
Post-head injury	4.7
Post-infectious	3.7–11.7
Other	4.4–19.6

References [2–4]

body cavity for CSF absorption. The most commonly used distal reservoir is the peritoneal cavity because it is easily accessed in surgery, has a large surface area, and allows for the placement of excess catheter to accommodate patient growth. When the peritoneal cavity is unusable due to scarring from a ruptured viscus or infection, the right atrium or the pleural cavity is typically used as an alternative.

Most CSF shunts are placed for the treatment of hydrocephalus and the most common etiologies in pediatric patients are listed in Table 10.1. When patients with these conditions accumulate CSF faster than they can absorb it, surgical treatment is indicated and the mainstay of treatment for more than 60 years is the implantable CSF shunt. The surgical procedure takes approximately 60–90 min to perform but signifies in most cases a lifelong commitment to the implant. Shunt failure is common, unfortunately, with 30–40% of first shunts failing within 1 year [5]. Failures are usually due to obstruction from scar tissue encasing the catheter and blocking the flow of CSF as well as postoperative infections.

Epidemiology

Infection complicates 5–20% of CSF shunts in children with a degree of variability across institutions [6, 7]. Most contemporary literature in the United States report shunt infections developing in 10–11% of surgical cases [6, 8]. Furthermore, the risk of shunt infections is dynamic with decreasing risk of infection with increasing time since shunt placement or revision [9]. Most shunt infections present with symptoms within the first 2–3 weeks of placement but may be longer in the setting of infection with less virulent organisms; over 90% of first infections present within 1 year of implantation [6, 10]. Much work has been done by many investigators to determine risk factors for infection of CSF shunts in children. In a series of 442 children with ventriculoperitoneal shunts (VPS) at Duke University, a history of prematurity, previous shunt infection, young age and the use of a neuroendoscope by the performing surgeon were independently associated with risk of developing a VPS infection [6]. These same investigators reported that specifically *Staphylococcus aureus* shunt infection was associated with hospitalization >3 days prior to shunt placement and/or previous *S. aureus* shunt infection. The need for shunt revision has been well associated with risk of infection and in fact increases with each subsequent revision [11]. The Hydrocephalus Clinical Research Network (HCRN), a collaboration of pediatric neurosurgical centers, reported a threefold increased risk of infection following one shunt revision and a greater than 13-fold increased risk following two or more revisions [8]. This group also reported an association with shunt infection and the presence of a gastrostomy tube, although the significance of this is not entirely clear and may be a consequence of medical complexity or disability in these patients. Some investigators have noted an association with higher rates of infection when shunts are placed in the summer months corresponding to the performance of operations by new surgical trainees [12]; however, this has not been a consistent finding.

Notably, repeat infections of shunts are common and occur in up to 25% of patients after first shunt infection [13, 14]. Reinfection is due to the same organism as the initial infection in up to 67% of cases [13, 15]. Risk for reinfection following an initial shunt infection has been associated with complex shunts, ventriculoatrial shunts (VAS), and the need for multiple shunt revisions [11, 16].

Clinical Features

Patients with shunt infection can present with a variety of non-specific symptoms and signs. Most commonly patients will have headaches or irritability, anorexia, nausea, and lethargy. Fever is not always present, so its absence does not exclude the diagnosis [17, 18]. Because a variety of illnesses can present with this constellation of findings, the clinician must take into account other factors when determining the likelihood of shunt infection.

In most patients who develop infection, inoculation with the offending microorganism occurs at the time of shunt insertion, and, therefore, these patients present within a few weeks to months of surgery. Patients who have not required shunt surgery in over 12 months have a very low likelihood of primary shunt infection [19]. Shunts can also become secondarily infected due to bacteremia; VAS are particularly susceptible to hematogenous seeding by microorganisms. A ruptured viscus (e.g., appendix) is a common cause of distal shunt infection in VP shunts, but infections can also occur after surgical procedures such as a gastric tube insertion.

The majority of shunt infections are caused by low-virulence organisms (e.g., coagulase-negative staphylococcus, *Propionibacterium acnes*) which result in minimal inflammation and an indolent clinical course prior to presentation; however, the virulence of the organism and the location of the primary site of infection determine the severity of symptoms. Infections involving the external surface of the shunt present with swelling and erythema along the shunt track and incisions. These infections usually arise shortly after surgery. Distal catheter infections are associated with the formation of a CSF pseudocyst. As these cysts enlarge with the accumulation of CSF, they cause abdominal distention and pain. As abdominal pressure increases, intracranial pressure will increase leading to headaches, nausea, and vomiting. Infections associated with the proximal end of the catheter result in ventriculitis, and the majority of these patients will present with symptoms of shunt failure due to catheter occlusion. Severe infections can spread and result in meningitis or rarely empyema and/or abscess formation.

Diagnosis

The diagnosis of shunt infection is based on the clinical presentation along with culture of CSF, surgical wounds, fluid from the distal reservoir (e.g., pseudocyst fluid in patients with a VPS; blood in patients with a VAS), and explanted shunt hardware. It is not always possible to definitively identify an infecting organism, especially in cases of CSF pseudocyst; even in the absence of positive cultures, most clinicians still consider these infections and treat with antimicrobials, erring on the side of caution.

The definition of a shunt infection varies across studies and institutions. This variation can explain differences in infection rates across institutions and can make studying the problem challenging. The HCRN has adopted the following definition for infection and uses it for all epidemiological reporting and quality improvement projects aimed at reducing the incidence of infection:

Shunt infection is defined as [20, 21]:

1. Identification of organisms on culture or gram stain from CSF, wound swab, or pseudocyst fluid
2. Shunt erosion (defined as wound breakdown with visible shunt hardware)
3. Abdominal pseudocyst (even in the absence of positive cultures)
4. Positive blood cultures in a child with a ventriculoatrial shunt

Microbiology

Identification of a causative pathogen is important in order to provide directed antimicrobial therapy as well as minimization of unnecessarily broad-spectrum therapy. As stated above, the vast majority of shunt infections are a consequence of microorganisms being introduced at the time of shunt insertion. As such, most published literature emphasizes the predominance of gram-positive organisms in these infections (Table 10.2). Most series report a predominance of coagulase-negative staphylococci (CoNS) which as a group account for 32–53% of all shunt infections [6, 7, 10, 22]. Among CoNS, the most consistently reported species is *Staphylococcus epidermidis*. *S. aureus* comprises the second most common cause of CSF shunt infection contributing to 23–38% of all infections [7, 10, 22]. The proportion of *S. aureus* cases secondary to methicillin-resistant *S. aureus* (MRSA) reported in the literature ranges from 28.6% to 87% [7, 26] and would be expected to vary based on local epidemiology.

Table 10.2 Relative frequency of microorganisms in CSF shunt infections based on published literature

Organism	% of cases
Coagulase-negative staphylococci	32–53
Staphylococcus aureus	23–38
Escherichia coli	2.9–5.4
Pseudomonas spp.	4–5.4
Klebsiella spp.	5.1
Other *Enterobacteriaceae*	9
Propionibacterium acnes	4–17
Enterococcus spp.	1–4
Haemophilus spp.	<1–1.4
Streptococcus pneumoniae	<1
Candida	<1
Mycobacteria	<1

References: [6, 7, 10, 22–25]

Gram-negative bacilli including both *Enterobacteriaceae* and *Pseudomonas* spp. account for 8–16% of pediatric CSF shunt infections [6, 7, 22]. In a series of specifically gram-negative VPS infections in children, the most common organisms were *Escherichia coli* (52%) and *Klebsiella pneumoniae* (22%); *Pseudomonas* was seen in 4% of cases [27]. Other pediatric series have reported a higher frequency of *Pseudomonas,* however, constituting up to 4–5% of all shunt infections [22]. Notably, gram-negative bacilli account for a much larger proportion of shunt infections in adults, contributing up to 82% of all cases [28]. *Propionibacterium acnes* has been described in 4–17% of pediatric shunt infections [6, 23]. *P. acnes* infections are typically associated with few systemic symptoms, presentation many months removed from shunt placement, with little local inflammation, as well as infection of the distal catheter [23, 29]. *P. acnes* may be more readily isolated in anaerobic culture and/or with prolonged incubation [30].

Late-onset shunt infections (usually, but not consistently, defined as those occurring more than a year after surgical implantation) represent a diverse group of pathologies and etiologies. Older literature reports a high frequency of relatively low-virulence pathogens among late-onset (>6 months after placement) shunt infections such as *S. epidermidis* and *P. acnes* [31]. Late-onset infections may involve primarily the distal end of the catheter and be a consequence of pseudocyst formation, peritonitis (such as from appendicitis), direct inoculation from abdominal surgery or trauma, or perforation of the bowel with the distal end of the catheter [24, 25]. Such infections involve gram-negative bacilli in approximately 50% of cases but may also include anaerobes, enterococci, *P. acnes*, and staphylococci [25].

CSF shunts infections may also occur through secondary seeding of the meninges and/or shunt hardware after hematogenous dissemination of microorganisms. Such infections have been described due to *Streptococcus pneumoniae* as well as *Haemophilus influenzae* [25, 32]. Prior to advent of the *H. influenzae* type B (HIB) vaccine, this organism was not infrequently described to contribute to CSF shunt infections in children [33]. In the post-vaccine era, HIB shunt infections are extremely uncommon but should be considered in unvaccinated populations. Notably, hematogenous shunt infections due to *S. pneumoniae* and/or *H. influenzae* may be able to be managed with medical therapy alone with shunt retention [32].

Fungi, principally *Candida* species, have rarely been implicated in CSF shunt infection with available data limited to nested reports within single-center series of shunt infections; most authors report these organisms in ≤1% of cases [22]. In a series from Taiwan, 8/37 patients with shunt infection had fungi isolated of which five cases were due to *C. albicans* [34]. The reported symptoms of *Candida* shunt infection were subtle with the most common symptom being vomiting and only a third of patients reporting fever or change in activity level/mental status. *Candida* are, however, well recognized as agents capable of infecting external ventricular drains (EVD) [35].

Nontuberculous mycobacteria, notably *Mycobacterium fortuitum* and *M. abscessus*, have very rarely been implicated in CSF shunt infections [36–38]. Such infections invariably require removal of neurosurgical hardware/devices as well as prolonged anti-mycobacterial therapy. Therapy must be guided by the susceptibilities of the individual mycobacterial isolate, and, given the paucity of literature, consultation with an expert in mycobacteria disease is recommended.

Medical Management

Essential to medical management of CSF shunt infections is the early initiation of intravenous antimicrobial therapy after obtaining CSF cultures but prior to availability of results. As such, empiric antibiotic choice should provide coverage for both the most common and serious pathogens as well as penetrate into CSF (Fig. 10.1). The Infectious Diseases Society of America (IDSA) published clinical practice guidelines for the management of healthcare-associated ventriculitis (including CSF shunt infections) and meningitis in 2017 [39]. The IDSA guidelines recommend a combination of vancomycin and a CNS-active antipseudomonal β-lactam (cefepime, ceftazidime, or meropenem) for empiric therapy pending culture results. In cases of allergy or intolerance to β-lactams, aztreonam or ciprofloxacin are viable substitutes.

Once the microbiologic etiology has been identified, antimicrobial therapy should be tailored to the specific organism. For methicillin-susceptible *S. aureus* (MSSA) or methicillin-susceptible CoNS, the drugs of choice are nafcillin or oxacillin. For MRSA or methicillin-resistant CoNS, vancomycin is the preferred agent. Current guidelines recommend administration of vancomycin in order to achieve serum trough concentrations of 15–20 µg/ml in adult patients [39–41]. There is no data available which support this practice in children; however, studies are extremely limited. Vallejo et al. [26], in a retrospective series of children with *S. aureus* CNS infections, reported eight children with MRSA ventriculitis and vancomycin serum trough concentrations measured who were treated successfully; the median trough among these patients was 10.6 µg/ml (range: 5.4–15.7 µg/ml), suggesting that lower trough values may be adequate in children. Some experts recommend using alternative agents to vancomycin (such as linezolid, daptomycin, or trimethoprim-sulfamethoxazole) for infections

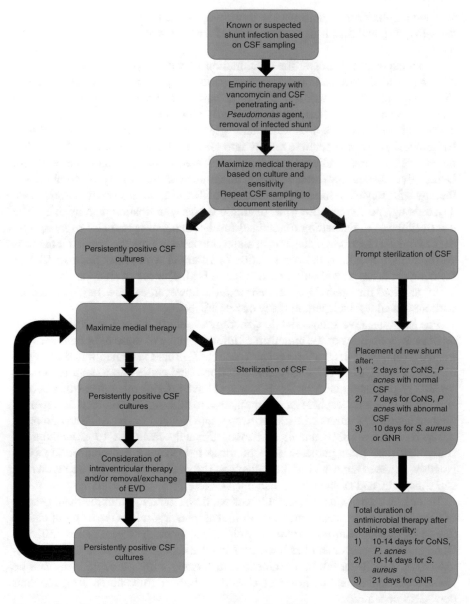

Fig. 10.1 Schematic overview of the management of CSF shunt infection based on IDSA guidelines [39]. Disclaimer: The presented framework is to serve as a general guideline and is no substitute for sound clinical judgment

caused by MRSA isolates with vancomycin MIC >1 µg/ml [41]. Linezolid has been used to successfully treat CSF shunt infections in children with MRSA or vancomycin-resistant *Enterococcus* (VRE) in the face of clinical failure or intolerance to other agents [42, 43]. Limited data exists for the use of ceftaroline, a cephalosporin with activity against MRSA, in pediatric shunt infection. Case reports describe its successful utilization in adults with healthcare-associated meningitis and shunt infections [44, 45], and thus it may serve as an alternative when other agents cannot be used.

Some experts recommend the combination of vancomycin (or oxacillin) with rifampin in staphylococcal shunt infection, particularly when hardware is left in situ [39]. In the presence of medical devices or hardware, certain bacteria may adhere and develop biofilm, a relatively metabolically inert state in which cell wall-active antimicrobials (such as β-lactams and glycopeptides) have reduced activity. Rifampin is known to penetrate readily into CSF as well as biofilms, and as such it may serve as a useful adjunct particularly when all hardware cannot be removed. Descriptive studies have described treatment success and safety of combination therapy with vancomycin and rifampin for CoNS and *S. aureus* shunt infection [46, 47], although no comparative trials of single versus combination therapy exist. The use of rifampin in the setting of retained foreign material is partially supported by the orthopedic literature; in the case of staphylococcal orthopedic implant infections with retention in adults, the combination of rifampin with either flucloxacillin or vancomycin is associated with improved cure [48]. The use of rifampin is not routinely required for staphylococcal ventriculitis, however, as cure may be achieved without this additional agent in many cases [26, 39].

For gram-negative shunt infection, therapy should in general be directed based on the susceptibilities of the organism of interest. Many of these infections are well treated with a third-generation cephalosporin [27]. There is some limited literature to suggest however that *Enterobacter* infections (and conceivably other organisms capable of producing an AmpC β-lactamase) have inferior outcomes when treated with third-generation cephalosporins compared to other agents. Foster et al. reported the outcomes of 19 adults with *Enterobacter* spp. isolated from CSF. They reported a success rate of 83% among patients ultimately switched to trimethoprim-sulfamethoxazole compared to 54% of those treated with a cephalosporin [49]. Notably, however almost all of the patients in the study were initially treated with a cephalosporin, and as such these data must be interpreted with caution.

In the rare case of *Candida* shunt infection, IDSA guidelines for the management of *Candida* infections recommend liposomal amphotericin B as the agent of choice due to its broad-spectrum activity as well as excellent CNS penetration [50, 51]. Once clinical improvement has been evidenced and culture and susceptibility testing results have been finalized, transition to therapy with a triazole agent can be considered. Echinocandins, however, should not be used for ventriculitis given their poor CNS penetration.

Role of Intraventricular Therapy

While rigorous data are limited, in the event of failure to sterilize CSF with intravenous antimicrobials alone, consideration could be given the use of intraventricular (IVT) antibiotics [39]. In general, IVT antibiotics should be given along with concomitant intravenous agents. The most commonly utilized and studied antibiotics for intraventricular administration are vancomycin and aminoglycosides. In one small randomized trial of adults with staphylococcal ventriculitis associated with an EVD, IVT vancomycin was associated with a faster clearance of CSF than the intravenous form; no adverse events related to IVT vancomycin were noted in this study [52]. In studies of adults with gram-negative rod post-neurosurgical ventriculitis, the addition of IVT gentamicin to intravenous antibiotics was associated with a more rapid sterilization of CSF (6.6 vs. 12.9 days) [53], a higher cure rate, and lower relapse rate than IV antibiotics alone [54]. One major challenge of administering IVT antibiotics in children is determining the appropriate dosing given their much smaller ventricular volume compared to adults. Studies of adults have used IVT vancomycin doses of 5–20 mg followed by clamping of the ventricular drain for 15–60 min. Investigators at the University of Tennessee reported the use of IVT vancomycin in 17 children at doses of 5–10 mg. The mean maximal CSF vancomycin trough concentration was 18.4 ± 21.8 µg/ml in this study; notably CSF troughs were much lower in adolescents (2 ± 1.4 µg/ml), than school-age children (13.5 ± 7.7 µg/ml) or infants ≤10 kg (29.1 ± 26.3 µg/ml) [55]. Thus, while large studies are lacking, many experts recommend an IVT vancomycin dose of 5 mg for infants, 10 mg for older children, and 20 mg for adolescents or adults. In children, gentamicin doses of 1–2 mg have been associated with therapeutic CSF trough levels (~ 15 µg/ml) and clinical success [56]. In general, β-lactam antibiotics should not be administered IVT because of the risk of provoking seizures. Additionally, IVT amphotericin has been used for refractory fungal CNS infections, particularly *Cryptococcus* [57], and may have a role in the treatment of shunt infections/ventriculitis due to these organisms that do not clear following removal of hardware, albeit the literature on this specific topic is sparse. It should be noted, however, that the more commonly used IVT antimicrobials are not without some risk including the development of CSF eosinophilia and aseptic meningitis [55, 58]. Patients receiving IVT antimicrobials have been reported to have seizures, focal neurologic findings (such as nystagmus), and hearing loss, although to what degree these findings are directly attributable to IVT antibiotics is unclear, given the underlying CNS pathology [59]. Furthermore, in one study an increased mortality was noted among infants and neonates with gram-negative enteric meningitis and/or ventriculitis who received IVT gentamicin although the exact impact of medication administration on this outcome is a bit unclear [60]. There are few reports of other minor side effects with IVT antibiotics (such as headache or irritability which may be attributable to chemical/aseptic meningitis); however, the condition of the patients receiving treatment (i.e., a CNS infection in the setting of an underlying neurologic comorbidity) may make the ascertainment of such minor adverse events challenging. Given these considerations, the decision to use IVT and the dose/frequency must be individualized and based on clinical judgment and patient response.

Duration of Therapy

There are very limited high-quality data available on which to base recommendations for duration of therapy in shunt infection. The duration of therapy is typically guided by clinical response to surgical and medical therapy. For patients with EVDs in place, current national guidelines recommend regular sampling of CSF for culture in order to document time to CSF sterility [39]. For patients with infection caused by *P. acnes* or CoNS with minimal symptoms, no/minimal pleocytosis, and normal CSF glucose, a treatment duration of 10 days is recommended by IDSA guidelines; by contrast, those patients with more significant clinical symptoms or abnormal laboratory values should be treated for 14 days. Infections due to *S. aureus* are recommended to be treated for 14 days, while those with gram-negative infection should be treated for 21 days [39]. Many experts in the field begin "counting" duration of therapy from the time of the first negative CSF culture, particularly in the case of repeatedly positive cultures. As national guidelines are based on very limited data, however, clinical judgment must take priority and duration of therapy guided in large part by individual patient response.

Surgical Management

Considerable variation exists in the surgical management of the infected CSF shunt and multiple procedures are usually necessary [61, 62]. Generally, when an implant becomes infected, it is removed; however, most patients with hydrocephalus will not tolerate the lack of CSF drainage and require some form of continued CSF diversion while the infection is being cleared. Surgical practices include (1) the complete removal of the infected CSF shunt and placement of an EVD, followed by replacement of the shunt when the CSF is sterile; (2) shunt externalization at the distal end through a small incision over the catheter, followed by shunt replacement when CSF is sterile; and (3) nonsurgical management. These procedures can be performed in the operating room or at the bedside depending on the clinical circumstances and available resources. When CSF fluid samples continue to show evidence of active infection while on antibiotic therapy (i.e., persistently positive cultures), additional EVD changes or removal of externalized shunts are required. Despite numerous attempts, no study has been able to show a convincing advantage to any approach and reinfection rates remain unacceptably high in pediatric patients (15–25%) [6, 10, 13, 14, 16, 61, 62]. Despite a lack of high-quality evidence, experts strongly recommend the removal of infected hardware in patients who will tolerate the procedure [39].

Timing of Shunt Replacement

Once the CSF infection has cleared, surgical practices vary with regard to the reimplantation of a shunt [61]. Recent recommendations from the IDSA are based on infecting organism although the evidence to support these recommendations is limited (Fig. 10.1). In the event of a distal infection due to abdominal pseudocyst, most experts agree that the distal catheter can be replaced into the peritoneum at a new entry site after completion of antibiotic therapy and resolution of the pseudocyst on imaging [63]. Recurrence rates of 4–18% have been reported in these cases [64, 65].

Prognosis

The prognosis after shunt insertion will vary with the virulence of the infecting organism and the effectiveness of treatment. Mortality due to infection is unusual, but rates between 13% and 34% have been reported [66–68]. Increasing evidence suggests that shunt infections in young patients are associated with a higher risk of long-term cognitive effects which are not seen with simple shunt failure without infection [66, 69]. These data highlight the importance of taking active steps to reduce the rate of shunt infection.

Postoperative Meningitis, Intracranial Abscesses, and Skull Osteomyelitis Following Craniotomy

Epidemiology

A variety of surgical site infections (SSI) complicating craniotomy exist and can include superficial infections, subgaleal abscesses, bone flap/skull osteomyelitis, intracranial abscesses, and postoperative meningitis. Rates of infection have varied from 1% to 8% and differ by institution, surgical technique, indication for surgery, and age group [70–73]. Postoperative meningitis is most frequently reported in the literature [70] although it is likely that other less severe infections (such as superficial SSI) are under reported. Identified risk factors for developing postcraniotomy infection include perioperative steroid use, CSF leak, the need for emergent surgery, and the presence of an EVD [73, 74].

Clinical Features

Little data is available regarding the specificity and sensitivity of common signs and symptoms of infection in postoperative cases. It can also be difficult to obtain accurate information in these patients when mental status is affected by surgery or the underlying pathology. Fever is not a specific sign in the postoperative period and can be driven by a variety of factors (e.g., drugs, anesthesia, thrombophlebitis, hypothalamic abnormalities, chemical meningitis, etc.). A high clinical suspicion for infection is warranted in the setting of headache, declining mental status, meningismus, and/or fever in the postoperative neurosurgical patient.

Diagnosis

The diagnosis of postoperative infections relies heavily on cultures from the suspected area. CSF profiles, including white blood cells, can be elevated after surgical procedures, and therefore cannot be relied upon for definitive diagnosis. Magnetic resonance imaging (MRI) with and without gadolinium enhancement and diffusion-weighted imaging can aid in the diagnosis of brain abscesses and fluid collections associated with infected bone flaps.

Microbiology

The microbiology of postcraniotomy surgical site infections is similar to that of other SSIs with a predominance of *S. aureus*, accounting for 51–60% of cases [70, 71]. CoNS have been reported in approximately 5–20% of cases and *Enterobacteriaceae* in 8–17% of cases [70, 71]. *Pseudomonas* spp. have also been identified in these infections although their exact incidence is not well defined. Group A streptococci have also been well described as causes of SSI in general; however, their incidence is fairly low in post-neurosurgical SSI.

Medical Management

The prompt initiation of antimicrobial therapy is imperative in the management of postcraniotomy SSI. For known or suspected superficial surgical site infection, oral antimicrobial therapy directed against staphylococci may be a reasonable and effective treatment option. While there is no specific literature to suggest an optimal duration of therapy for superficial SSI in this scenario, a course of therapy of 7–14 days guided by clinical response may be reasonable. It is essential, however, that the provider's clinical index of suspicion for more severe infection (i.e., deep SSI) be high and extremely close follow-up of such patients is encouraged. Empiric broad-spectrum therapy directed against the most likely causative organisms and utilizing agents with good CSF penetration is appropriate when deeper infection is suspected. Current management guidelines published by the IDSA recommend a combination of vancomycin along with an antipseudomonal β-lactam (ceftazidime, cefepime, or a carbapenem) for postoperative meningitis [39]. Once a causative pathogen is identified, therapy should be tailored to this specific organism. A 4–6 week course of directed intravenous antimicrobial therapy is recommended by many experts for intracranial abscesses or skull osteomyelitis following surgical drainage/debridement.

Surgical Management

Surgical management in the setting of postoperative meningitis involves the removal of any device or hardware in the infected cistern or operative space; most cases require only medical management. Rarely, cases of meningitis may transiently or permanently develop hydrocephalus and CSF diversion is required. The presence of a brain abscess or empyema requires reoperation to drain the infection and obtain cultures to define the offending organism. In approximately 25% of cases, repeat drainage or aspiration of an abscess is required to clear the infection. Skull osteomyelitis following craniotomy requires bone flap removal followed by delayed cranioplasty [75].

Prognosis

Prognosis varies based on the infecting organism(s) and the effectiveness of treatment. Mortality is rarely reported in the United States, but rates appear to be low (<1%) when promptly treated [76, 77].

Infections Involving Intrathecal Baclofen Pumps

Epidemiology

Intrathecal pumps provide a mechanism to administer medications directly into the CSF, allowing for the achievement of higher drug levels than is possible with oral medications. Infection complicates approximately 10% of baclofen pumps placed for spasticity [78]. Subcutaneous placement of the pump is associated with a much higher rate of infection (up to 20%) than subfascial implantation (~4%) [79]. Notably, there is a higher incidence of infection following baclofen pump placement in children than adults [80]. Sixty-nine percent of infections present within 1 month of placement and may be superficial SSI or deeper infection [81]. The presence of a gastrostomy has been identified as risk factor for infection in some studies although this may more accurately reflect malnutrition and medical complexity [81]. In one large study, young age, a history of wound dehiscence and number of surgical revisions were independently associated with risk of infection [82].

Clinical Features

Clinical features vary based on the location of the infection. Superficial infections at incision sites commonly present with local signs of inflammation (erythema, tenderness, swelling) and purulence. Fever is rarely present [83, 84]. Deep infections involving the surgical pouch created for the pump more commonly are associated with fever as well as pain, tenderness, erythema, and swelling at the operative site. When the CSF is infected, patients commonly have fever, meningismus, purulent drainage from the surgical incisions, declining mental status and/or display signs of sepsis.

Diagnosis

The diagnosis of infection is based on a combination of the presence of signs and symptoms suggestive of infection (as above) and the culture of organisms from the infected site. The obtainment of cultures from the pocket, surrounding tissue, catheter tip, and/or CSF is essential in establishing a microbiologic diagnosis. The majority of infections occur early, within 30 days of implantation, but late infections over a year after insertion do occur.

Microbiology

Over 50% of all infections are reportedly caused by *S. aureus* with MRSA contributing to approximately 15% of cases [78, 81]. CoNS are reported in approximately 15% of cases with *Pseudomonas* (8–30%) and *E. coli* (7–10%) and other *Enterobacteriaceae* being the next most commonly reported pathogens [78, 81, 82, 85]. Group B streptococci are also occasionally reported as causes of these infections.

Medical Management

Antibiotic management of baclofen pump-related infections is challenging, and empiric antibiotic choice should be directed toward the most likely pathogens (*S. aureus*, CoNS, and *Pseudomonas*) and include drugs with adequate CNS penetration. While disease may be limited to a superficial surgical site infection, efforts should be made to ensure that infection does not extend into deeper structures utilizing physical exam and laboratory evaluations as well as imaging studies when appropriate. Oral antimicrobial therapy, however, may be sufficient for many cases of superficial infection. In one series 24/25 patients with superficial infection were cured with oral antibiotics alone [85]. With deep infections including those involving the pump, pump pocket, catheter, or meninges, medical therapy alone is rarely successful and most often requires explantation of the pump and all associated hardware to achieve clinical cure [78, 85].

Surgical Management

Given that these patients are often dependent on intrathecal baclofen and the challenges of pump implantation and removal, much interest exists in attempts to salvage infected pumps. A number of case reports exist of successful salvage of pumps with wound washout and instillation of antibiotic into the pump reservoir along with intravenous antibiotics [86–88]. Such attempts appear to be rarely successful in a pediatric population based on available literature. Hester et al. described 11 patients with cerebral palsy who developed deep baclofen pump infections [85]. Among eight initially managed with antibiotics alone, all ultimately required pump removal; among the other three patients managed with IV antibiotics following washout procedures, 2/3 required subsequent pump removal due to difficulty eradicating infection. A similar low rate of success was reported by Dickey et al. when attempting to salvage severely infected pumps with pump sterilization and wound washout; only 2 of 7 attempts were successful in avoiding pump explantation [84]. Thus, it is advisable to proceed with hardware removal when at all possible for deep CNS pump-related infections followed by approximately 2 weeks of intravenous therapy (similar to that for gram-positive meningitis). For cases in which infected devices cannot be removed, consideration should be given to prolonged oral antimicrobial suppression following a course of intravenous antimicrobial therapy.

Prognosis

With prompt diagnosis and treatment, baclofen pump infections are associated with good outcomes. The majority of patients elect to undergo reimplantation of the device after the infection is clear. Recurrent infections have been reported sporadically [84, 89].

Infection Involving Vagal Nerve Stimulators

Epidemiology

While modern antiepileptic drugs are typically very effective in managing seizures, almost a third of patients will not completely have seizures controlled with medications alone [90]. For patients with refractory epilepsy, the use of a vagus nerve stimulator (VNS) is one option to achieve seizure control and improve quality of life. As with any medical device, however, VNS are associated with a small but important risk of infection. Infections complicating VNS are rare, occurring in <1–4% of devices in most series [91, 92]. Notably, the proportion of cases experiencing infection in children (4.5–7%) are twice as high as that in adults (2.1%) [92, 93]. The mean time from insertion to infection has been reported at 14 days with 75% of cases occurring within 3 months of implantation [94].

Clinical Features

Clinical features are similar to those associated with other implant-associated infections including erythema, swelling, pain, and purulence around the surgical insertion site. Fever is inconsistently present. The diagnosis of VNS infections is typically based both on clinical suspicion and wound cultures taken at the time of surgical explantation.

Microbiology

While literature which discusses the specific microbiology of these infections is limited, there is a tremendous predominance of *S. aureus* in those infections that are reported [93, 95, 96]. It is conceivable, however, that other common skin flora (such as CoNS) and healthcare-associated pathogens (such as *Pseudomonas* spp.) could be potential causes of these infections, and this should be considered when selecting empiric therapy.

Medical Management

Given the rarity of these infections, it is difficult to provide high-quality evidence-based treatment guidance specific to this disease entity. Similar to the case of intra-thecal baclofen pump infections, superficial wound infections may be adequately treated with a short course of oral antimicrobial therapy alone [92]. Rare case reports exist of treatment success of nerve stimulator infections without removal of the device [95]. Most studies report that the majority of patients ultimately undergo removal of the generator with or without leads followed by a course of intravenous antimicrobial therapy. The proportion of cases requiring device removal ranges from 58% to 73% [92, 94]. Patel and Edwards [96] reported two cases of VNS pocket infection that were treated initially with device in situ; both cases experienced treatment failure while on appropriate antibiotics ultimately requiring removal of device. Specific antibiotic choice in these infections should be guided by culture data and directed toward *S. aureus* and other healthcare-associated pathogens while awaiting culture data. The reported duration of therapy for these infections has ranged from 3 to 6 weeks in the setting of device removal [96].

Surgical Management

Standard surgical therapy consists of complete hardware removal. Complete removal does require redo dissection in the cervical region within the carotid sheath with manipulation of the vagal nerve. This can be a difficult dissection. Due to the risk involved from repeat surgery during explantation and future replacement in this delicate area, attempts at lead salvage within the cervical region have been attempted with reasonable success in small numbers. Wozniak et al. report success in three out of four patients with infections of the VNS [97]. The technique involves the opening of the chest incision and removal of the generator; the cervical leads are disconnected from the generator and kept in place. The ends of the leads are placed into a newly created surgical pocket lateral to the infected surgical bed. Intravenous antibiotics are given for 3–4 weeks. Approximately 4 weeks after antibiotics are discontinued, if there is no evidence of recurrence, the generator is replaced. Recovery after prompt medical treatment for VNS infections is excellent; there have been no long-term consequences associated with VNS infections reported in the literature.

Prevention of Infections Associated with Neurosurgery

The principles of infection prevention for neurosurgical procedures are very similar to that recommended for other surgeries and are discussed elsewhere in this text (Chap. 2). Antibiotic prophylaxis has been demonstrated to reduce rates of postoperative meningitis in patients undergoing craniotomy [98]. Antibiotic prophylaxis should be administered within 60 min before surgical incision. Cefazolin is the drug of choice for prophylaxis and should be administered in 2–3 g doses in adults and 30 mg/kg in children; cefazolin should be re-dosed in 4 h if needed based on the length of the surgery [99]. For patients with β-lactam allergies, clindamycin and vancomycin are acceptable substitutes for cefazolin. Additionally, in patients with known MRSA colonization or recent history of MRSA infection, addition of vancomycin to prophylaxis should be considered.

Guidelines developed by a collaboration of the American Society of Health-System Pharmacists (ASHP), the IDSA, the Surgical Infection Society (SIS) and the Society for Healthcare Epidemiology of America (SHEA) could reach no consensus on the use (or duration of use) of antimicrobial prophylaxis in patients with EVDs [99]. There have been conflicting reports of the benefits of prophylaxis for patients with EVDs in place [100, 101]. Systematic reviews have found benefit to the use of systemic antimicrobial prophylaxis in patients with EVDs although individual studies examining this are heterogeneous and frequently underpowered, making interpretation challenging [102]. Prophylaxis may be particularly useful when the incidence of infection in an individual center is high [102]. If used, the optimal duration of prophylaxis is also unclear. Notably, the use of antimicrobial prophylaxis (typically cefazolin) may select for resistant pathogens not treated by the prophylactic regimen [100, 103]. The recent IDSA guidelines for the management of healthcare-associated meningitis/ventriculitis [39] discourage antimicrobial prophylaxis for the entire duration of an external ventricular drain, in part to reduce the emergence of drug-resistant infections. Perhaps related in part to the discrepancies in the literature, variability exists across institutions with regard to how often and for how long prophylaxis is administered in patients with EVDs.

Bathing with an antiseptic solution (such as chlorhexidine gluconate) the evening prior to or the morning of elective surgery is generally recommended [104], although specific data for pediatric neurosurgery are limited. The use of chlorhexidine hair wash was associated with a reduction of shunt infections in one series [105]. Other interventions associated with reductions in shunt infections in children include double gloving by the surgeon, with removal of the outer set of gloves prior to handling of the shunt [106, 107]. Not shaving of the scalp or limited shaving has been associated with some observed reduction in SSI and VPS infection in children compared to shaving; however most studies are small and use historical controls [108, 109]. Studies in both adults and children have illustrated that the use of antibiotic (usually rifampin/minocycline)-impregnated shunt catheters is associated with a reduction in shunt infection [110, 111]. In one very large study, including 1770 pediatric shunt patients, the use of antibiotic-impregnated catheters was associated with a reduced infection incidence even when controlling for other confounders [112]. While their use is supported by national guidelines [39], further research is needed to understand the optimal role of antibiotic-impregnated catheters for infection prevention. The use of intraventricular injection of antibiotics at the time of shunt surgery (e.g., vancomycin and gentamycin) is also associated with a decline in shunt infection rates [113].

The use of quality improvement techniques to lower infection rates has been successfully applied to the problem of neurosurgical infections. The implementation of a standardized protocol or checklist with steps known to or believed to reduce infections, analogous to infection prevention bundles for other HAIs, has been shown to significantly lower infection rates in shunt surgery and baclofen pump insertion surgery [20, 21, 114]. A HCRN study examined compliance and outcomes associated with an infection prevention protocol at time of shunt placement which included antibiotic-impregnated catheters, perioperative antibiotics (as described above), hand scrub, double gloving, and application of antimicrobial impregnated drapes to the surgical field (i.e., Ioban©, 3 M). The study found that compliance with this protocol was associated with a reduced incidence of infection (8.7% vs. 5%) [21]. These data underscore the importance of continued quality improvements efforts to minimize SSI in this vulnerable patient population.

References

1. Greenblatt H, Dagi T, Epstein M. A history of neurosurgery. Park Ridge: American Association of Neurological Surgeons Publishing; 1997.
2. Riva-Cambrin J, Kestle JR, Holubkov R, Butler J, Kulkarni AV, Drake J, et al. Risk factors for shunt malfunction in pediatric hydrocephalus: a multicenter prospective cohort study. J Neurosurg Pediatr. 2016;17(4):382–90.
3. Schrander-Stumpel C, Fryns JP. Congenital hydrocephalus: nosology and guidelines for clinical approach and genetic counselling. Eur J Pediatr. 1998;157(5):355–62.
4. Gmeiner M, Wagner H, Zacherl C, Polanski P, Auer C, van Ouwerkerk WJ, et al. Long-term mortality rates in pediatric hydrocephalus-a retrospective single-center study. Childs Nerv Syst. 2017;33(1):101–9.
5. Kulkarni AV, Riva-Cambrin J, Butler J, Browd SR, Drake JM, Holubkov R, et al. Outcomes of CSF shunting in children: comparison of hydrocephalus clinical research network cohort with historical controls: clinical article. J Neurosurg Pediatr. 2013;12(4):334–8.
6. McGirt MJ, Zaas A, Fuchs HE, George TM, Kaye K, Sexton DJ. Risk factors for pediatric ventriculoperitoneal shunt infection and predictors of infectious pathogens. Clin Infect Dis. 2003;36(7):858–62.
7. Lee JK, Seok JY, Lee JH, Choi EH, Phi JH, Kim SK, et al. Incidence and risk factors of ventriculoperitoneal shunt infections in children: a study of 333 consecutive shunts in 6 years. J Korean Med Sci. 2012;27(12):1563–8.
8. Simon TD, Butler J, Whitlock KB, Browd SR, Holubkov R, Kestle JR, et al. Risk factors for first cerebrospinal fluid shunt infection: findings from a multi-center prospective cohort study. J Pediatr. 2014;164(6):1462–1468.e2.
9. McGirt MJ, Leveque JC, Wellons JC 3rd, Villavicencio AT, Hopkins JS, Fuchs HE, et al. Cerebrospinal fluid shunt survival and etiology of failures: a seven-year institutional experience. Pediatr Neurosurg. 2002;36(5):248–55.
10. Odio C, McCracken GH Jr, Nelson JD. CSF shunt infections in pediatrics. A seven-year experience. Am J Dis Child. 1984;138(12):1103–8.
11. Simon TD, Whitlock KB, Riva-Cambrin J, Kestle JR, Rosenfeld M, Dean JM, et al. Revision surgeries are associated with significant increased risk of subsequent cerebrospinal fluid shunt infection. Pediatr Infect Dis J. 2012;31(6):551–6.
12. Kestle JR, Cochrane DD, Drake JM. Shunt insertion in the summer: is it safe? J Neurosurg. 2006;105(3 Suppl):165–8.
13. Kestle JR, Garton HJ, Whitehead WE, Drake JM, Kulkarni AV, Cochrane DD, et al. Management of shunt infections: a multicenter pilot study. J Neurosurg. 2006;105(3 Suppl):177–81.
14. Kulkarni AV, Rabin D, Lamberti-Pasculli M, Drake JM. Repeat cerebrospinal fluid shunt infection in children. Pediatr Neurosurg. 2001;35(2):66–71.

15. Tuan TJ, Thorell EA, Hamblett NM, Kestle JR, Rosenfeld M, Simon TD. Treatment and microbiology of repeated cerebrospinal fluid shunt infections in children. Pediatr Infect Dis J. 2011;30(9):731–5.
16. Simon TD, Mayer-Hamblett N, Whitlock KB, Langley M, Kestle JR, Riva-Cambrin J, et al. Few patient, treatment, and diagnostic or microbiological factors, except complications and intermittent negative cerebrospinal fluid (CSF) cultures during first CSF shunt infection, are associated with reinfection. J Pediatric Infect Dis Soc. 2014;3(1):15–22.
17. Kontny U, Hofling B, Gutjahr P, Voth D, Schwarz M, Schmitt HJ. CSF shunt infections in children. Infection. 1993;21(2):89–92.
18. Mancao M, Miller C, Cochrane B, Hoff C, Sauter K, Weber E. Cerebrospinal fluid shunt infections in infants and children in mobile, Alabama. Acta Paediatr. 1998;87(6):667–70.
19. Kestle J, Drake J, Milner R, Sainte-Rose C, Cinalli G, Boop F, et al. Long-term follow-up data from the Shunt Design Trial. Pediatr Neurosurg. 2000;33(5):230–6.
20. Kestle JR, Riva-Cambrin J, Wellons JC 3rd, Kulkarni AV, Whitehead WE, Walker ML, et al. A standardized protocol to reduce cerebrospinal fluid shunt infection: the hydrocephalus clinical research network quality improvement initiative. J Neurosurg Pediatr. 2011;8(1):22–9.
21. Kestle JR, Holubkov R, Douglas Cochrane D, Kulkarni AV, Limbrick DD Jr, Luerssen TG, et al. A new hydrocephalus clinical research network protocol to reduce cerebrospinal fluid shunt infection. J Neurosurg Pediatr. 2016;17(4):391–6.
22. Davis SE, Levy ML, McComb JG, Masri-Lavine L. Does age or other factors influence the incidence of ventriculoperitoneal shunt infections? Pediatr Neurosurg. 1999;30(5):253–7.
23. Arnell K, Cesarini K, Lagerqvist-Widh A, Wester T, Sjolin J. Cerebrospinal fluid shunt infections in children over a 13-year period: anaerobic cultures and comparison of clinical signs of infection with Propionibacterium acnes and with other bacteria. J Neurosurg Pediatr. 2008;1(5):366–72.
24. Baird C, O'Connor D, Pittman T. Late shunt infections. Pediatr Neurosurg. 1999;31(5):269–73.
25. Vinchon M, Lemaitre MP, Vallee L, Dhellemmes P. Late shunt infection: incidence, pathogenesis, and therapeutic implications. Neuropediatrics. 2002;33(4):169–73.
26. Vallejo JG, Cain AN, Mason EO, Kaplan SL, Hulten KG. Staphylococcus aureus central nervous system infections in children. Pediatr Infect Dis J. 2017;36(10):947–51.
27. Stamos JK, Kaufman BA, Yogev R. Ventriculoperitoneal shunt infections with gram-negative bacteria. Neurosurgery. 1993;33(5):858–62.
28. Lyke KE, Obasanjo OO, Williams MA, O'Brien M, Chotani R, Perl TM. Ventriculitis complicating use of intraventricular catheters in adult neurosurgical patients. Clin Infect Dis. 2001;33(12):2028–33.
29. Viraraghavan R, Jantausch B, Campos J. Late-onset central nervous system shunt infections with Propionibacterium acnes: diagnosis and management. Clin Pediatr (Phila). 2004;43(4):393–7.
30. Konen E. Anaerobic gram-positive nonsporulating bacilli. In: Mandell GL, Bennett JE, Dolin R, editors. Principles and practice of infectious diseases. 7th ed. Philadelphia: Elsevier; 2010. p. 3125–8.
31. Schiff SJ, Oakes WJ. Delayed cerebrospinal-fluid shunt infection in children. Pediatr Neurosci. 1989;15(3):131–5.
32. Shurtleff DB, Loeser JD, Avellino AM, Duguay S, Englund JA, Marcuse EK, et al. Haemophilus influenzae and Streptococcus pneumoniae infections in children with cerebrospinal fluid shunts. Pediatr Neurosurg. 2009;45(4):276–80.
33. Schoenbaum SC, Gardner P, Shillito J. Infections of cerebrospinal fluid shunts: epidemiology, clinical manifestations, and therapy. J Infect Dis. 1975;131(5):543–52.
34. Chiou CC, Wong TT, Lin HH, Hwang B, Tang RB, Wu KG, et al. Fungal infection of ventriculoperitoneal shunts in children. Clin Infect Dis. 1994;19(6):1049–53.
35. O'Brien D, Stevens NT, Lim CH, O'Brien DF, Smyth E, Fitzpatrick F, et al. Candida infection of the central nervous system following neurosurgery: a 12-year review. Acta Neurochir. 2011;153(6):1347–50.

36. Montero JA, Alrabaa SF, Wills TS. Mycobacterium abscessus ventriculoperitoneal shunt infection and review of the literature. Infection. 2016;44(2):251–3.
37. Cadena G, Wiedeman J, Boggan JE. Ventriculoperitoneal shunt infection with mycobacterium fortuitum: a rare offending organism. J Neurosurg Pediatr. 2014;14(6):704–7.
38. Midani S, Rathore MH. Mycobacterium fortuitum infection of ventriculoperitoneal shunt. South Med J. 1999;92(7):705–7.
39. Tunkel AR, Hasbun R, Bhimraj A, Byers K, Kaplan SL, Michael Scheld W, et al. 2017 Infectious diseases Society of America's Clinical Practice Guidelines for healthcare-associated ventriculitis and meningitis. Clin Infect Dis. 2017; 64(6): e34–65.
40. Rybak M, Lomaestro B, Rotschafer JC, Moellering R Jr, Craig W, Billeter M, et al. Therapeutic monitoring of vancomycin in adult patients: a consensus review of the American Society of Health-System Pharmacists, the Infectious Diseases Society of America, and the Society of Infectious Diseases Pharmacists. Am J Health Syst Pharm. 2009;66(1):82–98.
41. Liu C, Bayer A, Cosgrove SE, Daum RS, Fridkin SK, Gorwitz RJ, et al. Clinical practice guidelines by the infectious diseases society of america for the treatment of methicillin-resistant Staphylococcus aureus infections in adults and children. Clin Infect Dis. 2011;52(3):e18–55.
42. Yilmaz A, Dalgic N, Musluman M, Sancar M, Colak I, Aydin Y. Linezolid treatment of shunt-related cerebrospinal fluid infections in children. J Neurosurg Pediatr. 2010;5(5):443–8.
43. Cook AM, Ramsey CN, Martin CA, Pittman T. Linezolid for the treatment of a heteroresistant Staphylococcus aureus shunt infection. Pediatr Neurosurg. 2005;41(2):102–4.
44. Kuriakose SS, Rabbat M, Gallagher JC. Ceftaroline CSF concentrations in a patient with ventriculoperitoneal shunt-related meningitis. J Antimicrob Chemother. 2015; 70(3):953–4.
45. Balouch MA, Bajwa RJ, Hassoun A. Successful use of ceftaroline for the treatment of MRSA meningitis secondary to an infectious complication of lumbar spine surgery. J Antimicrob Chemother. 2015;70(2):624–5.
46. Gombert ME, Landesman SH, Corrado ML, Stein SC, Melvin ET, Cummings M. Vancomycin and rifampin therapy for Staphylococcus epidermidis meningitis associated with CSF shunts: report of three cases. J Neurosurg. 1981;55(4):633–6.
47. Vichyanond P, Olson LC. Staphylococcal CNS infections treated with vancomycin and rifampin. Arch Neurol. 1984;41(6):637–9.
48. Zimmerli W, Widmer AF, Blatter M, Frei R, Ochsner PE. Role of rifampin for treatment of orthopedic implant-related staphylococcal infections: a randomized controlled trial. Foreign-Body Infection (FBI) Study Group. JAMA. 1998;279(19):1537–41.
49. Foster DR, Rhoney DH. Enterobacter meningitis: organism susceptibilities, antimicrobial therapy and related outcomes. Surg Neurol. 2005;63(6):533–7; discussion 537.
50. Groll AH, Giri N, Petraitis V, Petraitiene R, Candelario M, Bacher JS, et al. Comparative efficacy and distribution of lipid formulations of amphotericin B in experimental Candida albicans infection of the central nervous system. J Infect Dis. 2000;182(1):274–82.
51. Pappas PG, Kauffman CA, Andes DR, Clancy CJ, Marr KA, Ostrosky-Zeichner L, et al. Clinical practice guideline for the management of candidiasis: 2016 update by the Infectious Diseases Society of America. Clin Infect Dis. 2016;62(4):e1–50.
52. Pfausler B, Spiss H, Beer R, Kampl A, Engelhardt K, Schober M, et al. Treatment of staphylococcal ventriculitis associated with external cerebrospinal fluid drains: a prospective randomized trial of intravenous compared with intraventricular vancomycin therapy. J Neurosurg. 2003;98(5):1040–4.
53. Wang JH, Lin PC, Chou CH, Ho CM, Lin KH, Tsai CT, et al. Intraventricular antimicrobial therapy in postneurosurgical Gram-negative bacillary meningitis or ventriculitis: a hospital-based retrospective study. J Microbiol Immunol Infect. 2014;47(3):204–10.
54. Tangden T, Enblad P, Ullberg M, Sjolin J. Neurosurgical gram-negative bacillary ventriculitis and meningitis: a retrospective study evaluating the efficacy of intraventricular gentamicin therapy in 31 consecutive cases. Clin Infect Dis. 2011;52(11):1310–6.
55. Al-Jeraisy M, Phelps SJ, Christensen ML, Einhaus S. Intraventricular vancomycin in pediatric patients with cerebrospinal fluid shunt infections. J Pediatr Pharmacol Ther. 2004;9(1):36–42.

56. Pickering LK, Ericsson CD, Ruiz-Palacios G, Blevins J, Miner ME. Intraventricular and parenteral gentamicin therapy for ventriculitis in children. Am J Dis Child. 1978;132(5):480–3.
57. Nakama T, Yamashita S, Hirahara T, Okamoto S, Honda S, Watanabe M, et al. Usefulness of intraventricular infusion of antifungal drugs through Ommaya reservoirs for cryptococcal meningitis treatment. J Neurol Sci. 2015;358(1–2):259–62.
58. Haase KK, Lapointe M, Haines SJ. Aseptic meningitis after intraventricular administration of gentamicin. Pharmacotherapy. 2001;21(1):103–7.
59. Remes F, Tomas R, Jindrak V, Vanis V, Setlik M. Intraventricular and lumbar intrathecal administration of antibiotics in postneurosurgical patients with meningitis and/or ventriculitis in a serious clinical state. J Neurosurg. 2013;119(6):1596–602.
60. McCracken GH Jr, Mize SG, Threlkeld N. Intraventricular gentamicin therapy in gram-negative bacillary meningitis of infancy. Report of the Second Neonatal Meningitis Cooperative Study Group. Lancet. 1980;1(8172):787–91.
61. Whitehead WE, Kestle JR. The treatment of cerebrospinal fluid shunt infections. Results from a practice survey of the American Society of Pediatric Neurosurgeons. Pediatr Neurosurg. 2001;35(4):205–10.
62. Simon TD, Hall M, Dean JM, Kestle JR, Riva-Cambrin J. Reinfection following initial cerebrospinal fluid shunt infection. J Neurosurg Pediatr. 2010;6(3):277–85.
63. Roitberg BZ, Tomita T, McLone DG. Abdominal cerebrospinal fluid pseudocyst: a complication of ventriculoperitoneal shunt in children. Pediatr Neurosurg. 1998;29(5):267–73.
64. Gutierrez FA, Raimondi AJ. Peritoneal cysts: a complication of ventriculoperitoneal shunts. Surgery. 1976;79(02):188–92.
65. Hahn YS, Engelhard H, DG ML. Abdominal CSF pseudocyst. Clinical features and surgical management. Pediatr Neurosci. 1985;12(2):75–9.
66. Vinchon M, Dhellemmes P. Cerebrospinal fluid shunt infection: risk factors and long-term follow-up. Childs Nerv Syst. 2006;22(7):692–7.
67. George R, Leibrock L, Epstein M. Long-term analysis of cerebrospinal fluid shunt infections. A 25-year experience. J Neurosurg. 1979;51(6):804–11.
68. Walters BC, Hoffman HJ, Hendrick EB, Humphreys RP. Cerebrospinal fluid shunt infection. Influences on initial management and subsequent outcome. J Neurosurg. 1984;60(5):1014–21.
69. Kulkarni AV, Drake JM, Lamberti-Pasculli M. Cerebrospinal fluid shunt infection: a prospective study of risk factors. J Neurosurg. 2001;94(2):195–201.
70. Korinek AM. Risk factors for neurosurgical site infections after craniotomy: a prospective multicenter study of 2944 patients. The French study Group of Neurosurgical Infections, the SEHP, and the C-CLIN Paris-Nord. Service Epidemiologie Hygiene et Prevention. Neurosurgery. 1997;41(5):1073–9; discussion 1079–81.
71. Mollman HD, Haines SJ. Risk factors for postoperative neurosurgical wound infection. A case-control study. J Neurosurg. 1986;64(6):902–6.
72. Blomstedt GC. Infections in neurosurgery: a retrospective study of 1143 patients and 1517 operations. Acta Neurochir. 1985;78(3–4):81–90.
73. Campbell E, Beez T, Todd L. Prospective review of 30-day morbidity and mortality in a paediatric neurosurgical unit. Childs Nerv Syst. 2017;33(3):483–9.
74. Kourbeti IS, Vakis AF, Ziakas P, Karabetsos D, Potolidis E, Christou S, et al. Infections in patients undergoing craniotomy: risk factors associated with post-craniotomy meningitis. J Neurosurg. 2015;122(5):1113–9.
75. Baumeister S, Peek A, Friedman A, Levin LS, Marcus JR. Management of postneurosurgical bone flap loss caused by infection. Plast Reconstr Surg. 2008;122(6):195e–208e.
76. Reichert MC, Medeiros EA, Ferraz FA. Hospital-acquired meningitis in patients undergoing craniotomy: incidence, evolution, and risk factors. Am J Infect Control. 2002;30(3):158–64.
77. McClelland S 3rd, Hall WA. Postoperative central nervous system infection: incidence and associated factors in 2111 neurosurgical procedures. Clin Infect Dis. 2007;45(1):55–9.
78. Bayhan IA, Sees JP, Nishnianidze T, Rogers KJ, Miller F. Infection as a complication of intrathecal baclofen treatment in children with cerebral palsy. J Pediatr Orthop. 2016;36(3):305–9.

79. Motta F, Antonello CE. Analysis of complications in 430 consecutive pediatric patients treated with intrathecal baclofen therapy: 14-year experience. J Neurosurg Pediatr. 2014;13(3):301–6.
80. Vender JR, Hester S, Waller JL, Rekito A, Lee MR. Identification and management of intrathecal baclofen pump complications: a comparison of pediatric and adult patients. J Neurosurg. 2006;104(1 Suppl):9–15.
81. Fjelstad AB, Hommelstad J, Sorteberg A. Infections related to intrathecal baclofen therapy in children and adults: frequency and risk factors. J Neurosurg Pediatr. 2009;4(5):487–93.
82. Spader HS, Bollo RJ, Bowers CA, Riva-Cambrin J. Risk factors for baclofen pump infection in children: a multivariate analysis. J Neurosurg Pediatr. 2016;17(6):756–62.
83. Horan TC, Andrus M, Dudeck MA. CDC/NHSN surveillance definition of health care-associated infection and criteria for specific types of infections in the acute care setting. Am J Infect Control. 2008;36(5):309–32.
84. Dickey MP, Rice M, Kinnett DG, Lambert R, Donauer S, Gerber MA, et al. Infectious complications of intrathecal baclofen pump devices in a pediatric population. Pediatr Infect Dis J. 2013;32(7):715–22.
85. Hester SM, Fisher JF, Lee MR, Macomson S, Vender JR. Evaluation of salvage techniques for infected baclofen pumps in pediatric patients with cerebral palsy. J Neurosurg Pediatr. 2012;10(6):548–54.
86. Bennett MI, Tai YM, Symonds JM. Staphylococcal meningitis following Synchromed intrathecal pump implant: a case report. Pain. 1994;56(2):243–4.
87. Boviatsis EJ, Kouyialis AT, Boutsikakis I, Korfias S, Sakas DE. Infected CNS infusion pumps. Is there a chance for treatment without removal? Acta Neurochir. 2004;146(5):463–7.
88. Zed PJ, Stiver HG, Devonshire V, Jewesson PJ, Marra F. Continuous intrathecal pump infusion of baclofen with antibiotic drugs for treatment of pump-associated meningitis. Case report. J Neurosurg. 2000;92(2):347–9.
89. Nichols KR, Knoderer CA, Jackson NG, Manaloor JJ, Christenson JC. Success with extended-infusion meropenem after recurrence of baclofen pump-related achromobacter xylosoxidans meningitis in an adolescent. J Pharm Pract. 2015;28(4):430–3.
90. Kwan P, Brodie MJ. Early identification of refractory epilepsy. N Engl J Med. 2000;342(5):314–9.
91. Elliott RE, Rodgers SD, Bassani L, Morsi A, Geller EB, Carlson C, et al. Vagus nerve stimulation for children with treatment-resistant epilepsy: a consecutive series of 141 cases. J Neurosurg Pediatr. 2011;7(5):491–500.
92. Revesz D, Rydenhag B, Ben-Menachem E. Complications and safety of vagus nerve stimulation: 25 years of experience at a single center. J Neurosurg Pediatr. 2016;18(1):97–104.
93. Smyth MD, Tubbs RS, Bebin EM, Grabb PA, Blount JP. Complications of chronic vagus nerve stimulation for epilepsy in children. J Neurosurg. 2003;99(3):500–3.
94. Kahlow H, Olivecrona M. Complications of vagal nerve stimulation for drug-resistant epilepsy: a single center longitudinal study of 143 patients. Seizure. 2013;22(10):827–33.
95. Ortler M, Luef G, Kofler A, Bauer G, Twerdy K. Deep wound infection after vagus nerve stimulator implantation: treatment without removal of the device. Epilepsia. 2001;42(1):133–5.
96. Patel NC, Edwards MS. Vagal nerve stimulator pocket infections. Pediatr Infect Dis J. 2004;23(7):681–3.
97. Wozniak SE, Thompson EM, Selden NR. Vagal nerve stimulator infection: a lead-salvage protocol. J Neurosurg Pediatr. 2011;7(6):671–5.
98. Barker FG 2nd. Efficacy of prophylactic antibiotics against meningitis after craniotomy: a meta-analysis. Neurosurgery. 2007;60(5):887–94; discussion 887–94.
99. Bratzler DW, Dellinger EP, Olsen KM, Perl TM, Auwaerter PG, Bolon MK, et al. Clinical practice guidelines for antimicrobial prophylaxis in surgery. Am J Health Syst Pharm. 2013;70(3):195–283.
100. Alleyne CH Jr, Hassan M, Zabramski JM. The efficacy and cost of prophylactic and perioprocedural antibiotics in patients with external ventricular drains. Neurosurgery. 2000;47(5):1124–7; discussion 1127–9.

101. Poon WS, Ng S, Wai S. CSF antibiotic prophylaxis for neurosurgical patients with ventriculostomy: a randomised study. Acta Neurochir Suppl. 1998;71:146–8.
102. Sonabend AM, Korenfeld Y, Crisman C, Badjatia N, Mayer SA, Connolly ES Jr. Prevention of ventriculostomy-related infections with prophylactic antibiotics and antibiotic-coated external ventricular drains: a systematic review. Neurosurgery. 2011;68(4):996–1005.
103. Lozier AP, Sciacca RR, Romagnoli MF, Connolly ES Jr. Ventriculostomy-related infections: a critical review of the literature. Neurosurgery. 2008;62(Suppl 2):688–700.
104. O'Hara LM, Thom KA, Preas MA. Update to the Centers for Disease Control and Prevention and the Healthcare Infection Control Practices Advisory Committee Guideline for the Prevention of Surgical Site Infection (2017): a summary, review, and strategies for implementation. Am J Infect Control. 2018;46:602–9.
105. Hommelstad J, Madso A, Eide PK. Significant reduction of shunt infection rate in children below 1 year of age after implementation of a perioperative protocol. Acta Neurochir. 2013;155(3):523–31.
106. Rehman AU, Rehman TU, Bashir HH, Gupta V. A simple method to reduce infection of ventriculoperitoneal shunts. J Neurosurg Pediatr. 2010;5(6):569–72.
107. Tulipan N, Cleves MA. Effect of an intraoperative double-gloving strategy on the incidence of cerebrospinal fluid shunt infection. J Neurosurg. 2006;104(1 Suppl):5–8.
108. Horgan MA, Piatt JH Jr. Shaving of the scalp may increase the rate of infection in CSF shunt surgery. Pediatr Neurosurg. 1997;26(4):180–4.
109. Ratanalert S, Musikawat P, Oearsakul T, Saeheng S, Chowchuvech V. Non-shaved ventriculoperitoneal shunt in Thailand. J Clin Neurosci. 2005;12(2):147–9.
110. Govender ST, Nathoo N, van Dellen JR. Evaluation of an antibiotic-impregnated shunt system for the treatment of hydrocephalus. J Neurosurg. 2003;99(5):831–9.
111. Zabramski JM, Whiting D, Darouiche RO, Horner TG, Olson J, Robertson C, et al. Efficacy of antimicrobial-impregnated external ventricular drain catheters: a prospective, randomized, controlled trial. J Neurosurg. 2003;98(4):725–30.
112. Parker SL, McGirt MJ, Murphy JA, Megerian JT, Stout M, Engelhart L. Comparative effectiveness of antibiotic-impregnated shunt catheters in the treatment of adult and pediatric hydrocephalus: analysis of 12,589 consecutive cases from 287 US hospital systems. J Neurosurg. 2015;122(2):443–8.
113. Ragel BT, Browd SR, Schmidt RH. Surgical shunt infection: significant reduction when using intraventricular and systemic antibiotic agents. J Neurosurg. 2006;105(2):242–7.
114. Desai VR, Raskin JS, Mohan A, Montojo J, Briceno V, Curry DJ, et al. A standardized protocol to reduce pediatric baclofen pump infections: a quality improvement initiative. J Neurosurg Pediatr. 2018;21(4):395–400.

Infections Complicating Cardiothoracic Surgery and Cardiac Devices

11

Jesus G. Vallejo, J. Chase McNeil, and Judith R. Campbell

Surgical site infections (SSIs) are a common postoperative complication in children undergoing cardiac surgery [1]. SSIs have a significant impact on patient outcomes, including increased duration of hospitalization, healthcare costs, and increased risk for death [2, 3]. Consensus criteria for SSIs have been developed by the Centers for Disease Control and Prevention (CDC) to standardize data collection for the National Healthcare Safety Network (NHSN) program [4]. SSIs are classified as incisional superficial, incisional deep, or organ/space infection. According to this classification, postoperative mediastinitis is considered an organ/space SSI.

Superficial and Deep Surgical Site Infections

Epidemiology and Risk Factors

The reported incidence of SSIs following pediatric cardiac surgery has ranged from 0.5% to 6% [5–7]. In series of pediatric patients undergoing cardiac surgery, incisional superficial SSIs have accounted for 3–94% of reported SSIs and incisional deep infections for 1–8.5% [5, 6, 8, 9]. Allpress et al. [5] reported that a longer duration of surgery and age <1 month were independent predictors for SSI (superficial and deep) in hospitalized patients after cardiovascular surgery. Murray et al. [10] reported that in addition to young age, incorrect timing of preoperative antibiotics and excessive bleeding within 24 h of surgery were predictors for superficial and deep SSIs.

J. G. Vallejo (✉) · J. C. McNeil · J. R. Campbell
Department of Pediatrics, Section of Infectious Diseases, Baylor College of Medicine and Texas Children's Hospital, Houston, TX, USA
e-mail: jvallejo@bcm.edu

© Springer Nature Switzerland AG 2019
J. C. McNeil et al. (eds.), *Healthcare-Associated Infections in Children*,
https://doi.org/10.1007/978-3-319-98122-2_11

Pathogenesis and Microbiology

SSI requires microbial contamination of the surgical wound to occur. The microorganisms may originate from either endogenous or exogenous sources. Sources of endogenous flora include the patient's skin, mucous membranes, or hollow viscera. Typically >10^5 microorganisms per gram of tissue must be present for an SSI to develop [11]. However, if foreign material is present in the surgical site, the inoculum required may be much lower.

In three pediatric series, the most commonly isolated pathogens from superficial incisional and deep incisional SSIs were *Staphylococcus aureus*, coagulase-negative staphylococci (CoNS), and gram-negative bacteria [5, 6, 10].

Clinical Manifestations and Diagnosis

Superficial incisional SSI occurs within 30 days after the operative procedure and involves only the skin and subcutaneous tissue of incision. In addition, at least one of these criteria must be met:

1. Purulent drainage from the incision.
2. Isolation of pathogen from an aseptically collected incision culture.
3. Presence of pain, tenderness, swelling, or redness.
4. The diagnosis of superficial SSI is made by the surgeon at the time of exploration [4].

Deep incisional infection occurs within 30 or 90 days after the operative procedure and involves deep soft tissues of the incision (e.g., fascial and muscle layers). In addition, at least one of the following criteria must be met:

1. Purulent drainage is noted from the deep incision but not the mediastinum.
2. The deep incision dehisces, or it is opened by the surgeon in a febrile (>38 °C) patient in the presence of localized pain or tenderness.
3. The presence of an abscess at the time of exploration or on imaging.
4. The diagnosis of infection is made by the surgeon [4].

In one pediatric series, the median time to onset of superficial SSIs after cardiac surgery was 6 days, with a range of 6–30 days [12]. Mehta et al. [6] reported that the most common presenting features in patients with superficial or deep SSIs included fever (80%), incision swelling (10%), purulent drainage of the sternal incision (80%), and sternal instability (10%). It should be noted that the presence of sternal instability should prompt an evaluation to exclude extension of infection to the mediastinum [12].

Management

Superficial incisional infections may be treated topically or with oral antibiotics alone. An aseptically collected incision culture should be obtained whenever possible to help guide antibiotic management. Initial antibiotic therapy is directed against staphylococci, including methicillin-resistant *S. aureus* (MRSA), and gram-negative organisms. In one pediatric series, superficial SSIs were treated with 7–10 days of antibiotics [12]. Deep incisional SSI typically requires opening of the suture line and drainage of accumulated pus. If the infection is superficial to the sternum, it can typically be treated for 10–14 days.

Postoperative Mediastinitis

The mediastinum is a division of the thoracic cavity that contains the heart, thymus gland, portions of the esophagus and trachea, and other structures. Mediastinitis is a retrosternal wound infection frequently associated with sternal osteomyelitis. Organ/space infections (e.g., mediastinitis) occur within 30 or 90 days after the operative procedure and involve any part of the anatomy in organs and spaces other than the incision, which was opened or manipulated during cardiac surgery [4].

Epidemiology and Risk Factors

Poststernotomy mediastinitis is an uncommon but serious complication of thoracic surgery. In pediatric patients undergoing cardiac surgery, the reported incidence of mediastinitis has ranged from 0.1% to 1.4% [13–15]. In a review of over 30,000 procedures, Barker et al. [16] reported mediastinitis in 0.3% of cases. In pediatric patients undergoing cardiac transplantation, an incidence rate of 3% has been reported [13].

Some of the well-described risk factors (e.g., obesity and diabetes mellitus) for the development of poststernotomy mediastinitis in adults are not frequently seen in children. In a case-control study, Kagen et al. [17] compared 43 children with postoperative mediastinitis to 184 uninfected controls. The presence of a known or suspected genetic syndrome, American Society of Anesthesiologists (ASA) score >3, and presence of intracardiac pacing wires for >3 days were each associated with the development of postoperative mediastinitis. In a matched case-control study, Costello et al. [18] found that aortic cross-clamp time greater than 85 min and postoperative exposure to at least three separate red blood cell transfusions were independent risk factors for organ space infection/mediastinitis. However, when only potential risk factors known before surgery were considered, the need for preoperative hospitalization independently predicted the subsequent development of mediastinitis. Delayed sternal closure has also been reported as a risk factor associated with the development of mediastinitis in some reports [19] but not in others [15].

Pathogenesis and Microbiology

The pathogenesis of postoperative mediastinitis is multifactorial; however, the most important factor is intraoperative wound contamination. Host-related factors, such as the adequacy of local blood supply, nutrition, and immunologic status, also play an important role.

In children, *S. aureus* is isolated in 38–75% and CoNS in 7–52% of cases of mediastinitis [13]. In a series by Long et al. [13], 30% of mediastinitis cases were caused by gram-negative organisms, with *Pseudomonas aeruginosa* being the most common isolate. *Candida* spp. should be considered in any patient with infection of the mediastinum, particularly when broad-spectrum antimicrobial agents have been used. Heart transplant patients are prone to acquisition of infection with less common and more resistant pathogens, such as *Aspergillus fumigatus* and *Burkholderia cepacia* [13].

Clinical Manifestations

Postoperative mediastinitis may follow a fulminant or subacute clinical course. In three pediatric series, the median time to onset of infection after surgery was 10–14 days, with a range of 4–50 days [13–15]. The presenting features include fever, erythema of the incision, purulent drainage or tenderness of the sternal incision, wound dehiscence, and sternal instability [6, 14, 15]. Although signs of sternal wound infection can precede or follow the recognition of mediastinitis, fever and systemic toxicity appeared first in most patients.

Diagnosis

The diagnosis of postoperative mediastinitis is not challenging in patients presenting with the characteristic clinical pattern of fever, leukocytosis, and sternal instability and/or sternal wound drainage. Bacteremia is common in postoperative mediastinitis, occurring in 53–81% of pediatric patients [6, 14, 15]. Shah et al. [20] reported that postoperative mediastinitis caused by *S. aureus* was an independent risk factor for the development of bacteremia. Thus, a positive blood culture for *S. aureus* in the post-cardiac surgery patient should prompt a careful examination of the sternal incision. In a study of 5500 adult patients, the detection of *S. aureus* bacteremia had a likelihood ratio of 25 for the diagnosis of mediastinitis [21]. In contrast, patients with negative blood cultures were significantly less likely to have mediastinitis.

Computed tomography (CT) of the chest can be useful in patients with systemic symptoms or bacteremia in the absence of sternal wound drainage. Imaging abnormalities may include mediastinal soft tissue swelling, pleural effusion, and sternal dehiscence or erosion, but CT does not always reveal abnormalities [22]. The later imaging is performed after surgery, the more likely the findings will be highly indicative of mediastinitis. In adult studies, the sensitivity and specificity of chest CT for mediastinitis have been reported to be 100% and 85%, respectively, if the study is performed ≥14 days after surgery [23, 24]. The utility of magnetic resonance imaging (MRI) in children with possible postoperative mediastinitis has not been defined. The use of MRI of the chest may be limited when sternal wires are still in place or if the patient has artificial valves, a cardiac pacemaker or vascular clips.

Management

The treatment of mediastinitis following cardiac surgery requires aggressive surgical drainage/debridement and parenteral antibiotics. When feasible all necrotic tissue should be debrided and foreign material (e.g., sternal wires) removed. After wound debridement, continuous irrigation and vacuum-assisted closure or simple primary closed drainage have been reported to be effective management options in pediatric patients [25, 26]. Open wound packing and delayed rectus abdominis flap, pectoralis muscle flap, or omental reconstruction may be required in some children, especially neonates [14, 27].

The selection of empiric antibiotics should be based on the institution's epidemiology of pathogens causing cardiac surgical site infections. Typically, therapy is directed against staphylococci, including MRSA, and gram-negative organisms. The combination of vancomycin and a third- or fourth-generation cephalosporin is commonly recommended. Once definitive culture results are available, antibiotics should be targeted to the pathogen isolated. Although studies have not evaluated the optimal duration of therapy for mediastinitis, 3–6 weeks of intravenous antibiotics is generally recommended [28]. The duration of treatment is determined by the severity and depth of infection. When sternal osteomyelitis is associated with mediastinitis, a minimum of 4–6 weeks of therapy is highly recommended. Thus, systemic antibiotics must be given for at least 3–6 weeks for children with postoperative mediastinitis and/or sternal osteomyelitis.

Cardiac Implantable Electronic Device Infections

Cardiac implantable electronic devices (CIEDs), including both pacemakers (PM) and implantable cardioverter-defibrillators (ICD), are increasingly utilized in adults for the management of rhythm disturbances [29]. As with any medical device, the use of CIEDs are associated with the potential risk of infection. Such infection may be superficial in nature (typical superficial SSI) or involve the device pocket (pocket infection) or the leads (pacemaker endocarditis). Importantly, pocket site infections may coexist with lead and/or valvular endocarditis. There is a relative paucity of literature regarding the epidemiology and management of such infections in children, and recommendations must largely be gleaned from studies of adult patients.

Epidemiology

Based on data reported in the mid-2000s [30], in adults the incidence of CIED infection is estimated as 1.9/1000 device-years with a much higher rate of infection among ICDs (8.9/1000 device-years) than PMs (1/1000 device-years). Independent risk factors for infection in adults include dual-chamber devices, device revision, long-term steroid use, and the need for >2 pacing leads [31, 32]. Other patient-level risk factors associated with infection in adults have included diabetes, end-stage renal disease, malignancy, heart failure, skin disorders, and previous device infection [33]. In a series of specifically pediatric patients, revision procedures (as opposed to primary implantation) and an underlying diagnosis of Down syndrome have been identified as independent risk factors for pacemaker infections [34]. Compliance with antimicrobial prophylaxis prior to device implantation has been associated with reduced risk of infection [31] in adults. Notably, in a recent survey of pediatric cardiac electrophysiologists, only 7% consistently followed the 2010 American Heart Association (AHA) guidelines regarding antibiotic prophylaxis [35].

Microbiology

In series of adult patients with CIED infections, staphylococci are isolated from 69% to 90% of patients [31, 32, 36, 37] with approximately equal distribution between S. aureus and CoNS. The incidence of MRSA among such cases would be expected to vary geographically with the general epidemiology of MRSA; in one series from the Cleveland Clinic, nearly 20% of all CIED infections were due to MRSA [37]. Viridans group streptococci account for approximately 15% of cases [38]. Gram-negative pathogens cause a minority of cases, contributing to 3–15% of CIED infections [30, 36]. Interestingly, in 1 pediatric series [34], gram-negative bacilli caused 4/9 cases (44.4%) of deep pocket infections. Fungi and mycobacteria rarely cause CIED infections with data limited largely to case reports.

Clinical Features

Infections involving the device pocket typically present with local signs of inflammation including erythema, warmth, pain/tenderness, drainage, or even dehiscence with device exposure [37]. When the device has eroded through the overlying soft tissues and is exposed, it must be assumed to be infected. Patients with lead infection/lead endocarditis typically present with systemic symptoms referable to bacteremia and include fever, chills, rigors, weight loss, or even stigmata of sub-acute endocarditis. Notably, similar to valvular endocarditis, the acuity of disease presentation may be influenced by the causative organism, with *S. aureus* often described as having a more fulminant presentation, a longer duration of bacteremia, and a higher mortality (up to 25%) [39, 40].

Diagnosis

Guidelines available from the Heart Rhythm Society (HRS) and developed in col-laboration with the AHA and the Infectious Diseases Society of America (IDSA) recommend the obtainment of at least two sets of blood cultures (including both aerobic and anaerobic cultures) prior to initiating antibiotics in patients with sus-pected CIED infection [41]. The presence of a positive blood culture in a patient with a CIED creates a branch point in clinical decision-making as bacteremia may reflect direct CIED infection, seeding of leads from an unrelated focus, or bactere-mia from a nonvascular focus without involvement of the CIED. Transesophageal echocardiogram (TEE) is recommended in adults with known or suspected CIED infection to evaluate for lead vegetation; TEE has enhanced sensitivity for diagnos-ing lead vegetation over transthoracic echocardiography (TTE, sensitivity 33% compared to TEE) in adults [42]. TEE should also be strongly considered in patients presenting with obvious pocket infection; in one study, lead involvement was noted in 88% of patients with pocket infection despite lack of systemic symptoms [43]. While data in CIED infection specifically are limited, TEE may not be completely necessary in the pediatric population. TTE has enhanced sensitivity in children compared to adults due to differences in thoracic diameter and body habitus. Furthermore, the need to definitively diagnose or exclude lead endocarditis in chil-dren must be balanced with the potential risks of TEE and the physical limitations of performing this procedure due to the small size of many children with CIEDs.

In patients with suspected pocket infection, ultrasound can help define the extent of purulent collections. PET/CT may be a useful adjunct in the diagnosis of pocket infection in adults, particularly in complex or unclear cases [44].

To establish a microbiologic diagnosis, in addition to blood cultures, obtaining cultures of any purulent collections around the generator or leads as well as cultures of the surrounding tissue is crucial.

Management

As a rule, devices (including leads) should be removed when CIED infection is confirmed or considered highly probable [41]. A multidisciplinary approach (infec-tious diseases, cardiology, cardiac surgery) is essential to the optimum management of CIED infections. The vast majority of adult patients can be cured of either pocket infection or lead endocarditis with a combination of antimicrobial therapy and device removal [37, 45]. In at least one study, failure to remove the device was associated with a sevenfold increase in mortality; in this same study, delayed device removal after trial of medical therapy was associated with a higher mortality compared to immediate device removal [46]. Furthermore, there exists a significant risk of relapse following discontinuation of antimicrobial therapy when devices are retained. Similarly, in patients who develop valvular endocarditis who also have a CIED in place, device removal is recommended to minimize potential recurrence from a nidus within the leads.

In general, broad-spectrum empiric therapy is warranted in patients with known or suspected CIED infection [41]. An effective anti-staphylococcal agent (i.e., vancomycin) should be included empirically given the high prevalence of these organisms in CIED infections. Similar to the treatment of infective endocarditis, bactericidal agents are preferred over bacteriostatic ones. In general, a minimum 2-week course of therapy is recommended for pocket infections following device removal assuming there is no evidence of lead involvement. When lead vegetations are present or there is a high suspicion of lead endocarditis, a 4-week course of therapy following device removal is recommended for *S. aureus* infections with a shorter course of therapy (2 weeks) for disease due to other organisms (again, assuming all foreign material has been removed). When valvular endocarditis exists in tandem with either pocket or lead infection, duration of therapy should be extended as dictated in AHA's endocarditis guidelines [47, 48].

In the presence of ongoing bacteremia, without an identifiable source, a high index of suspicion must exist for CIED infections even when echocardiography does not reveal lead vegetation. In such patients with bacteremia due to *S. aureus*, CoNS, *Propionibacterium acnes*, or *Candida*, removal of the device along with a course of antimicrobial therapy is recommended [41]. In patients with bacteremia due to viridans streptococci, Group B streptococcus, or *Enterococcus* spp., current guidelines recommend either complete removal or a period of observation with device in situ along with targeted antimicrobial therapy. In patients with bacteremia due to gram-negative enterics or pneumococci, observation is recommended given the rarity of these organisms to cause CIED infection. For any patient given a trial with device in situ, all hardware should be removed if bacteremia recurs or continues despite appropriate therapy.

While current available guidelines recommend removal of all hardware, some practitioners attempt to salvage devices/leads with medical therapy alone. The likelihood of success, however, with such attempts at salvage is quite low. In one multicenter study, 127 adult patients with CIED infections underwent attempted management with device in situ [49]. Among these 74 (58%) experienced early salvage failure and had the device removed at a median of 3 days. Among the remaining 53 patients, 51% experienced treatment failure over a 6-month period. The authors were unable to identify any clinical or laboratory variables to predict successful salvage. Some patients with retained devices have been managed with chronic antimicrobial suppression therapy. In a recent series from the Mayo Clinic of 37 patients with CIED infection with device retention managed with chronic suppressive therapy, 18% experienced infection relapse within 1 year [38]. Based on very limited data, in extenuating circumstances, patients may be managed with chronic oral antimicrobial suppression following a period of intravenous therapy. However, a substantial risk of relapse and treatment failure exists in these patients.

For patients requiring continued pacing, the optimal timing for placement of a new CIED following removal for infection is unclear. Current guidelines recommend delaying the placement of a new device until blood cultures have been negative for at least 72 h and until all purulent foci of infection have been drained [41]. Additionally, new devices should be placed in locations different from that of the original device (such as the contralateral side).

Ventricular Assist Device (VAD) Infections

Mechanical circulatory support devices have been utilized to improve the survival of patients with end-stage heart failure since 1964 [50]. In 1994, the Food and Drug Administration (FDA) approved left ventricular assist devices (VAD) as a bridge to transplantation. The technological advances of these devices over the last two decades come primarily from their use as a bridge to transplant in adult patients [51]. Despite improvement in the mechanics and management of these devices, infection remains a significant complication. These device-related infections can involve the surgical site, the driveline, the device pocket, the pump itself, or multiple sites. A basic schematic of a VAD is provided in Fig. 11.1. Whether VAD is used as bridge to transplantation or destination therapy (a palliative measure for patients not eligible for transplant), infection contributes to increased hospital stay, morbidity, and mortality [52].

Prior to the use of VADs in children, almost 50% of children with severe heart failure died or required heart transplantation [53]. Given the limitation of donor cardiac grafts for transplantation, children awaiting heart transplantation have a high waiting list mortality rate, reported as high as 17% of 3098 children in a large multicenter cohort study [54]. As VADs evolved from pulsatile pump to continuous flow devices and smaller sizes became available, VAD use in pediatrics increased [55]. VAD implantation as bridge to transplant is now the standard of care for critically ill children awaiting cardiac transplantation and has improved survival of children with severe heart failure [55–57]. VADs are now used in children from infancy

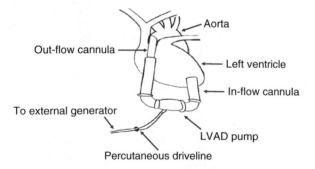

Fig. 11.1 Basic schematic of a generic left ventricular assist device (LVAD). In young children, paracorporeal LVADs are commonly used with the pump outside the body and the cannulas entering the body percutaneously

to adolescence; however, published literature and recommendations on the management of VAD infections in children are limited.

Epidemiology

Early reports on the epidemiology of VAD-associated infections came from a small number of adult patients in single institutions with the incidence of infection ranging from 20% to 80%. In that era, there was variation in definitions and diagnostic evaluation for VAD patients with suspected infection [58–61]. Recognizing the substantial infection-related morbidity and mortality in VAD patients, the International Society for Heart and Lung Transplantation (ISHLT) formed the Infectious Disease Working Group, consisting of experts in infectious diseases, cardiology, pathology, and cardiothoracic surgery, to develop criteria for definitions of infections in VAD patients, which were the basis for consensus guidelines published in 2011 [62]. Subsequent publications have employed these definitions (Table 11.1), thus providing opportunity to compare epidemiology and outcomes data.

In a multicenter cohort study of 247 adults who underwent left ventricular assist device (LVAD) implantation, LVAD-associated infections (LVADI) were reviewed using the ISHLT definitions. The overall incidence of LVADI was 33 per 100 person-years of LVAD support with driveline infections and VAD-related bloodstream infection being the two most common infections. Most LVADI events occurred between 2 weeks and 2 months of implantation. As is the case in many device-associated infections, the cumulative risk of infection increases with duration of ventricular assist device use. Several adult studies have identified host risk factors that contribute to overall risk of infection in these patients including advanced age, poor nutrition, duration of intensive care unit stay, and duration of ventilator

Table 11.1 ISHLT Infectious Disease Working Group classification of infection in patients using ventricular assist devices

VAD-specific infections
Pump and/or cannula infection
Pocket infection
Percutaneous driveline infections (superficial or deep)
VAD-related infections
Infective endocarditis
Bloodstream infection (CVC-associated or non-CVC associated)
Mediastinitis
VAD-related (sternal wound infection, extension of pocket infection)
Non-VAD related (i.e., perforation of esophagus)
Non-VAD infections (examples below)
Lower respiratory tract infection
Clostridium difficile infection
Urinary tract infection

support. Comorbid conditions such as diabetes mellitus and renal insufficiency (some requiring hemodialysis) were also factors that increased the risk of VAD infection [52, 58, 59].

Epidemiologic data in pediatric VAD patients are limited. Early study of pulsatile-flow VAD in children reported infection in 50% [55]. Cabrera and colleagues reviewed the outcomes of a cohort of 51 children who underwent VAD implantation over a 10-year period at a single institution. They employed the ISHTL definitions to evaluate infectious complications in this cohort and reported a VAD infection rate for patients supported with a pulsatile device of 8 per 1000 device-days and for continuous flow device of 7 per 1000 device-days. Time to infection was similar for both types of devices at 39 and 37 days, respectively [56]. In 2012, the Pediatric Interagency Registry for Mechanical Circulatory Support (Pedimacs), the pediatric component of the Interagency Registry for Mechanically Assisted Circulatory Support (Intermacs), was formed and began to prospectively collect data relevant to VAD support in patients less than 19 years. Blume et al. reported data on the first 364 patients, their pre-implant characteristics, outcomes, and adverse events [57]. Device type differed by age with the median age of patients with paracorporeal pulsatile and paracorporeal continuous flow devices being 1.7 years compared with a median age of 14.9 years for intracorporeal continuous flow devices. This difference is attributed to limitations in the size of devices that could be implanted in young infants. In contrast to the adult data in Intermacs, only 6% of children had significant renal dysfunction at the time of implantation; however, liver dysfunction was present in 28%. Overall survival at 6 months was 72% but only 47% in patients <1 year compared to 81% in those who were aged 11–19 years. Major early adverse events, defined as occurring in the first 3 months after device implantation, included bleeding, infection, and stroke. Some infections, however, occurred as late as 6–9 months postimplant. The early infection rate was 13–33 per 100 patient-months and varied by device; the late infection rate was 5–23 per 100 patient-months. Of the 73 patients that died after implant, only 3 (4%) were due to infection [57]. Retrospective and prospective reports of infections in pediatric VAD recipients are reported to range between 39% and 63% [55, 57, 63, 64]. In a recent analysis of the Pedimacs data on 222 patients enrolled between 2012 and 2015, 27 patients had at least 1 infectious adverse event (AE). Infections were the most common AE, accouting for 17% of all AEs. Of the infections, 50% were non-device infection (e.g., urinary tract infection) and 24% sepsis, and 25% involved external or internal pump components.

Microbiology

LVAD infections in adults are most often due to gram-positive organisms, typically staphylococci, with *S. aureus* (including MRSA) and CoNS reported in nearly 24–56% of cases [52]. Enterococci have also been reported in these patients. Gram-negative organisms may be isolated from LVAD infections as well; in early series from single institutions, *P. aeruginosa* was the predominant gram-negative bacillus. More recent multicenter reports note VAD infections due to healthcare-associated Enterobacteriaceae, such as *Enterobacter* spp. and *Klebsiella* spp. [59]; these infections have been associated with poor outcome. Fungal infections, typically due to *Candida* spp., have been reported in as high as 36% of LVAD infections in one study and are associated with substantial mortality [52, 56, 60]. Limited pediatric series have noted similar microbiology of VAD infections in children compared to adults but with worse outcome in children with infection due to *Candida* spp. or gram-negative infections [56]. In the Pedimacs report of infectious complications of VAD in children, bacterial and fungal etiologies were identified in 73% and 12%, respectively, but specific organisms were not provided [63].

Clinical Features

In general, patients with VAD may present with a broad spectrum of infectious complications. Patients may have a range of symptoms including non-specific symptoms such as fever, lethargy and local signs of inflammation to fulminant sepsis with systemic inflammatory response syndrome. The ISHLT has categorized and defined these for consistent reporting of outcomes (Table 11.1). *VAD-specific infections* are those related to the hardware, specifically the pump, cannula, and percutaneous driveline, or the body sites that contain the device components, such as pocket that holds the pump or percutaneous tunnel of the driveline. Driveline infections are the most common VAD-specific infection in both adult and pediatric patients. Signs of driveline and pocket infections range from erythema and warmth to purulent drainage from or fluid collection along the percutaneous tunnel or pocket with wound dehiscence. Ideally, diagnosis and treatment of localized superficial infections occur early in the course before progression to sepsis and deep-seated infection.

VAD-related infections include endocarditis, bloodstream infection including sepsis, central line-associated bloodstream infection, or deep organ space infections such as mediastinitis arising from extension of pocket infection. Postimplantation sepsis is a risk factor for mortality in adults [52, 59, 61], but there is insufficient data on postimplantation sepsis in children to draw conclusion regarding outcome. VAD-related endocarditis involves the inner components of the device that are in contact with the bloodstream [52]. Nienaber et al. reported an incidence of VAD endocarditis of 1.6 per 100 person-years in a multicenter retrospective review of 247 adults with continuous flow VAD [60]. Patients with endocarditis presented earlier and with fever and systemic inflammatory response symptoms. Additionally, evidence of embolic lesions or dissemination to the central nervous system or other organs may be evident. Although less common, VAD endocarditis and associated embolic events were associated with up to 50% mortality.

Given that VAD patients are hospitalized in intensive care units pre- and postimplantation, they are at risk for non-VAD infections such as healthcare-associated lower respiratory tract infection, *C. difficile* infection, or urinary tract infection, which are discussed in Chaps. 7, 12, and 13, respectively.

Diagnosis

The ISHLT guidelines provide a framework for diagnostic evaluation of infections in VAD patients based on defined categories of VAD infection [60]. A careful physical examination and assessment of VAD function is essential. Daily assessment of surgical wounds and percutaneous driveline exit site is critical to early detection and treatment of localized infectious processes. Patients with suspected VAD infection should have laboratory evaluation that includes complete blood count, inflammatory markers (i.e., C-reactive protein), and at least 2–3 sets of blood cultures (including both aerobic and anaerobic cultures) prior to initiating antibiotics. In patients with suspected driveline or pocket infection, ultrasound or CT scan may be helpful to characterize the extent of fluid collections. To establish a microbiologic diagnosis, in addition to obtaining blood cultures, cultures of any fluid collections around the driveline site or pocket should be obtained. Any surgical debridement of tissue in these areas should also be sent for culture. As with any patient in the intensive care unit, evaluation for suspected VAD infection also includes evaluation for other common healthcare-associated infections such as catheter-associated urinary tract infection, ventilator-associated pneumonia, and central line-associated bloodstream infection (CLABSI). Furthermore, these patients are at risk for *Clostridium difficile* infection (CDI), due to their underlying critically ill condition and receipt of perioperative antimicrobial agents (and often antimicrobials for other indications as well). Thus, if diarrhea or significant change in stool output develops, specimens should be sent to evaluate for the presence of *Clostridium difficile* toxin (see Chap. 12). Other diagnostic tests should be performed based on local and hospital epidemiology, for example, testing for respiratory viruses (RSV, influenza) during respiratory viral season (see Chap. 14).

Management

Although standardized definitions have been developed to guide understanding of the spectrum of infectious complications in VAD patients, practice guidelines are limited for management of these complications in adult patients [52, 60]. The American Heart Association and Infectious Diseases Society of America developed a proposed management algorithm for LVADI based in large part on multicenter studies in adults. An overview of general guideline considerations is provided in Fig. 11.2 [60].

A multidisciplinary approach with infectious diseases, cardiology, critical care, cardiac surgery, diagnostic imaging, and interventional radiology expertise is valuable for optimal evaluation and definitive management of VAD infections.

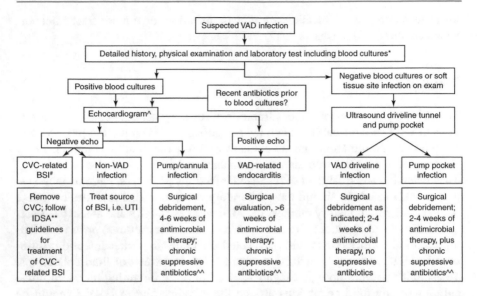

Fig. 11.2 Guidelines for the management of ventricular assist device-associated infections based on adult literature and adapted from Nienaber et al. [60]. Management decisions should be individualized based on clinical presentation and patient factors. *2–3 sets of blood cultures. ^Echocardiogram: transesophageal (TEE) or transthoracic if TEE is not possible. ^^Chronic suppressive antimicrobial therapy is recommended if treatment failure or recurrence Abbreviations: #BSI bloodstream infection, **IDSA Infectious Diseases Society of America

Medical Management

Empiric antibiotic therapy should be broad spectrum with inclusion of an effective anti-staphylococcal agent (i.e., vancomycin) given the high prevalence of these organisms in VAD infections. Antimicrobial agents effective against gram-negative organisms should be added pending culture results and with consideration of local epidemiology for multidrug-resistant organisms in a given unit or history of such in the specific patient. In some instances, empiric antifungal therapy is warranted if the patient has previously received prolonged courses of broad-spectrum antibiotics which predisposes to invasive *Candida* disease. Once specific culture data is available, therapy should be tailored based on susceptibility results of isolated pathogens. If cultures are negative, therapy should be chosen based on local epidemiology and antibiotic susceptibility patterns of the given unit and/or patient population. In the multicenter study by Nienaber et al., 76% of patients were managed without surgical intervention, and the median duration of therapy was 28 days [60]. Duration of therapy may be shorter for localized superficial driveline or pocket infections provided blood cultures prior to antibiotics were negative. Patients with pump and cannula infection or VAD-related endocarditis are treated longer, up to 6 weeks [60]. In general, chronic suppressive therapy is recommended if the VAD is believed to be seeded. This may manifest as failure to clear bloodstream infection despite appropriate antimicrobial therapy in instances of VAD-related endocarditis, pump or cannula infection, or pump pocket infection [60].

Surgical Management

In general, indications for surgical evaluation and debridement of VAD-associated infections include failure of conservative management, pump/cannula infection, VAD-related endocarditis, and driveline or pocket infections with fluid collections [60]. In some instances, replacement of the device is necessary to eradicate the infection although associated with the risk of recurrence of infection in the new device and nontrivial operative risks.

In summary, as VADs have increased in utilization, the mortality of severe cardiac failure pending transplantation has decreased. Devices are now small enough to implant in young infants as well as children and adolescents, thus improving outcomes in children waiting for cardiac transplantation. Infection remains one of the most common adverse events associated with these devices and is associated with significant morbidity and mortality. Early diagnosis and treatment have been successful without adversely affecting outcomes posttransplantation in limited studies. While gram-positive organisms cause most infections, those secondary to gram-negative bacilli or yeast and those associated with sepsis have worse clinical outcomes.

Prevention of Infections Associated with Cardiovascular Surgery

The foundation of prevention of surgical site infections (SSI) is appropriate perioperative antimicrobial prophylaxis and skin antisepsis. National guidelines provide evidence-based recommendations for the prevention of SSI for specific procedures [65–67]. Typically, agents effective against skin flora (i.e., *S. aureus*) should be administered a minimum of 60 min prior to incision such that bactericidal concentrations of the agents are achieved in serum and tissues when the incision is made. The perioperative antibiotic prophylaxis of choice for cardiovascular procedures is cefazolin; in patients known to be colonized with MRSA, cefazolin should be used in combination with vancomycin. New CDC Guidelines for Prevention of SSI recommend an alcohol-based skin antiseptic, either chlorhexidine-alcohol (e.g., ChloraPrep®, Becton Dickinson) or iodophor-alcohol (e.g., DuraPrep®, 3M) products [68]. When comparing chlorhexidine-alcohol to iodophor-alcohol, no differences were noted in SSI outcomes; however, differences exist in the recommended contact time for effectiveness of these two products (30 s and 3 min, respectively) [69]. Recently, institutions have implemented preoperative screening for MRSA and MSSA colonization and decolonization protocols with chlorhexidine (CHG)-based product for bathing and mupirocin ointment for colonized patients [70]. In a randomized controlled trial of >800 adults, the *S. aureus* SSI rate was 2.5% in the group receiving mupirocin-chlorhexidine decolonization compared to 7.9% in the placebo group [70]. Preoperative surgical site antisepsis should be as that outlined in published SSI prevention guidelines [67].

Preoperatively optimizing nutritional status and achieving glycemic control may be helpful, as several studies have indicated increased infection in those with poor nutrition and diabetes mellitus [52]. Similarly, those with comorbidities, such as renal insufficiency, had worse outcomes; thus optimizing management of those conditions prior to surgery is preferred [52, 71].

For prevention of VAD-specific infections, postimplantation securement of the driveline is recommended, as driveline infections are increased in patients with trauma around the driveline site [71–73]. In addition, meticulous attention to daily exit site care with CHG or other antiseptic agents has reduced driveline tunnel site infections in some centers; however this practice has not been evaluated in a multicenter study.

The basic principles of outbreak investigation used in the hospital in general are applicable to cardiac surgery patients as well. The investigation of clusters of infections in cardiac ICU or in postsurgical patients, whether common (such as CLABSIs) or exotic, is imperative given the medically fragile status of many of these patients. This is underscored by a recent worldwide outbreak of *Mycobacterium chimaera* among post-cardiac surgery patients associated with contaminated heater-cooler devices [74].

References

1. Levy I, Ovadia B, Erez E, Rinat S, Ashkenazi S, Birk E, et al. Nosocomial infections after cardiac surgery in infants and children: incidence and risk factors. J Hosp Infect. 2003;53(2):111–6.
2. Klevens RM, Edwards JR, Richards CL Jr, Horan TC, Gaynes RP, Pollock DA, et al. Estimating health care-associated infections and deaths in U.S. hospitals, 2002. Public Health Rep. 2007;122(2):160–6.
3. Edwards JR, Peterson KD, Mu Y, Banerjee S, Allen-Bridson K, Morrell G, et al. National Healthcare Safety Network (NHSN) report: data summary for 2006 through 2008, issued December 2009. Am J Infect Control. 2009;37(10):783–805.
4. Horan TC, Andrus M, Dudeck MA. CDC/NHSN surveillance definition of health care-associated infection and criteria for specific types of infections in the acute care setting. Am J Infect Control. 2008;36(5):309–32.
5. Allpress AL, Rosenthal GL, Goodrich KM, Lupinetti FM, Zerr DM. Risk factors for surgical site infections after pediatric cardiovascular surgery. Pediatr Infect Dis J. 2004;23(3):231–4.
6. Mehta PA, Cunningham CK, Colella CB, Alferis G, Weiner LB. Risk factors for sternal wound and other infections in pediatric cardiac surgery patients. Pediatr Infect Dis J. 2000;19(10):1000–4.
7. Sohn AH, Schwartz JM, Yang KY, Jarvis WR, Guglielmo BJ, Weintrub PS. Risk factors and risk adjustment for surgical site infections in pediatric cardiothoracic surgery patients. Am J Infect Control. 2010;38(9):706–10.
8. McNeil JC, Ligon JA, Hulten KG, Dreyer WJ, Heinle JS, Mason EO, et al. Staphylococcus aureus infections in children with congenital heart disease. J Pediatric Infect Dis Soc. 2013;2(4):337–44.
9. Sarvikivi E, Lyytikainen O, Nieminen H, Sairanen H, Saxen H. Nosocomial infections after pediatric cardiac surgery. Am J Infect Control. 2008;36(8):564–9.

10. Murray MT, Krishnamurthy G, Corda R, Turcotte RF, Jia H, Bacha E, et al. Surgical site infections and bloodstream infections in infants after cardiac surgery. J Thorac Cardiovasc Surg. 2014;148(1):259–65.
11. Krizek TJ, Robson MC. Evolution of quantitative bacteriology in wound management. Am J Surg. 1975;130(5):579–84.
12. Edwards MS, Baker CJ. Median sternotomy wound infections in children. Pediatr Infect Dis. 1983;2(2):105–9.
13. Long CB, Shah SS, Lautenbach E, Coffin SE, Tabbutt S, Gaynor JW, et al. Postoperative mediastinitis in children: epidemiology, microbiology and risk factors for Gram-negative pathogens. Pediatr Infect Dis J. 2005;24(4):315–9.
14. Tortoriello TA, Friedman JD, McKenzie ED, Fraser CD, Feltes TF, Randall J, et al. Mediastinitis after pediatric cardiac surgery: a 15-year experience at a single institution. Ann Thorac Surg. 2003;76(5):1655–60.
15. Al-Sehly AA, Robinson JL, Lee BE, Taylor G, Ross DB, Robertson M, et al. Pediatric post-sternotomy mediastinitis. Ann Thorac Surg. 2005;80(6):2314–20.
16. Barker GM, O'Brien SM, Welke KF, Jacobs ML, Jacobs JP, Benjamin DK Jr, et al. Major infection after pediatric cardiac surgery: a risk estimation model. Ann Thorac Surg. 2010;89(3):843–50.
17. Kagen J, Lautenbach E, Bilker WB, Matro J, Bell LM, Dominguez TE, et al. Risk factors for mediastinitis following median sternotomy in children. Pediatr Infect Dis J. 2007;26(7):613–8.
18. Costello JM, Graham DA, Morrow DF, Morrow J, Potter-Bynoe G, Sandora TJ, et al. Risk factors for surgical site infection after cardiac surgery in children. Ann Thorac Surg. 2010;89(6):1833–41; discussion 1841–2
19. Harder EE, Gaies MG, Yu S, Donohue JE, Hanauer DA, Goldberg CS, et al. Risk factors for surgical site infection in pediatric cardiac surgery patients undergoing delayed sternal closure. J Thorac Cardiovasc Surg. 2013;146(2):326–33.
20. Shah SS, Lautenbach E, Long CB, Tabbutt S, Gaynor JW, Bilker WB, et al. Staphylococcus aureus as a risk factor for bloodstream infection in children with postoperative mediastinitis. Pediatr Infect Dis J. 2005;24(9):834–7.
21. Fowler VG Jr, Kaye KS, Simel DL, Cabell CH, McClachlan D, Smith PK, et al. Staphylococcus aureus bacteremia after median sternotomy: clinical utility of blood culture results in the identification of postoperative mediastinitis. Circulation. 2003;108(1):73–8.
22. Exarhos DN, Malagari K, Tsatalou EG, Benakis SV, Peppas C, Kotanidou A, et al. Acute mediastinitis: spectrum of computed tomography findings. Eur Radiol. 2005;15(8):1569–74.
23. Jolles H, Henry DA, Roberson JP, Cole TJ, Spratt JA. Mediastinitis following median sternotomy: CT findings. Radiology. 1996;201(2):463–6.
24. Yamashiro T, Kamiya H, Murayama S, Unten S, Nakayama T, Gibo M, et al. Infectious mediastinitis after cardiovascular surgery: role of computed tomography. Radiat Med. 2008;26(6):343–7.
25. Ugaki S, Kasahara S, Arai S, Takagaki M, Sano S. Combination of continuous irrigation and vacuum-assisted closure is effective for mediastinitis after cardiac surgery in small children. Interact Cardiovasc Thorac Surg. 2010;11(3):247–51.
26. Anslot C, Hulin S, Durandy Y. Postoperative mediastinitis in children: improvement of simple primary closed drainage. Ann Thorac Surg. 2007;84(2):423–8.
27. Ohye RG, Maniker RB, Graves HL, Devaney EJ, Bove EL. Primary closure for postoperative mediastinitis in children. J Thorac Cardiovasc Surg. 2004;128(3):480–6.
28. Siegman-Igra Y, Shafir R, Weiss J, Herman O, Schwartz D, Konforti N. Serious infectious complications of midsternotomy: a review of bacteriology and antimicrobial therapy. Scand J Infect Dis. 1990;22(6):633–43.
29. Cabell CH, Heidenreich PA, Chu VH, Moore CM, Stryjewski ME, Corey GR, et al. Increasing rates of cardiac device infections among Medicare beneficiaries: 1990-1999. Am Heart J. 2004;147(4):582–6.

30. Uslan DZ, Sohail MR, St Sauver JL, Friedman PA, Hayes DL, Stoner SM, et al. Permanent pacemaker and implantable cardioverter defibrillator infection: a population-based study. Arch Intern Med. 2007;167(7):669–75.
31. Sohail MR, Uslan DZ, Khan AH, Friedman PA, Hayes DL, Wilson WR, et al. Risk factor analysis of permanent pacemaker infection. Clin Infect Dis. 2007;45(2):166–73.
32. Nery PB, Fernandes R, Nair GM, Sumner GL, Ribas CS, Menon SM, et al. Device-related infection among patients with pacemakers and implantable defibrillators: incidence, risk factors, and consequences. J Cardiovasc Electrophysiol. 2010;21(7):786–90.
33. Polyzos KA, Konstantelias AA, Falagas ME. Risk factors for cardiac implantable electronic device infection: a systematic review and meta-analysis. Europace. 2015;17(5):767–77.
34. Cohen MI, Bush DM, Gaynor JW, Vetter VL, Tanel RE, Rhodes LA. Pediatric pacemaker infections: twenty years of experience. J Thorac Cardiovasc Surg. 2002;124(4):821–7.
35. Chen SY, Ceresnak SR, Motonaga KS, Trela A, Hanisch D, Dubin AM. Antibiotic prophylaxis practices in pediatric cardiac implantable electronic device procedures: a survey of the pediatric and congenital electrophysiology society (PACES). Pediatr Cardiol. 2018;39(6):1129–33.
36. Sohail MR, Uslan DZ, Khan AH, Friedman PA, Hayes DL, Wilson WR, et al. Management and outcome of permanent pacemaker and implantable cardioverter-defibrillator infections. J Am Coll Cardiol. 2007;49(18):1851–9.
37. Tarakji KG, Chan EJ, Cantillon DJ, Doonan AL, Hu T, Schmitt S, et al. Cardiac implantable electronic device infections: presentation, management, and patient outcomes. Heart Rhythm. 2010;7(8):1043–7.
38. Tan EM, DeSimone DC, Sohail MR, Baddour LM, Wilson WR, Steckelberg JM, et al. Outcomes in patients with cardiovascular implantable electronic device infection managed with chronic antibiotic suppression. Clin Infect Dis. 2017;64(11):1516–21.
39. Le KY, Sohail MR, Friedman PA, Uslan DZ, Cha SS, Hayes DL, et al. Clinical features and outcomes of cardiovascular implantable electronic device infections due to staphylococcal species. Am J Cardiol. 2012;110(8):1143–9.
40. Hussein AA, Baghdy Y, Wazni OM, Brunner MP, Kabbach G, Shao M, et al. Microbiology of cardiac implantable electronic device infections. JACC Clin Electrophysiol. 2016;2(4):498–505.
41. Kusumoto FM, Schoenfeld MH, Wilkoff BL, Berul CI, Birgersdotter-Green UM, Carrillo R, et al. 2017 HRS expert consensus statement on cardiovascular implantable electronic device lead management and extraction. Heart Rhythm. 2017;14(12):e503–51.
42. Fowler VG Jr, Li J, Corey GR, Boley J, Marr KA, Gopal AK, et al. Role of echocardiography in evaluation of patients with Staphylococcus aureus bacteremia: experience in 103 patients. J Am Coll Cardiol. 1997;30(4):1072–8.
43. Klug D, Lacroix D, Savoye C, Goullard L, Grandmougin D, Hennequin JL, et al. Systemic infection related to endocarditis on pacemaker leads: clinical presentation and management. Circulation. 1997;95(8):2098–107.
44. Granados U, Fuster D, Pericas JM, Llopis JL, Ninot S, Quintana E, et al. Diagnostic accuracy of 18F-FDG PET/CT in infective endocarditis and implantable cardiac electronic device infection: a cross-sectional study. J Nucl Med. 2016;57(11):1726–32.
45. Deharo JC, Quatre A, Mancini J, Khairy P, Le Dolley Y, Casalta JP, et al. Long-term outcomes following infection of cardiac implantable electronic devices: a prospective matched cohort study. Heart. 2012;98(9):724–31.
46. Le KY, Sohail MR, Friedman PA, Uslan DZ, Cha SS, Hayes DL, et al. Impact of timing of device removal on mortality in patients with cardiovascular implantable electronic device infections. Heart Rhythm. 2011;8(11):1678–85.
47. Baddour LM, Wilson WR, Bayer AS, Fowler VG Jr, Tleyjeh IM, Rybak MJ, et al. Infective endocarditis in adults: diagnosis, antimicrobial therapy, and management of complications: a scientific statement for healthcare professionals from the American Heart Association. Circulation. 2015;132(15):1435–86.
48. Baltimore RS, Gewitz M, Baddour LM, Beerman LB, Jackson MA, Lockhart PB, et al. Infective endocarditis in childhood: 2015 update: a scientific statement from the American Heart Association. Circulation. 2015;132(15):1487–515.

49. Peacock JE Jr, Stafford JM, Le K, Sohail MR, Baddour LM, Prutkin JM, et al. Attempted salvage of infected cardiovascular implantable electronic devices: are there clinical factors that predict success? Pacing Clin Electrophysiol. 2018;41(5):524–31.
50. Hogness JR, Van Antwer M. The artificial heart program: current status and history. In: Hogness JR, Van Antwer M, editors. The artificial heart: prototypes, policies and patients. Washington, DC: National Academy Press; 1991. p. 14–25.
51. Rose EA, Gelijns AC, Moskowitz AJ, Heitjan DF, Stevenson LW, Dembitsky W, et al. Long-term use of a left ventricular assist device for end-stage heart failure. N Engl J Med. 2001;345(20):1435–43.
52. Gordon RJ, Quagliarello B, Lowy FD. Ventricular assist device-related infections. Lancet Infect Dis. 2006;6(7):426–37.
53. Towbin JA, Lowe AM, Colan SD, Sleeper LA, Orav EJ, Clunie S, et al. Incidence, causes, and outcomes of dilated cardiomyopathy in children. JAMA. 2006;296(15):1867–76.
54. Almond CSD, Thiagarajan RR, Piercey GE, Gauvreau K, Blume ED, Bastardi HJ, et al. Waiting list mortality among children listed for heart transplantation in the United States. Circulation. 2009;119(5):717–27.
55. Fraser CD Jr, Jaquiss RD, Rosenthal DN, Humpl T, Canter CE, Blackstone EH, et al. Prospective trial of a pediatric ventricular assist device. N Engl J Med. 2012;367(6):532–41.
56. Cabrera AG, Khan MS, Morales DL, Chen DW, Moffett BS, Price JF, et al. Infectious complications and outcomes in children supported with left ventricular assist devices. J Heart Lung Transplant. 2013;32(5):518–24.
57. Blume ED, VanderPluym C, Lorts A, Baldwin JT, Rossano JW, Morales DLS, et al. Second annual pediatric interagency registry for mechanical circulatory support (Pedimacs) report: pre-implant characteristics and outcomes. J Heart Lung Transplant. 2018;37(1):38–45.
58. Malani PN, Dyke DB, Pagani FD, Chenoweth CE. Nosocomial infections in left ventricular assist device recipients. Clin Infect Dis. 2002;34(10):1295–300.
59. Gordon RJ, Weinberg AD, Pagani FD, Slaughter MS, Pappas PS, Naka Y, et al. Prospective, multicenter study of ventricular assist device infections. Circulation. 2013;127(6):691–702.
60. Nienaber JJ, Kusne S, Riaz T, Walker RC, Baddour LM, Wright AJ, et al. Clinical manifestations and management of left ventricular assist device-associated infections. Clin Infect Dis. 2013;57(10):1438–48.
61. Topkara VK, Kondareddy S, Malik F, Wang IW, Mann DL, Ewald GA, et al. Infectious complications in patients with left ventricular assist device: etiology and outcomes in the continuous-flow era. Ann Thorac Surg. 2010;90(4):1270–7.
62. Hannan MM, Husain S, Mattner F, Danziger-Isakov L, Drew RJ, Corey GR, et al. Working formulation for the standardization of definitions of infections in patients using ventricular assist devices. J Heart Lung Transplant. 2011;30(4):375–84.
63. Auerbach SR, Richmond ME, Schumacher KR, Lopez-Colon D, Mitchell MB, Turrentine MW, et al. Infectious complications of ventricular assist device use in children in the United States: data from the pediatric interagency registry for mechanical circulatory support (Pedimacs). J Heart Lung Transplant. 2018;37(1):46–53.
64. Rosenthal DN, Almond CS, Jaquiss RD, Peyton CE, Auerbach SR, Morales DR, et al. Adverse events in children implanted with ventricular assist devices in the United States: data from the pediatric interagency registry for mechanical circulatory support (PediMACS). J Heart Lung Transplant. 2016;35(5):569–77.
65. Berrios-Torres SI, Umscheid CA, Bratzler DW, Leas B, Stone EC, Kelz RR, et al. Centers for Disease Control and Prevention guideline for the prevention of surgical site infection, 2017. JAMA Surg. 2017;152(8):784–91.
66. Bratzler DW, Dellinger EP, Olsen KM, Perl TM, Auwaerter PG, Bolon MK, et al. Clinical practice guidelines for antimicrobial prophylaxis in surgery. Am J Health Syst Pharm. 2013;70(3):195–283.
67. Mangram AJ, Horan TC, Pearson ML, Silver LC, Jarvis WR. Guideline for prevention of surgical site infection, 1999. Centers for Disease Control and Prevention (CDC) hospital infection control practices advisory committee. Am J Infect Control. 1999;27(2):97–132; quiz 133–4; discussion 196.

68. O'Hara LM, Thom KA, Preas MA. Update to the Centers for Disease Control and Prevention and the Healthcare Infection Control Practices Advisory Committee guideline for the prevention of surgical site infection (2017): a summary, review, and strategies for implementation. Am J Infect Control. 2018;46(6):602–9.
69. Darouiche RO, Wall MJ Jr, Itani KM, Otterson MF, Webb AL, Carrick MM, et al. Chlorhexidine-alcohol versus povidone-iodine for surgical-site antisepsis. N Engl J Med. 2010;362(1):18–26.
70. Bode LG, Kluytmans JA, Wertheim HF, Bogaers D, Vandenbroucke-Grauls CM, Roosendaal R, et al. Preventing surgical-site infections in nasal carriers of Staphylococcus aureus. N Engl J Med. 2010;362(1):9–17.
71. Goldstein DJ, Naftel D, Holman W, Bellumkonda L, Pamboukian SV, Pagani FD, et al. Continuous-flow devices and percutaneous site infections: clinical outcomes. J Heart Lung Transplant. 2012;31(11):1151–7.
72. Kusne S, Staley L, Arabia F. Prevention and infection management in mechanical circulatory support device recipients. Clin Infect Dis. 2017;64(2):222–8.
73. Saraswat MK, Magruder JT, Crawford TC, Gardner JM, Duquaine D, Sussman MS, et al. Preoperative Staphylococcus Aureus screening and targeted decolonization in cardiac surgery. Ann Thorac Surg. 2017;104(4):1349–56.
74. Ninh A, Weiner M, Goldberg A. Healthcare-associated mycobacterium chimaera infection subsequent to heater-cooler device exposure during cardiac surgery. J Cardiothorac Vasc Anesth. 2017;31(5):1831–5.

Healthcare-Associated Gastrointestinal Infections

12

Jonathan D. Crews

Epidemiology

Nosocomial Diarrhea

Diarrhea is a frequent occurrence in community settings. In the United States alone, there are an estimated 179 million episodes of acute diarrhea per year [1]. Children less than 5 years old experience the greatest burden of community-acquired diarrhea, of which the majority is from enteric infections [2].

For hospitalized patients, diarrhea is relatively common. Prevalence studies estimate that 1–5% of pediatric hospitalizations are complicated by nosocomial diarrhea [3–5]. Such estimates vary based on several factors. Publications from developing countries generally report a higher incidence of nosocomial diarrhea than developed countries [6]. Children under 2 years of age have the highest rate of nosocomial diarrhea [7, 8]. Additionally, certain pediatric subpopulations are more susceptible to developing diarrhea during inpatient stays, including children with chronic gastrointestinal disorders, malignancy, or hematopoietic stem cell transplant (HSCT) recipients. Overall, the burden of nosocomial diarrhea is likely underestimated, however, as short-lived episodes may go unreported.

Healthcare-associated (HA) diarrhea is traditionally defined as the acute onset of diarrhea ($\geq$ 3 unformed stools in a 24-hour period) beginning $\geq$72 h after hospital admission. Hospitalized children can develop diarrhea for various reasons, but it is typically as a consequence of the therapies to which they are exposed or from a gastrointestinal infection acquired in the hospital setting.

J. D. Crews
Department of Pediatrics, Section of Infectious Diseases, Baylor College of Medicine, Houston, TX, USA

Pediatric Infectious Diseases, The Children's Hospital of San Antonio, San Antonio, TX, USA
e-mail: crews@bcm.edu

© Springer Nature Switzerland AG 2019
J. C. McNeil et al. (eds.), *Healthcare-Associated Infections in Children*,
https://doi.org/10.1007/978-3-319-98122-2_12

Healthcare-Associated Gastrointestinal Infections

The organisms most frequently implicated in HA gastrointestinal infections in children are *Clostridium difficile*, norovirus, and rotavirus. The epidemiology of these organisms has changed substantially in recent years. *Clostridium difficile*, a frequent cause of antibiotic-associated diarrhea in adults, has emerged globally as an important healthcare-associated pathogen in children, with an increasing number of infections occurring among hospitalized children [9]. Norovirus and rotavirus are the primary causes of community-acquired viral gastroenteritis in children and consequently are frequently introduced into hospital settings by infected children requiring hospital admission. The rotavirus vaccine has resulted in dramatic reductions in community-onset infections, with attendant declines in nosocomial disease [10]. Norovirus, an important cause of hospital diarrheal outbreaks, is now the leading cause of acute gastroenteritis in countries with widespread rotavirus vaccination [11]. Occasionally, bacteria other than *C. difficile* can spread within hospitals. *Salmonella,* diarrheagenic *Escherichia coli*, and *Campylobacter* can cause foodborne outbreaks or person-to-person spread and appear to be a more common cause of nosocomial disease in developing countries [6, 12]. Parasitic pathogens, like *Cryptosporidium* and *Giardia*, are rare causes of nosocomial disease.

The burden of nosocomial gastrointestinal infections in children's hospitals is not inconsequential [4, 13, 14]. For example, a 2009 point prevalence study performed at 30 pediatric inpatient facilities in Canada found viral gastrointestinal infections to be the third most common healthcare-associated infection [14]. In studies conducted prior to the rotavirus vaccine, 20–35% of children hospitalized with rotavirus infections acquired their disease in the healthcare setting [15]. General pediatric wards are especially prone to nosocomial gastrointestinal infections given that children with community-acquired infections are frequently admitted to these units [13]. Patients admitted to shared hospital rooms have been found to have an increased risk of acquiring enteric infections [7, 16].

Patient factors can increase the risk of gastrointestinal infections among hospitalized children, including weakened immunity, diminished gastric acidity, and alterations in intestinal motility or flora. Infants and young children may be more susceptible because of their inability to contain body fluids and the close physical contact that occurs with their care. Antibiotics, which disrupt intestinal flora, are an important risk factor for *C. difficile* infection [17].

The majority of nosocomial enteric infections that occur in pediatric healthcare settings develop when an infected patient transmits the pathogen to a susceptible patient. Transmission occurs either through direct person-to-person contact or indirectly through contamination of the hospital environment. Molecular data has shown that the majority of nosocomial viral gastroenteritis is from community strains brought into the hospital from infected patients and subsequently spread to susceptible individuals [18]. Infected healthcare workers – whether ill or merely short-term carriers – may spread organisms to susceptible patients through direct patient care or indirectly via the hospital environment. Additionally, contaminated goods – whether food, water, medicine, or medical instruments – can lead to common source outbreaks.

Clinical Features

Diarrhea is the most common symptom of HA gastrointestinal infections. Patients typically have watery or loose stools with increased stool frequency. Vomiting can occur, especially with norovirus infection. Evident hematochezia is uncommon and, if present, should prompt consideration of a bacterial pathogen. Additional signs and symptoms include low-grade fever, nausea, loss of appetite, and abdominal cramps or pain. Dehydration, hemodynamic instability, and electrolytes abnormalities are potential complications of nosocomial diarrhea.

Norovirus, rotavirus, and other enteric viruses cause abrupt onset of watery diarrhea associated with low-grade fever, nausea, and vomiting. Vomiting is especially prominent with norovirus infection. Symptoms typically last for 2–4 days. Norovirus can cause prolonged symptoms in immunocompromised children, particularly HSCT or solid organ transplant recipients [19].

Clostridium difficile infection (CDI) causes diarrhea with colitis. Bowel movements can contain mucous or occult blood. Low-grade fever and lower abdominal pain or cramping are common. Severe disease can develop, leading to profuse diarrhea, severe abdominal pain or distention, leukocytosis, elevated serum creatinine, or hypoalbuminemia [20]. Fulminant disease, characterized by ileus, toxic megacolon, hypotension, or shock, is uncommon, occurring in 2–7% of children with CDI [20, 21].

Diagnosis

The hospitalized child with nosocomial diarrhea should undergo evaluation to determine the source of their symptoms. An important first step is to verify the presence of clinically significant diarrhea. As patients and families (even, healthcare providers) may use the term "diarrhea" inconsistently, one should clarify the onset, frequency, and consistency of bowel movements. A common definition of diarrhea is the passage of ≥3 loose stools per day, although it is important to recognize that this description may be inadequate for young children, particularly neonates, who can have multiple stools per day in the absence of illness. Any deviation from the child's typical stooling pattern should be noted; but an increase in stool frequency with loose or watery stools generally characterizes enteric infections.

A significant portion of nosocomial diarrhea, particularly mild episodes, is related to medical interventions common to hospital settings ("iatrogenic diarrhea") (see section "Noninfectious Etiologies"). The medication history should be reviewed, focusing on agents that are known to cause diarrhea – laxatives, stool

Table 12.1 Diagnostic tests for selected enteric pathogens

Organism	Test	Comment
Clostridium difficile	NAAT Toxin A/B EIA Multi-step algorithms: 1. GDH antigen followed by toxin A/B EIA 2. GDH antigen followed by NAAT	NAAT are very sensitive and may identify incidental carriers of *C. difficile*
Norovirus	NAAT	
Rotavirus	EIA NAAT	
Salmonella, Shigella, Campylobacter	Routine stool culture	
Shiga toxin-producing *Escherichia coli*	Stool culture for *E. coli* 0157:H7 Shiga toxin immunoassay NAAT	NAAT detects Shiga toxin genes, which can also be found in *Shigella* species

Adapted from reference [22]

NAAT nucleic acid amplification test, *EIA* enzyme immunoassay, *GDH* glutamate dehydrogenase

softeners, antibiotics, and chemotherapeutics. For patients receiving enteral feeding, the feeding regimen should be reviewed and optimized, considering the formula composition, site of infusion (gastric versus post-pyloric), type of infusion (continuous versus bolus), and the rate of infusion. The medical and surgical history should be reviewed as diarrhea can be a symptom of an underlying gastrointestinal disorder.

After confirming the presence of clinically significant diarrhea and determining that stool testing is indicated, many providers will target testing toward the most likely pathogen (see Table 12.1) [22]. *Clostridium difficile* should be considered in patients >12 months with risk factors and clinically significant diarrhea. Enteric viruses, especially norovirus, should be considered when vomiting is a prominent symptom. Routine stool cultures – which detect *Salmonella*, *Shigella*, *Campylobacter*, *Yersinia*, and Shiga toxin-producing *Escherichia coli* – have a very low yield and are not cost-effective when routinely performed for nosocomial diarrhea. Several publications recommend that microbiology laboratories reject orders for stool cultures after the third hospital day, except from immunocompromised patients or during a suspected nosocomial outbreak ("3-day rule") [23, 24].

Recently, multiplex gastrointestinal panels have become available that detect a broad range of bacteria, viruses, and parasites from a single stool specimen. These molecular-based assays allow for a variety of enteric pathogens to be tested in a few hours' time. Since they are more sensitive than conventional testing methodologies, they yield a higher positivity rate. Clinical interpretation of these panels, however, can be challenging due to their ability to detect low-level colonization or nonviable organisms as well as their tendency to detect multiple pathogens. The gastrointestinal panels may, however, prove promising for immunocompromised patients or for rapid investigation of suspected outbreaks. Further research is needed to guide the clinical use of these new diagnostic panels [25].

Causes of Healthcare-Associated Diarrhea

Norovirus

Norovirus is the most common cause of sporadic and epidemic gastroenteritis in the United States [11, 26]. The noroviruses are single-stranded RNA viruses comprised of six genogroups. The 2 genogroups that commonly cause human disease, GI and GII, are further divided into 9 and 22 genotypes, respectively. The GII.4 virus is the most prevalent in human disease. It is strongly associated with person-to-person transmission, outbreaks in healthcare settings, and more severe disease [27, 28]. Genogroup I viruses are associated with foodborne and waterborne outbreaks [28].

Norovirus outbreaks have been reported in restaurants, schools, military barracks, and cruise ships; however, the majority of outbreaks occur in healthcare facilities [28]. Their low infectious dose, high viral load in feces, and environmental stability render noroviruses particularly effective at spreading within semi-enclosed settings [29]. In the United States, the majority of norovirus outbreaks within healthcare institutions occur in long-term care facilities [29]. Norovirus outbreaks can spread rapidly within hospitals. A recent study estimated that the average time from the infection of one patient to another during norovirus outbreaks was 1.86 days [16]. According to a 2010 systematic review, the median number of affected patients in hospital outbreaks was 30 (range: 3–95 patients), and the median outbreak duration was 19 days (range: 6–92 days) [30]. Healthcare workers are often infected during outbreaks, though their role in the propagation of hospital outbreaks remains unclear.

Norovirus was initially described as the "winter vomiting disease" due to its seasonality and tendency to cause vomiting as a major symptom. The incubation period is relatively short (24–48 h), and the onset of symptoms is typically abrupt. Children with hospital-acquired norovirus infection tend to have a more severe and protracted illness than children with community-acquired disease [31]. Immunocompromised children can have symptoms for weeks to months [19]. Asymptomatic norovirus infection can occur, though asymptomatic shedders, whether patient or healthcare staff, rarely contribute to hospital outbreaks [32].

The preferred method for laboratory detection of norovirus infection is reverse transcriptase polymerase chain reaction (RT-PCR). Testing can be performed with a stand-alone assay or as part of a multiplex gastrointestinal panel. Since children with norovirus infection can have viral shedding for weeks after their illness (and immunocompromised children for months), a positive RT-PCR test may not establish norovirus as the etiology of the illness. Therefore, the results of diagnostic testing should be interpreted with epidemiology and clinical factors. If norovirus diagnostic tests are unavailable, an effective tool at identifying outbreaks is the Kaplan criteria – vomiting in >50% of patients, mean incubation period of 24–48 h, mean duration of illness of 12–60 h, and no bacterial pathogen detected [33].

The treatment of norovirus infection is supportive. Dehydration and electrolyte abnormalities should be managed in all patients. Antiemetics may be helpful for some patients. Several candidate norovirus vaccines are currently under development.

Rotavirus

Prior to the introduction of the rotavirus vaccine, rotavirus was estimated to cause around two million hospitalizations and 440,000 deaths worldwide in children less than 5 years of age [34]. Young children are particularly at risk of rotavirus infection, with severe infection and dehydration more likely in children <2 years [35].

Rotavirus is highly contagious. It has a small infectious dose and is excreted in high amounts in stool. The hospital environment can serve as a reservoir for rotavirus transmission, as the virus can survive up to 10 days on dry, nonporous surfaces [36].

Nosocomial infections represent a significant proportion of the overall burden of rotavirus disease. A 2012 meta-analysis estimates that the year-round nosocomial rotavirus incidence is 0.4 per 100 hospitalizations. The incidence was the highest for children under 2 years of age hospitalized during epidemic months (8.1 nosocomial rotavirus infections per 100 hospitalizations) [37]. Following introduction of the rotavirus vaccine, studies have documented a decline in the burden of nosocomial rotavirus disease [10, 38].

Rotavirus causes a watery diarrhea associated with vomiting and low-grade fever that can last for several days. Among nosocomial cases, asymptomatic infection appears to be common in neonates and young infants [39]. Nosocomial infection can prolong hospital stay, necessitate rehydration therapy, and increase hospital costs [40, 41].

Enzyme-linked immunosorbent assays (ELISA) or molecular-based assays can detect rotavirus in stool specimens. ELISA can detect virus in the 1–2 days prior to symptom onset and up to 2 weeks following the illness [42]. The treatment of rotavirus infection is supportive. Oral and intravenous rehydration therapy is used when indicated.

Other Enteric Viruses

Although norovirus and rotavirus cause the majority of hospital-acquired viral gastroenteritis in children, several other viruses are also implicated in childhood diarrhea. These viruses – the enteric adenoviruses (serotypes 40 and 41), astrovirus, and sapovirus – cause a clinical syndrome similar to norovirus and rotavirus and have been reported to cause nosocomial enteric infections. Laboratory detection of these viruses generally requires molecular-based assays, though an enzyme immunoassay (EIA) is available for the enteric adenoviruses [22].

Both sporadic and epidemic nosocomial diseases have been described with the enteric adenoviruses [18, 43]. An outbreak of adenovirus type 41 in a pediatric HSCT unit impacted six patients and was terminated only after enhanced infection control practices were implemented [44]. Astrovirus is the cause of <10% of viral gastroenteritis in children. It tends to affect young infants and can occasionally cause nosocomial disease in children's hospitals [45, 46]. Sapovirus, which is in the same Caliciviridae family as norovirus, can cause outbreaks in schools, childcare centers, and long-term care facilities [47, 48]. Sapovirus is an uncommon cause of hospital-acquired gastroenteritis in children [18, 49].

Clostridium difficile

Clostridium difficile is the most common bacterial cause of nosocomial diarrhea in children and adults. It is an important cause of antibiotic-associated diarrhea and one of the most common healthcare-associated pathogens in the United States [50].

Clostridium difficile is an anaerobic, toxin-producing, gram-positive bacillus. In the environment, it exists in a spore form, rendering it resistant to alcohol, gastric acid, antibiotics, and most disinfectants. Following ingestion, spores germinate into the vegetative form upon reaching the intestine. Toxin-producing ("toxigenic") strains are capable of producing disease through the expression of toxins A and B, which injure the mucosal epithelial cells of the large intestine. Non-toxigenic strains are not capable of causing intestinal disease.

A change in the frequency and severity of *Clostridium difficile* infection (CDI) occurred in the early 2000s. Hospital outbreaks of unusually severe disease were attributed to the emergence of a new strain, the hypervirulent NAP1/BI/027 strain [51]. Around this time, CDI incidence began to increase among hospitalized children [9, 52, 53]. A study of 22 children's hospitals in the United States found a 53% increase in pediatric CDI from 2001 to 2006 (2.6 to 4.0 cases per 1000 admissions) despite a constant rate of *C. difficile* testing [9]. CDI also occurs in children outside of hospital settings, with recent studies suggesting that community-acquired disease is increasing in children [21, 54]. *Clostridium difficile* can cause significant morbidity in children; hospitalized children with CDI have longer hospital stay, increased hospital costs, and greater risk of in-hospital mortality [55]

Exposure to antibiotics is the most important risk factor for CDI in children [17, 56, 57]. Multiple antibiotics have been implicated, particularly broad-spectrum antibiotics including cephalosporins, clindamycin, and fluoroquinolones. Gastric acid suppressants (both proton pump inhibitors and histamine-2 receptor antagonists) have also been associated with pediatric CDI [58, 59]. Several medical conditions are associated with pediatric CDI, including malignancy, solid organ transplantation, inflammatory bowel disease, and cystic fibrosis.

CDI can produce a spectrum of disease, ranging from asymptomatic colonization or mild watery diarrhea to severe colitis complicated by toxic megacolon and shock. Most patients have mild to moderate diarrhea. Fulminant disease, characterized by ileus, toxic megacolon, hypotension, or shock, is uncommon, occurring in 2–7% of children [20].

Multiple diagnostic tests are available for *C. difficile*. Toxin enzyme immunoassays (EIA) detect free toxin – either toxin A and/or B – in stool. They are relatively inexpensive and have a rapid turnaround time, though they are limited by poor sensitivity. Nucleic acid amplification tests (NAATs) detect the presence of toxin-producing *C. difficile*. They are highly sensitive and specific. Importantly, they cannot distinguish colonization from clinical infection and, as a consequence, may detect incidental *C. difficile* carriers. Multi-step algorithms may optimize testing performance and are endorsed by US and European guidelines [60, 61]. The algorithms generally include an EIA for glutamate dehydrogenase – an enzyme produced by toxigenic and non-toxigenic strains – as an initial screening test. If positive, additional testing is necessary to detect the presence of toxin or toxigenic organism.

Given that highly sensitive NAAT diagnostic tests may identify carriers of *C. difficile*, it is important to avoid testing in patients with a low likelihood of CDI [62–64]. Thus, several items should be considered before testing (see Table 12.2). Importantly, testing should only be performed in children with clinically significant diarrhea. Infants <12 months old should not be tested, since fecal carriage is highly prevalent during infancy and *C. difficile* has not been shown to be a pathogen in this population. Testing should only be performed on unformed stool. Repeat testing and "tests of cure" are unnecessary and may increase the risk of false-positive results [61, 62, 65]. Clinician education and computerized order alerts can decrease unnecessary *C. difficile* testing at children's hospitals [63, 64].

The initial management of CDI includes supportive care and the discontinuation of inciting antibiotics [61]. Metronidazole and vancomycin are effective for patients needing therapy directed at *C. difficile*. Both agents are effective at achieving clinical cure, although vancomycin may have a lower recurrence rate [66]. Either metronidazole or vancomycin is recommended for children with mild to moderate disease (Table 12.3); current guidelines, however, favor vancomycin or fidaxomicin over metronidazole for adults with mild to moderate disease [61]. Vancomycin is preferred for children with severe disease since studies indicate adults with severe CDI that receive vancomycin have a higher cure rate than those receiving metronidazole [62]. For children with severe disease that are unable to tolerate oral therapy, rectal installation of vancomycin and intravenous metronidazole is preferred.

Recurrent *C. difficile* infection – a return of infection after a period of symptom resolution – occurs in 15–25% of children with CDI [20, 67]. Recurrences may reflect a relapse from the previous infecting strain or reinfection with a new strain. Risk factors for recurrent CDI in children include underlying malignancy, exposure to multiple antibiotic classes, and receipt of concomitant antibiotics [67, 68]. The optimal management of *C. difficile* recurrences has not been determined. For the first recurrence, a second course with the same antibiotic used during the initial episode is generally preferred. For subsequent recurrences, vancomycin is the

Table 12.2 Considerations for *Clostridium difficile* testing in children

Only test patients with clinically significant diarrhea (≥3 unformed stools per day)
Only perform testing on loose or watery stool specimens
Avoid testing children that have received laxatives or stool softeners in the previous 48 h
Age-specific considerations: Children <12 months old: avoid testing   Children 12–36 months old: only test children with risk factors and after other causes have been excluded
Do not perform a "test of cure" after treatment
Do not perform multiple tests on a single patient

Adapted from references [62–64]

Table 12.3 Treatment of *Clostridium difficile* infection in children

	Treatment	Dose
Initial episode, mild to moderate disease	Metronidazole, OR	7.5 mg/kg/dose (max: 500 mg/dose) PO 3–4 times daily × 10 days
	Vancomycin	10 mg/kg/dose (max: 125 mg/dose) PO 4 times daily × 10 days
First recurrence	Vancomycin	10 mg/kg/dose (max: 125 mg/dose) PO 4 times daily × 10 days
Subsequent recurrences	Vancomycin taper/pulse regimen	10 mg/kg/dose (max: 125 mg/dose) PO 4 times daily × 10–14 days, then 2 times daily × 7 days, then daily × 7 days, then every 2–3 days for 2–8 weeks
	Fidaxomicin[a]	8 mg/kg/dose (max: 200 mg/dose) PO 2 times daily × 10 days
	Vancomycin with "rifaximin chaser"	Vancomycin: 10 mg/kg/dose (max: 125 mg/dose) PO 4 times daily × 10 days; then Rifaximin[b] 10 mg/kg/dose (max: 400 mg/dose) 3 times daily × 20 days.
	Fecal microbiota transplantation	
Severe or Fulminant disease[c]	Vancomycin	10 mg/kg/dose PO 4 times daily [max: 500 mg/dose] × 10 days
	Metronidazole (add when ileus or toxic megacolon is present)	10 mg/kg/dose IV 3 times daily [max: 500 mg/dose] × 10 days

Adapted from reference [61]
[a]Fidaxomicin is not FDA approved for children <18 years of age
[b]Rifaximin is not FDA approved for children <12 years of age. There is also limited data to guide pediatric dosing
[c]Rectal installation of vancomycin should be considered for patients with an ileus or toxic megacolon

preferred agent [61, 62]. A pulse-tapered regimen of vancomycin has been successful in observational studies and a clinical trial in adults [69, 70]. Prolonged or frequent courses of metronidazole are discouraged due to the potential for neurotoxicity. Additional agents used for recurrent CDI in children include fidaxomicin, rifaximin following a standard course of vancomycin ("rifaximin chaser"), and nitazoxanide. Fidaxomicin, which is currently only approved for individuals ≥18 years old, has been shown to have a lower recurrence rate compared to vancomycin in randomized trials in adults [71]. Fecal microbiota transplantation (FMT), the administration of donor fecal matter, was found effective in adults with recurrent CDI, but the pediatric experience remains limited to case reports and case series.

Bacterial Enteritis

Aside from *C. difficile*, bacterial enteropathogens are rarely implicated in nosocomial diarrhea. Yet given their ability to cause rapid (and dramatic) hospital outbreaks, it is critical to consider these organisms when evaluating a child with nosocomial diarrhea. *Salmonella*, *Shigella*, *Campylobacter*, and diarrheagenic *E. coli* can spread within healthcare facilities through contaminated food, person-to-person contact, or indirectly through contaminated medical equipment or an inadequately cleaned hospital environment.

Outbreaks due to nontyphoidal *Salmonella* species have occurred in acute care and long-term care facilities. The majority of hospital outbreaks are foodborne, with secondary cases occurring through person-to-person transmission. Egg products and undercooked meats are the most commonly implicated foods [72]. Powder infant formula contaminated with nontyphoidal *Salmonella* has caused an outbreak among hospitalized infants [73]. Additionally, inadequate decontamination of medical equipment, including gastrointestinal endoscopes and transesophageal echocardiography probes, has resulted in nosocomial salmonellosis [74, 75]. A review of 52 nosocomial *Salmonella* outbreaks between 1995 and 2011 found published outbreaks in 15 neonatal/maternity units and 7 pediatric wards [72]. *Salmonella* outbreaks are estimated to cost hospitals $1800 of direct costs per nosocomial infection [76].

Diarrheagenic *E. coli* can be an important hospital pathogen in pediatric facilities in developing countries [12, 77]. Enteropathogenic *E. coli* (EPEC) was previously recognized to cause outbreaks of severe diarrheal disease with high attack rates in newborn nurseries [78, 79]. Enterotoxigenic *E. coli* (ETEC) generally causes community-acquired diarrhea in children <2 years old in developing countries. Hospital outbreaks from ETEC attributed to contaminated formula have occurred in newborns and infants [80–82]. Shiga toxin-producing *E. coli* (STEC), including *E. coli* 0157, have been reported to be transmitted within healthcare settings. Contaminated homemade food brought into the hospital precipitated one published outbreak [83]. Person-to-person transmission following admission of an infected patient is probably the most common transmission route for nosocomial disease. Also, hospital personnel can acquire STEC from patients in the course of clinical care [84].

Additional bacterial pathogens have caused HA gastrointestinal infections. *Campylobacter* species have caused hospital outbreaks related to contamination of hospital food or water. Nursery outbreaks of *Campylobacter* diarrhea and meningitis have also been documented [85–87]. Hospital outbreaks of foodborne *Listeria monocytogenes* have been reported [88, 89]. *Shigella* species, despite its low infectious dose, is only rarely acquired in hospital settings [90, 91]. In developing countries, cholera can be transmitted within hospitals by contaminated water or by person-to-person spread [92].

Noninfectious Etiologies

Noninfectious factors can contribute to the development of diarrhea among inpatients. Medications and tube feeding are of particular importance. Diarrhea is a well-documented side effect for various medicines (see Table 12.4).

Table 12.4 Selected medications associated with diarrhea

Drug category	Comment
Antibiotics	Broad-spectrum antibiotics are most commonly implicated
Antineoplastics	Important examples include 5-fluorour acil, methotrexate, and cisplatin
Antiretrovirals	Protease inhibitors can cause steatorrhea
Gastric acid suppressants	Can occur with both protein pump inhibitors and H_2 receptor antagonists
Immunosuppressants	Examples include cyclophosphamide, mycophenolate mofetil, and sirolimus
Laxatives	Common cause of diarrhea in healthcare settings. Examples include osmotic agents (e.g., polyethylene glycol, lactulose, and magnesium salts) and stimulants (e.g., bisacodyl, senna)
NSAIDs	Long-term usage can lead to mucosal injury and diarrhea

Adapted from references [93, 94]

Antibiotics cause diarrhea in about 10–20% of children who receive them [95]. Broad-spectrum antibiotics – aminopenicillins (especially when administered with clavulanate), cephalosporins, and clindamycin – are particularly prone to causing diarrhea. Antibiotic-associated diarrhea occurs through several mechanisms – disruption of intestinal microbiota, overgrowth of enteric pathogens (i.e., *Clostridium difficile*), and alterations in metabolic function leading to colonic dysfunction [96].

Laxatives, given their frequent use within hospital settings, can be an overlooked cause of nosocomial diarrhea [97]. Sorbitol, when used as an excipient, can cause diarrhea due to its osmotic effects [93]. Medication classes that are recognized to cause diarrhea include chemotherapeutics, immunosuppressants, proton pump inhibitors, and nonsteroidal anti-inflammatory drugs. Additionally, diarrhea is a common symptom of opioid withdrawal in critically ill children who have received prolonged analgesics or sedatives [98].

The most common side effect from tube feeding is diarrhea. Advancing the amount of daily feed and too rapid of an infusion rate can cause diarrhea. Hyperosmolar feedings can also cause diarrhea [99].

Infection Prevention

General Prevention Measures

Sound infection control measures are critical to the prevention of healthcare-associated infections (see Chap. 1 for a discussion on the basic principles of infection control). In this section, we will highlight infection control practices as they relate to gastrointestinal infections.

Hand hygiene is the foundation of infection prevention. Its importance for HA gastrointestinal infections cannot be overemphasized since healthcare workers, hands are potential vehicles for transmitting enteric pathogens. One study found that a hospital-wide hand hygiene campaign at a children's hospital improved hand hygiene compliance and decreased rates of nosocomial rotavirus [100]. Alcohol-based hand disinfectants, though generally encouraged within healthcare facilities, are less effective at the removal of norovirus and *C. difficile* spores from hands [101, 102]. Thus, handwashing with soap and water is encouraged when caring for patients with a known or suspected infection from norovirus or *C. difficile*.

Contact precautions (gowns and gloves) should be observed for the duration of diarrheal symptoms. A longer duration of isolation may be warranted for immuno-compromised patients as they shed enteric pathogens for a greater period of time. Careful attention to routine environmental cleaning and disinfection of patient care areas is important as multiple enteric pathogens can survive for a long time on hospital surfaces. Standard cleaning products are appropriate for the majority of pathogens, though they are inadequate against norovirus and *C. difficile* spores. Sodium hypochlorite (bleach) solution has been shown to be effective against both agents [29, 103]. Alternative non-bleach-based, EPA-approved cleaning products are also available.

Antibiotic stewardship has become an important strategy in the prevention of hospital-acquired *C. difficile* infection. The restriction of high-risk antibiotics (i.e., clindamycin, cephalosporins, and fluoroquinolones) has been effective in decreasing *C. difficile* infection rates in outbreak settings [103]. (See Chap. 3 for a discussion on antimicrobial stewardship).

Outbreak Management

Hospital outbreaks of gastrointestinal infections can unfold rapidly. During outbreak settings, it is important to emphasize strict adherence to basic infection control practices and to implement enhanced prevention strategies. Norovirus is the most likely organism to cause a hospital outbreak of infectious diarrhea. Guidelines are available from the CDC on the prevention and management of norovirus outbreaks [104].

During outbreaks of *C. difficile* or norovirus, the use of soap and water, instead of alcohol-based disinfectants, for hand hygiene is recommended. Single occupancy rooms should be used for patients with infectious diarrhea when possible. Cohorting patients into separate groups – symptomatic, exposed and asymptomatic, and unexposed – is a measure to be considered to limit the potential for person-to-person transmission. Strict adherence to contact isolation should be followed for patients with infectious diarrhea. For norovirus, contact isolation should be extended for at least 48 h after symptom duration in outbreak settings, as per CDC guidelines [104]. Also, it is important to minimize the access of visitors and nonessential personnel to the affected unit.

Early recognition of hospital-based foodborne outbreaks allows for earlier interventions – whether removal of the contaminated food product and/or exclusion of an infected food handler. Ill food handlers should remain off work for at least 48 h. Adherence to the US Food and Drug Administration Food Code is important in the prevention of foodborne outbreaks.

References

1. Scallan E, Griffin PM, Angulo FJ, Tauxe RV, Hoekstra RM. Foodborne illness acquired in the United States--unspecified agents. Emerg Infect Dis. 2011;17:16–22.
2. Jones TF, McMillian MB, Scallan E, et al. A population-based estimate of the substantial burden of diarrhoeal disease in the United States; FoodNet, 1996–2003. Epidemiol Infect. 2007;135:293–301.
3. Brady MT, Pacini DL, Budde CT, Connell MJ. Diagnostic studies of nosocomial diarrhea in children: assessing their use and value. Am J Infect Control. 1989;17:77–82.
4. Ford-Jones EL, Mindorff CM, Langley JM, et al. Epidemiologic study of 4684 hospital-acquired infections in pediatric patients. Pediatr Infect Dis J. 1989;8:668–75.
5. Langley JM, LeBlanc JC, Hanakowski M, Goloubeva O. The role of Clostridium difficile and viruses as causes of nosocomial diarrhea in children. Infect Control Hosp Epidemiol. 2002;23:660–4.
6. Kamalaratnam CN, Kang G, Kirubakaran C, et al. A prospective study of nosocomial enteric pathogen acquisition in hospitalized children in South India. J Trop Pediatr. 2001;47:46–9.
7. Ford-Jones EL, Mindorff CM, Gold R, Petric M. The incidence of viral-associated diarrhea after admission to a pediatric hospital. Am J Epidemiol. 1990;131:711–8.
8. Sidler JA, Haberthur C, Dumoulin A, Hirsch HH, Heininger U. A retrospective analysis of nosocomial viral gastrointestinal and respiratory tract infections. Pediatr Infect Dis J. 2012;31:1233–8.
9. Kim J, Smathers SA, Prasad P, Leckerman KH, Coffin S, Zaoutis T. Epidemiological features of Clostridium difficile-associated disease among inpatients at children's hospitals in the United States, 2001–2006. Pediatrics. 2008;122:1266–70.
10. Anderson EJ, Rupp A, Shulman ST, Wang D, Zheng X, Noskin GA. Impact of rotavirus vaccination on hospital-acquired rotavirus gastroenteritis in children. Pediatrics. 2011;127:e264–70.
11. Payne DC, Vinje J, Szilagyi PG, et al. Norovirus and medically attended gastroenteritis in U.S. children. N Engl J Med. 2013;368:1121–30.
12. Chandra BK, Singh G, Taneja N, Pahil S, Singhi S, Sharma M. Diarrhoeagenic Escherichia coli as a predominant cause of paediatric nosocomial diarrhoea in India. J Med Microbiol. 2012;61:830–6.
13. Raymond J, Aujard Y. Nosocomial infections in pediatric patients: a European, multicenter prospective study. European Study Group. Infect Control Hosp Epidemiol. 2000;21:260–3.
14. Rutledge-Taylor K, Matlow A, Gravel D, et al. A point prevalence survey of health care-associated infections in Canadian pediatric inpatients. Am J Infect Control. 2012;40:491–6.
15. Fischer TK, Bresee JS, Glass RI. Rotavirus vaccines and the prevention of hospital-acquired diarrhea in children. Vaccine. 2004;22(Suppl 1):S49–54.
16. Harris JP, Lopman BA, Cooper BS, O'Brien SJ. Does spatial proximity drive norovirus transmission during outbreaks in hospitals? BMJ Open. 2013;3:e003060.
17. Sandora TJ, Fung M, Flaherty K, et al. Epidemiology and risk factors for Clostridium difficile infection in children. Pediatr Infect Dis J. 2011;30:580–4.
18. Cunliffe NA, Booth JA, Elliot C, et al. Healthcare-associated viral gastroenteritis among children in a large pediatric hospital, United Kingdom. Emerg Infect Dis. 2010;16:55–62.
19. Ye X, Van JN, Munoz FM, et al. Noroviruses as a cause of diarrhea in immunocompromised pediatric hematopoietic stem cell and solid organ transplant recipients. Am J Transplant. 2015;15:1874–81.
20. Crews JD, Koo HL, Jiang ZD, Starke JR, DuPont HL. A hospital-based study of the clinical characteristics of Clostridium difficile infection in children. Pediatr Infect Dis J. 2014;33:924–8.
21. Khanna S, Baddour LM, Huskins WC, et al. The epidemiology of Clostridium difficile infection in children: a population-based study. Clin Infect Dis. 2013;56:1401–6.

22. Shane AL, Mody RK, Crump JA, et al. 2017 Infectious Diseases Society of America clinical practice guidelines for the diagnosis and management of infectious diarrhea. Clin Infect Dis. 2017;65:1963–73.
23. Bauer TM, Lalvani A, Fehrenbach J, et al. Derivation and validation of guidelines for stool cultures for enteropathogenic bacteria other than Clostridium difficile in hospitalized adults. JAMA. 2001;285:313–9.
24. Zaidi AK, Macone A, Goldmann AD. Impact of simple screening criteria on utilization of low-yield bacterial stool cultures in a children's hospital. Pediatrics. 1999;103:1189–92.
25. Binnicker MJ. Multiplex molecular panels for diagnosis of gastrointestinal infection: performance, result interpretation, and cost-effectiveness. J Clin Microbiol. 2015;53:3723–8.
26. Ahmed SM, Hall AJ, Robinson AE, et al. Global prevalence of norovirus in cases of gastroenteritis: a systematic review and meta-analysis. Lancet Infect Dis. 2014;14:725–30.
27. Huhti L, Szakal ED, Puustinen L, et al. Norovirus GII-4 causes a more severe gastroenteritis than other noroviruses in young children. J Infect Dis. 2011;203:1442–4.
28. Vega E, Barclay L, Gregoricus N, Shirley SH, Lee D, Vinje J. Genotypic and epidemiologic trends of norovirus outbreaks in the United States, 2009–2013. J Clin Microbiol. 2014;52:147–55.
29. Barclay L, Park GW, Vega E, et al. Infection control for norovirus. Clin Microbiol Infect. 2014;20:731–40.
30. Harris JP, Lopman BA, O'Brien SJ. Infection control measures for norovirus: a systematic review of outbreaks in semi-enclosed settings. J Hosp Infect. 2010;74:1–9.
31. Munir N, Liu P, Gastanaduy P, Montes J, Shane A, Moe C. Norovirus infection in immunocompromised children and children with hospital-acquired acute gastroenteritis. J Med Virol. 2014;86:1203–9.
32. Sukhrie FH, Teunis P, Vennema H, et al. Nosocomial transmission of norovirus is mainly caused by symptomatic cases. Clin Infect Dis. 2012;54:931–7.
33. Turcios RM, Widdowson MA, Sulka AC, Mead PS, Glass RI. Reevaluation of epidemiological criteria for identifying outbreaks of acute gastroenteritis due to norovirus: United States, 1998–2000. Clin Infect Dis. 2006;42:964–9.
34. Parashar UD, Hummelman EG, Bresee JS, Miller MA, Glass RI. Global illness and deaths caused by rotavirus disease in children. Emerg Infect Dis. 2003;9:565–72.
35. Parashar UD, Nelson EA, Kang G. Diagnosis, management, and prevention of rotavirus gastroenteritis in children. BMJ (Clinical research ed). 2013;347:f7204.
36. Gleizes O, Desselberger U, Tatochenko V, et al. Nosocomial rotavirus infection in European countries: a review of the epidemiology, severity and economic burden of hospital-acquired rotavirus disease. Pediatr Infect Dis J. 2006;25:S12–21.
37. Bruijning-Verhagen P, Quach C, Bonten M. Nosocomial rotavirus infections: a meta-analysis. Pediatrics. 2012;129:e1011–9.
38. Zlamy M, Kofler S, Orth D, et al. The impact of Rotavirus mass vaccination on hospitalization rates, nosocomial Rotavirus gastroenteritis and secondary blood stream infections. BMC Infect Dis. 2013;13:112.
39. Gianino P, Mastretta E, Longo P, et al. Incidence of nosocomial rotavirus infections, symptomatic and asymptomatic, in breast-fed and non-breast-fed infants. J Hosp Infect. 2002;50:13–7.
40. Gervasi G, Capanna A, Mita V, Zaratti L, Franco E. Nosocomial rotavirus infection: an up to date evaluation of European studies. Hum Vaccin Immunother. 2016;12:2413–8.
41. Verhagen P, Moore D, Manges A, Quach C. Nosocomial rotavirus gastroenteritis in a Canadian paediatric hospital: incidence, disease burden and patients affected. J Hosp Infect. 2011;79:59–63.
42. Pickering LK, Bartlett AV 3rd, Reves RR, Morrow A. Asymptomatic excretion of rotavirus before and after rotavirus diarrhea in children in day care centers. J Pediatr. 1988;112:361–5.
43. Carraturo A, Catalani V, Tega L. Microbiological and epidemiological aspects of rotavirus and enteric adenovirus infections in hospitalized children in Italy. New Microbiol. 2008;31:329–36.

44. Mattner F, Sykora KW, Meissner B, Heim A. An adenovirus type F41 outbreak in a pediatric bone marrow transplant unit: analysis of clinical impact and preventive strategies. Pediatr Infect Dis J. 2008;27:419–24.
45. Galdiero E, Marinelli A, Pisciotta MG, Pagliara I, Di Monteforte ES, Liguori G. Reverse transcriptase-PCR for the detection of Astrovirus in children with nosocomial acute diarrhoea in Naples, Italy. Med Mal Infect. 2005;35:213–7.
46. Shastri S, Doane AM, Gonzales J, Upadhyayula U, Bass DM. Prevalence of astroviruses in a children's hospital. J Clin Microbiol. 1998;36:2571–4.
47. Lyman WH, Walsh JF, Kotch JB, Weber DJ, Gunn E, Vinje J. Prospective study of etiologic agents of acute gastroenteritis outbreaks in child care centers. J Pediatr. 2009;154:253–7.
48. Pang XL, Lee BE, Tyrrell GJ, Preiksaitis JK. Epidemiology and genotype analysis of sapovirus associated with gastroenteritis outbreaks in Alberta, Canada: 2004–2007. J Infect Dis. 2009;199:547–51.
49. Brown JR, Shah D, Breuer J. Viral gastrointestinal infections and norovirus genotypes in a paediatric UK hospital, 2014–2015. J Clin Virol. 2016;84:1–6.
50. Lessa FC, Winston LG, McDonald LC, Emerging Infections Program CdST. Burden of Clostridium difficile infection in the United States. N Engl J Med. 2015;372:2369–70.
51. McDonald LC, Killgore GE, Thompson A, et al. An epidemic, toxin gene-variant strain of Clostridium difficile. N Engl J Med. 2005;353:2433–41.
52. Zilberberg MD, Tillotson GS, McDonald C. Clostridium difficile infections among hospitalized children, United States, 1997–2006. Emerg Infect Dis. 2010;16:604–9.
53. Nylund CM, Goudie A, Garza JM, Fairbrother G, Cohen MB. Clostridium difficile infection in hospitalized children in the United States. Arch Pediatr Adolesc Med. 2011;165:451–7.
54. Wendt JM, Cohen JA, Mu Y, et al. Clostridium difficile infection among children across diverse US geographic locations. Pediatrics. 2014;133:651–8.
55. Sammons JS, Localio R, Xiao R, Coffin SE, Zaoutis T. Clostridium difficile infection is associated with increased risk of death and prolonged hospitalization in children. Clin Infect Dis. 2013;57:1–8.
56. Crews JD, Anderson LR, Waller DK, Swartz MD, DuPont HL, Starke JR. Risk factors for community-associated Clostridium difficile-associated diarrhea in children. Pediatr Infect Dis J. 2015;34:919–23.
57. Adams DJ, Eberly MD, Rajnik M, Nylund CM. Risk factors for community-associated Clostridium difficile infection in children. J Pediatr. 2017;186:105–9.
58. Freedberg DE, Lamouse-Smith ES, Lightdale JR, Jin Z, Yang YX, Abrams JA. Use of acid suppression medication is associated with risk for C. difficile infection in infants and children: a population-based study. Clin Infect Dis. 2015;61:912–7.
59. Nylund CM, Eide M, Gorman GH. Association of Clostridium difficile infections with acid suppression medications in children. J Pediatr. 2014;165:979–84 e1.
60. Crobach MJ, Planche T, Eckert C, et al. European Society of Clinical Microbiology and Infectious Diseases: update of the diagnostic guidance document for Clostridium difficile infection. Clin Microbiol Infect. 2016;22(Suppl 4):S63–81.
61. McDonald LC, Gerding DN, Johnson S, et al. Clinical practice guidelines for Clostridium difficile infection in adults and children: 2017 update by the Infectious Diseases Society of America (IDSA) and Society for Healthcare Epidemiology of America (SHEA). Clin Infect Dis. 2018;66:e1–e48.
62. Schutze GE, Willoughby RE, Committee on Infectious D and American Academy of P. Clostridium difficile infection in infants and children. Pediatrics. 2013;131:196–200.
63. Nicholson MR, Freswick PN, Di Pentima MC, et al. The use of a computerized provider order entry alert to decrease rates of Clostridium difficile testing in young pediatric patients. Infect Control Hosp Epidemiol. 2017;38:542–6.
64. Kociolek LK, Bovee M, Carter D, et al. Impact of a healthcare provider educational intervention on frequency of Clostridium difficile polymerase chain reaction testing in children: a segmented regression analysis. J Pediatr Infect Dis Soc. 2017;6:142–8.

65. Deshpande A, Pasupuleti V, Patel P, et al. Repeat stool testing to diagnose Clostridium difficile infection using enzyme immunoassay does not increase diagnostic yield. Clin Gastroenterol Hepatol. 2011;9:665–9 e1.
66. Nelson RL, Suda KJ, Evans CT. Antibiotic treatment for Clostridium difficile-associated diarrhoea in adults. Cochrane Database Syst Rev. 2017;3:CD004610.
67. Nicholson MR, Thomsen IP, Slaughter JC, Creech CB, Edwards KM. Novel risk factors for recurrent Clostridium difficile infection in children. J Pediatr Gastroenterol Nutr. 2015;60:18–22.
68. Tschudin-Sutter S, Tamma PD, Milstone AM, Perl TM. Predictors of first recurrence of Clostridium difficile infections in children. Pediatr Infect Dis J. 2014;33:414–6.
69. Sirbu BD, Soriano MM, Manzo C, Lum J, Gerding DN, Johnson S. Vancomycin taper and pulse regimen with careful follow-up for patients with recurrent Clostridium difficile infection. Clin Infect Dis. 2017;65:1396–9.
70. Hota SS, Sales V, Tomlinson G, et al. Oral vancomycin followed by fecal transplantation versus tapering oral vancomycin treatment for recurrent Clostridium difficile infection: an open-label, randomized controlled trial. Clin Infect Dis. 2017;64:265–71.
71. Cornely OA, Crook DW, Esposito R, et al. Fidaxomicin versus vancomycin for infection with Clostridium difficile in Europe, Canada, and the USA: a double-blind, non-inferiority, randomised controlled trial. Lancet Infect Dis. 2012;12:281–9.
72. Lee MB, Greig JD. A review of nosocomial Salmonella outbreaks: infection control interventions found effective. Public Health. 2013;127:199–206.
73. Bornemann R, Zerr DM, Heath J, et al. An outbreak of Salmonella serotype Saintpaul in a children's hospital. Infect Control Hosp Epidemiol. 2002;23:671–6.
74. Robertson P, Smith A, Anderson M, et al. Transmission of Salmonella enteritidis after endoscopic retrograde cholangiopancreatography because of inadequate endoscope decontamination. Am J Infect Control. 2017;45:440–2.
75. Suleyman G, Tibbetts R, Perri MB, et al. Nosocomial outbreak of a novel extended-spectrum beta-lactamase Salmonella enterica Serotype Isangi among surgical patients. Infect Control Hosp Epidemiol. 2016;37:954–61.
76. Spearing NM, Jensen A, McCall BJ, Neill AS, McCormack JG. Direct costs associated with a nosocomial outbreak of Salmonella infection: an ounce of prevention is worth a pound of cure. Am J Infect Control. 2000;28:54–7.
77. Alrifai SB, Alsaadi A, Mahmood YA, Ali AA, Al-Kaisi LA. Prevalence and etiology of nosocomial diarrhoea in children < 5 years in Tikrit teaching hospital. East Mediterr Health J/La revue de sante de la Mediterranee orientale/al-Majallah al-sihhiyah li-sharq al-mutawassit. 2009;15:1111–8.
78. Gerards LJ, Hennekam RC, von Dijk WC, Roord JJ, Fleer A. An outbreak of gastroenteritis due to Escherichia coli 0142 H6 in a neonatal department. J Hosp Infect. 1984;5:283–8.
79. Boyer KM, Petersen NJ, Farzaneh I, Pattison CP, Hart MC, Maynard JE. An outbreak og gastroenteritis due to E. coli 0142 in a neonatal nursery. J Pediatr. 1975;86:919–27.
80. Ryder RW, Wachsmuth IK, Buxton AE, et al. Infantile diarrhea produced by heat-stable enterotoxigenic Escherichia coli. N Engl J Med. 1976;295:849–53.
81. Taneja N, Das A, Raman Rao DS, Jain N, Singh M, Sharma M. Nosocomial outbreak of diarrhoea by enterotoxigenic Escherichia coli among preterm neonates in a tertiary care hospital in India: pitfalls in healthcare. J Hosp Infect. 2003;53:193–7.
82. Zeng M, Shi W, Chang H, et al. Clonal spread of enterotoxigenic Escherichia coli O128:H45 strain in the neonate unit. Jpn J Infect Dis. 2016;69:127–30.
83. O'Brien SJ, Murdoch PS, Riley AH, et al. A foodborne outbreak of Vero cytotoxin-producing Escherichia coli O157:H-phage type 8 in hospital. J Hosp Infect. 2001;49:167–72.
84. Weightman NC, Kirby PJ. Nosocomial Escherichia coli O157 infection. J Hosp Infect. 2000;44:107–11.
85. Jelovcan S, Schmid D, Lederer I, et al. Cluster of nosocomial campylobacteriosis, Austria 2006. J Hosp Infect. 2008;69:97–8.

86. Morooka T, Umeda A, Fujita M, et al. Epidemiologic application of pulsed-field gel electrophoresis to an outbreak of Campylobacter fetus meningitis in a neonatal intensive care unit. Scand J Infect Dis. 1996;28:269–70.
87. Rautelin H, Koota K, von Essen R, Jahkola M, Siitonen A, Kosunen TU. Waterborne Campylobacter jejuni epidemic in a Finnish hospital for rheumatic diseases. Scand J Infect Dis. 1990;22:321–6.
88. Mazengia E, Kawakami V, Rietberg K, et al. Hospital-acquired listeriosis linked to a persistently contaminated milkshake machine. Epidemiol Infect. 2017;145:857–63.
89. Johnsen BO, Lingaas E, Torfoss D, Strom EH, Nordoy I. A large outbreak of Listeria monocytogenes infection with short incubation period in a tertiary care hospital. J Infect. 2010;61:465–70.
90. Centers for Disease C. Hospital-associated outbreak of Shigella dysenteriae type 2–Maryland. MMWR Morb Mortal Wkly Rep. 1983;32:250–2.
91. Beers LM, Burke TL, Martin DB. Shigellosis occurring in newborn nursery staff. Infect Control Hosp Epidemiol. 1989;10:147–9.
92. Bwire G, Malimbo M, Kagirita A, et al. Nosocomial cholera outbreak in a mental hospital: challenges and lessons learnt from Butabika National Referral Mental Hospital, Uganda. Am J Trop Med Hyg. 2015;93:534–8.
93. Philip NA, Ahmed N, Pitchumoni CS. Spectrum of drug-induced chronic diarrhea. J Clin Gastroenterol. 2017;51:111–7.
94. Abraham B, Sellin JH. Drug-induced diarrhea. Curr Gastroenterol Rep. 2007;9:365–72.
95. Johnston BC, Goldenberg JZ, Parkin PC. Probiotics and the prevention of antibiotic-associated diarrhea in infants and children. JAMA. 2016;316:1484–5.
96. McFarland LV. Antibiotic-associated diarrhea: epidemiology, trends and treatment. Future Microbiol. 2008;3:563–78.
97. Kinlay J, Sandora TJ. A qualitative study to identify reasons for Clostridium difficile testing in pediatric inpatients receiving laxatives or stool softeners. Am J Infect Control. 2017;45:539–41.
98. Ista E, van Dijk M, Gamel C, Tibboel D, de Hoog M. Withdrawal symptoms in critically ill children after long-term administration of sedatives and/or analgesics: a first evaluation. Crit Care Med. 2008;36:2427–32.
99. Blumenstein I, Shastri YM, Stein J. Gastroenteric tube feeding: techniques, problems and solutions. World J Gastroenterol. 2014;20:8505–24.
100. Zerr DM, Allpress AL, Heath J, Bornemann R, Bennett E. Decreasing hospital-associated rotavirus infection: a multidisciplinary hand hygiene campaign in a children's hospital. Pediatr Infect Dis J. 2005;24:397–403.
101. Tuladhar E, Hazeleger WC, Koopmans M, Zwietering MH, Duizer E, Beumer RR. Reducing viral contamination from finger pads: handwashing is more effective than alcohol-based hand disinfectants. J Hosp Infect. 2015;90:226–34.
102. Jabbar U, Leischner J, Kasper D, et al. Effectiveness of alcohol-based hand rubs for removal of Clostridium difficile spores from hands. Infect Control Hosp Epidemiol. 2010;31:565–70.
103. Dubberke ER, Carling P, Carrico R, et al. Strategies to prevent Clostridium difficile infections in acute care hospitals: 2014 update. Infect Control Hosp Epidemiol. 2014;35:628–45.
104. MacCannell T, Umscheid CA, Agarwal RK, et al. Guideline for the prevention and control of norovirus gastroenteritis outbreaks in healthcare settings. Infect Control Hosp Epidemiol. 2011;32:939–69.

Healthcare-Associated Urinary Tract Infections

13

Ann-Christine Nyquist

Introduction

Urinary tract infection is a common healthcare-associated infection (HAI) in the United States for the adult population and accounts for 12.9% of overall HAIs in acute care hospitals and 23% of infections in the ICU [1]. Although catheter-associated urinary tract infections (CAUTIs) predominate in adults, bloodstream infections (BSIs) are the most common HAIs in children. Approximately 70% of HAI UTIs occur in adult patients with an indwelling urinary catheter with most of the remaining cases having had instrumentation of the urinary tract [2]. The burden of healthcare-associated urinary tract infections and CAUTI in pediatric patients is not well defined, and our understanding of the most effective strategies to prevent CAUTI in children is limited due to the dearth of pediatric studies. Indirect evidence from adult studies and adaptation from evidence-based adult CAUTI prevention bundles [3] have been successfully and effectively deployed in the pediatric population [4].

Pathogenesis

Urethral catheterization allows entry of bacteria into the urinary tract via extraluminal and intraluminal routes. The extraluminal route is utilized either early, at the time of catheter insertion, or late, when endogenous organisms colonizing the patient's intestinal tract and perineum ascend along the outer surface of the catheter.

A.-C. Nyquist
Department of Pediatrics, Section of Infectious Diseases and Epidemiology, University of Colorado School of Medicine, Aurora, CO, USA

Infection Prevention and Control, Children's Hospital Colorado, Aurora, CO, USA
e-mail: chris.nyquist@childrenscolorado.org

© Springer Nature Switzerland AG 2019
J. C. McNeil et al. (eds.), *Healthcare-Associated Infections in Children*,
https://doi.org/10.1007/978-3-319-98122-2_13

Bacterial entry via the intraluminal route occurs when contaminated urine refluxes into the bladder from the collection bag or a break in the closed drainage system [5]. Biofilm formation on the catheter after placement into the bladder is crucial for the development and progression of CAUTI. Biofilm, composed of clusters of microorganisms and extracellular matrix, deposits on all surfaces of urinary catheters and allows for bacterial attachment. Although microorganisms grow more slowly in biofilms, the effects of many antimicrobials are diminished, and microorganisms may ascend the catheter to the bladder within 1–3 days [5]. Extraluminal routes of infection comprise approximately two-thirds of CAUTI episodes, and the remaining third result from intraluminal contamination.

Microbiology of CAUTI

The majority of organisms that cause CAUTI are commensal perineal flora, but bacteria acquired from the hands of healthcare personnel have also been implicated [6]. The microbiology of CAUTI in hospitalized children is similar to that reported for community-onset UTIs; enteric organisms such as *Klebsiella* and *Escherichia coli* are most common. Additional pathogens that have been frequently reported include *Pseudomonas, Enterococcus, and Enterobacter* [4, 7, 8]. There is a greater risk that a healthcare-associated CAUTI will be caused by a resistant organism compared to community-onset UTIs. Pediatric HAI infection data reported to the Centers for Disease Control and Prevention National Healthcare Safety Network (NHSN) from 2011 to 2014 described 2366 CAUTI pathogens, 83% were reported by PICUs, and 15% were reported by pediatric wards. Although pathogen distribution was similar between these two locations (*E. coli* and *P. aeruginosa* were the predominant pathogens), resistant organisms were more prevalent on the pediatric wards [8].

Epidemiology of CAUTI

Descriptive epidemiologic studies of pediatric CAUTI are limited. Many acute care hospitals who care for children are not required to report all HAIs in children to the NHSN [9, 10]. Furthermore, there are no high-quality data even in adult populations, where CAUTI is more common, suggesting that CAUTIs prolong a patient's length of stay or increases total costs. A meta-analysis of the financial impact of HAIs attributed relative costs to the following infections in descending order: surgical site infections (SSI, 34%), ventilator-associated pneumonia (VAP, 32%), central line-associated bloodstream infection (CLABSI, 19%), *C. difficile* (15%), and CAUTIs (0.3%) [11].

CAUTI in pediatric ICUs occurs at a rate of 0–3.4 UTI/1000 catheter-days; CAUTI rates in pediatric ICUs may not be decreasing as in other intensive care settings [12, 13]. In fact, despite lower device utilization ratios, CAUTI and CLABSI rates are higher in some pediatric unit types than corresponding adult units [12].

Risk Factors for CAUTI

In adult patient populations, almost all of the UTIs in ICUs are associated with an indwelling catheter. The duration of catheterization is the most important risk factor for CAUTI. The incidence of bacteriuria increases an average of 3–10% per day of catheterization. Other known modifiable risk factors in adults include nonadherence to aseptic catheter care, lower professional training of the inserter, catheter insertion outside the operating room, and catheter insertion after the sixth day of hospitalization. Nonmodifiable risk factors for CAUTI in adults include female sex, severe underlying illness, nonsurgical disease, age > 50 years, diabetes mellitus, and serum creatinine >2 mg/dL [14].

Risk factors for pediatric CAUTI are less well studied but, consistent with adult studies, also include duration of catheterization with an 8% increase in odds for developing infection with each consecutive day the catheter is left in place [7, 15]. Other risk factors in pediatric patients, described in a number of single-center studies, include female patients, chronic conditions, being on contact precautions, prior urinary catheterization, congenital anomalies of kidney and urinary tract, and structural or functional urinary tract abnormality [4, 7, 15]. According to NSHN data from 2009 to 2013, 5.2–6.1% of reported CAUTIs were complicated by a secondary bloodstream infection. Risk factors for bloodstream infections from a urinary source are incompletely understood [16].

Diagnosis of Urinary Tract Infection

Diagnosis of urinary tract infections in children, even without the presence of an indwelling urinary catheter, is challenging. For febrile infants and children from ages 2 to 24 months, the American Academy of Pediatrics recommends that the diagnosis of urinary tract infection be based on the presence of both pyuria (based on microscopy for WBCs and bacteria or dipstick leukocyte esterase) and a positive urine culture with at least 50,000 colony forming units (CFU) per mL of a single uropathogenic organism in an appropriately collected specimen of urine [17].

The Infectious Diseases Society of America (IDSA) published clinical practice guidelines for the diagnosis, prevention, and treatment of catheter-associated urinary tract infections in adults as the surveillance definition of CAUTI does not always reflect the clinical practices of infectious disease consultants or intensivists [18, 19]. The 2009 IDSA guideline for the diagnosis of CAUTI suggested that catheterized patients be thoroughly evaluated for alternative sources of infection, before attributing symptoms including fever to the urinary tract because of the high frequency of asymptomatic bacteriuria. Positive urine cultures often mislead, if not confuse, clinicians in the management of the catheterized patient. The American College of Critical Care Medicine (ACCCM) and the IDSA note that catheter-associated bacteriuria is typically indicative of colonization, is rarely symptomatic, and is an infrequent cause of fever or secondary bloodstream infection. Their joint guidance recommends that when evaluating fever in the critically ill, urine cultures should only be evaluated in patient populations at high risk of invasive infection: (1) those who are kidney transplantation recipients, (2) those who are neutropenic, (3) those who have recently had genitourinary surgery, or (4) those who demonstrate evidence of obstruction [20].

In a 2-year retrospective review from 2012 to 2013 at a large 1200 bed hospital with a 158 adult ICU bed, it was found that urine cultures obtained for the evaluation of fever form the basis for identification of CAUTIs in the ICU [21]. However, most patients with presumed CAUTIs were eventually found to have alternative explanations for fever, and CAUTI was associated with a low complication rate. Given the high frequency of fever in ICU, up to 50% in adult ICUs [22], the NHSN definition utilizing fever as the predominant symptom will cause the overestimation of the incidence of clinically significant CAUTI and is unlikely to be a good measure of hospital quality [21].

A recent study in an academic center, inclusive of the NICU and PICU, focused on a multifaceted approach to reduce ICU CAUTI. They placed an emphasis on best practices to prevent CAUTI followed by "stewardship of testing" consistent with published IDSA guidance [18] or evaluation of a fever prior to ordering a urine culture in a critically ill patient. This "stewardship of culturing" decreased the CAUTI rate by 33% without any increase in bloodstream infections attributed to *Enterobacteriaceae* [23]. Furthermore, concomitant urinalysis and microscopy are underutilized and may help distinguish bacteriuria versus infection in addition to careful utilization of urine culture [24].

Surveillance

Federal and state regulations address requirements for surveillance and reporting of HAIs. Many pediatric acute care hospitals do not report to NHSN. Only 72 children's hospitals, less than 2% of total hospitals reporting to NHSN, were included in the 2013 NHSN data summary [12]. The Joint Commission National Patient Safety Goals addresses surveillance and evidence-based practices to prevent CAUTI [25, 26].

The NHSN surveillance definition for HAI UTI has been the standard for inter-hospital comparison of CAUTI rates [25]. As part of this definition, an indwelling catheter is considered a drainage tube inserted into the urinary bladder through the urethra, left in place, and connected to a closed collection system. Thus, the NHSN definition excludes infections associated with straight catheters, suprapubic catheters, nephrostomy tubes, and condom catheters.

In 2015, two important modifications were made to the 2013 NHSN surveillance definition of CAUTI, excluding funguria and nonbacterial organisms as uropathogens and setting the threshold of organisms to $\geq 10^5$ CFU/mL for diagnosis. The current CAUTI definition is met by three simple criteria: (1) the presence of an indwelling urinary catheter for >2 days; (2) a urine culture growing $\geq 10^5$ CFU/mL of bacteria; and (3) signs or symptoms suggestive of a urinary tract infection (UTI) which may be met only by a temperature > 38 °C [27]. Notably, fever as the sole symptom, even if another source of fever is identified, occurs in almost 80% of CAUTI cases reported to the NHSN [28, 29].

Although UTI incidence per 1000 urinary catheter-days is the most accepted comparison measure, reducing unnecessary Foley use can actually increase a hospital's CAUTI rate by decreasing the rate's denominator of catheter-days. Some experts recommend utilizing rate of UTI per 10,000 patient-days as a more appropriate outcome measure of CAUTI prevention initiatives [30]. The widely accepted practice of using device-days as a method of risk adjustment to calculate device-associated infection rates may mask the impact of a successful quality improvement program and reward programs not actively engaged in reducing device usage. By contrast, the device utilization ratio (DUR) is patient-centered, objective, and currently captured as part of NHSN reporting and is easily obtainable from electronic medical records. The urinary catheter DUR is calculated by dividing the number of indwelling catheter-days by patient-days on the same unit. The DUR may provide a more direct reflection of overall improvement efforts focusing on reducing inappropriate urinary catheter use [27].

The use of electronic surveillance tools for CAUTI may decrease the time infection preventionists spend performing surveillance; however, efforts must be expended to ensure reliability of the data. Because error is easily introduced due to inaccurate or misidentified documentation, such as a patient receiving intermittent catheterization without an indwelling urinary catheter counting as a catheter-day, there must be attention to the validation of documentation between infection prevention and nursing to ensure the accuracy of surveillance reporting [31].

Prevention

Several guidelines, mainly focused on adult patients, have been developed for the prevention of CAUTI since the publication of the original 1981 CDC/ HICPAC guidelines [3, 32, 33].

Hand hygiene is the cornerstone in the prevention of all healthcare-associated infections, including CAUTI. Judicious use of antibiotics, as part of an overall antimicrobial stewardship program, is an additional important strategy to prevent the development of antimicrobial resistance in CAUTI. because inappropriate antibiotic treatment of bacteriuria is a significant risk for colonization with a multidrug-resistant organism [8]. Focused programs such as the adult-population comprehensive unit-based safety program (CUSP) [34] or the pediatric-patient-focused Solutions for Patient Safety (SPS) are important to develop an overall safety culture to prevent healthcare-associated conditions [35]. CUSP aimed to reduce CAUTI in ICUs and non-ICUs with a focus on technical factors (appropriate catheter use, aseptic insertion, proper maintenance) and socioadaptive factors, such as cultural and behavioral changes in hospital units. The program successfully reduced overall catheter use and CAUTI in non-ICUs but was not successful in reduction in the ICUs.

Two pediatric facilities have reported CAUTI reductions with a hospital-wide initiative [36] and a PICU-centered initiative [37], respectively. An engaged physician champion quality initiative also decreased urinary catheter DUR by 17% in a PICU that had CAUTI and DUR rates above the 90th percentile although this initiative did not show a reduction in CAUTI rates [38].

Davis et al. report a single-center pediatric observational study to assess impact of a CAUTI quality improvement bundle comprised of standardization of training for catheter insertions and maintenance practices, daily review of catheter necessity, and rapid review of all CAUTIs. Over a 3-year period, adoption of the bundle was associated with a 50% reduction in the mean monthly CAUTI rate from 5.41 to 2.49 per 1000 catheter-days although the median monthly catheter utilization ratio was unchanged [4].

Key evidence-based CAUTI prevention strategies for adults applicable to pediatric patients include the following: (1) avoid insertion of indwelling catheters and place only for appropriate indications; (2) remove indwelling catheters as soon as possible utilizing checklists, reminders, automatic stop orders, and nurse-based protocols; (3) utilize alternatives such as intermittent catheterization or condom catheters as possible; (4) ensure proper techniques for insertion and maintenance of catheters; and (5) implement a CAUTI prevention program that develops policy and implementation tools, provides education, and performs surveillance for catheter use and CAUTI [3, 14, 32, 33].

Placement of a urinary catheter should be avoided whenever possible. Pediatric providers should consider the use of in-and-out catheterization as an alternative to an indwelling urinary catheter for young boys who cannot use a condom catheter if they are continent and cooperative. In adult populations about 21–50% of indwelling urinary catheters are placed without an appropriate indication; estimates of catheters inappropriately retained account for 33–50% of total device days [39]. Prolonged catheterization is the primary risk factor for CAUTI, and reminder systems are effective interventions which can prompt the removal of unnecessary urinary catheters. A systemic review and meta-analysis by Meddings et al. found that urinary catheter reminders and stop orders in adult patient populations decreased CAUTI rates by 50% [40].

Universal use of a closed catheter drainage system with positioning of the bag below the level of the patient's bladder with the tubing from the catheter free of dependent loops is recommended [41]. Direct drainage into the urinary collecting system is often challenging in the pediatric population because the small size of some children makes redundant loops of tubing inevitable and thus increases the risk of reflux of urine from the collecting system backward into the bladder.

A number of evidence-based CAUTI prevention bundles have been developed for adult patients. Elements of these bundles in children have been utilized and published [4], and the Solutions for Patient Safety program has developed more comprehensive CAUTI prevention bundles [35]. Figure 13.1 illustrates a representative pediatric-focused CAUTI implementation bundle for catheter insertion, and Fig. 13.2 depicts a pediatric-focused CAUTI implementation bundle for catheter maintenance.

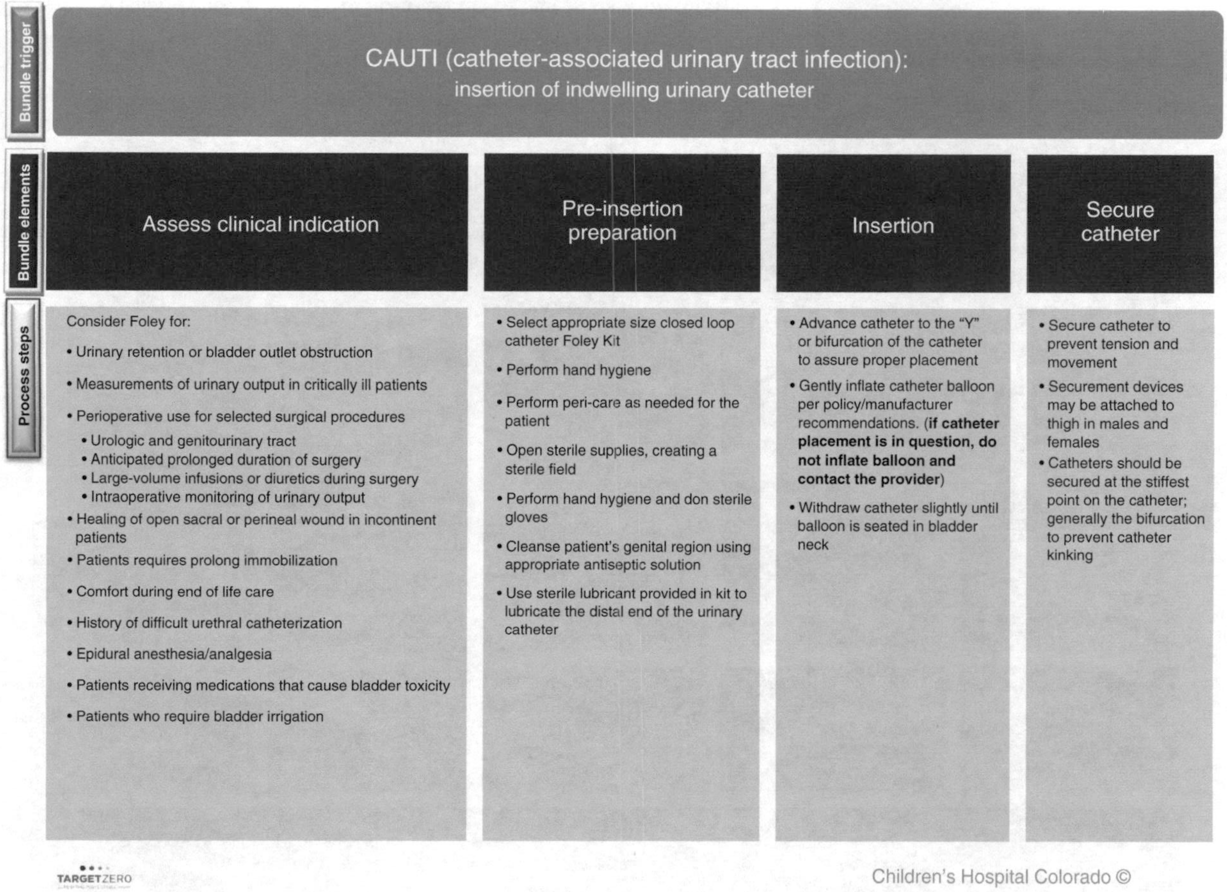

CAUTI (catheter-associated urinary tract infection):
insertion of indwelling urinary catheter

Bundle trigger

Bundle elements

Process steps

Assess clinical indication	Pre-insertion preparation	Insertion	Secure catheter
Consider Foley for: • Urinary retention or bladder outlet obstruction • Measurements of urinary output in critically ill patients • Perioperative use for selected surgical procedures • Urologic and genitourinary tract • Anticipated prolonged duration of surgery • Large-volume infusions or diuretics during surgery • Intraoperative monitoring of urinary output • Healing of open sacral or perineal wound in incontinent patients • Patients requires prolong immobilization • Comfort during end of life care • History of difficult urethral catheterization • Epidural anesthesia/analgesia • Patients receiving medications that cause bladder toxicity • Patients who require bladder irrigation	• Select appropriate size closed loop catheter Foley Kit • Perform hand hygiene • Perform peri-care as needed for the patient • Open sterile supplies, creating a sterile field • Perform hand hygiene and don sterile gloves • Cleanse patient's genital region using appropriate antiseptic solution • Use sterile lubricant provided in kit to lubricate the distal end of the urinary catheter	• Advance catheter to the "Y" or bifurcation of the catheter to assure proper placement • Gently inflate catheter balloon per policy/manufacturer recommendations. **(if catheter placement is in question, do not inflate balloon and contact the provider)** • Withdraw catheter slightly until balloon is seated in bladder neck	• Secure catheter to prevent tension and movement • Securement devices may be attached to thigh in males and females • Catheters should be secured at the stiffest point on the catheter; generally the bifurcation to prevent catheter kinking

TARGETZERO

Children's Hospital Colorado ©

Fig. 13.1 Example of an insertion bundle for catheter-associated urinary tract infection prevention

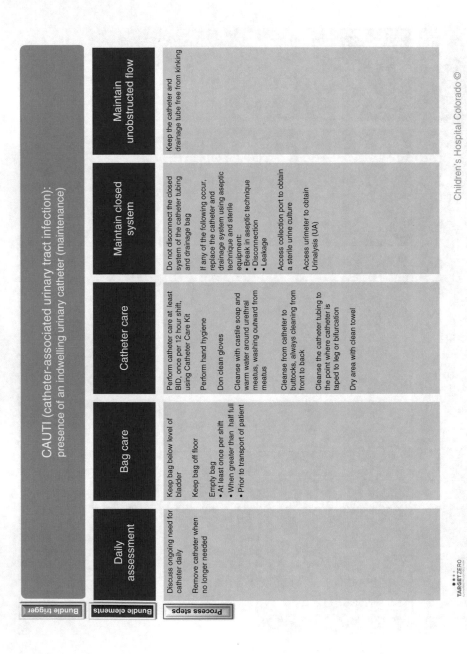

Fig. 13.2 Example of a maintenance bundle for catheter-associated urinary tract infection prevention

Management Strategies and Treatment

Significant gaps to guide management and treatment of CAUTI exist for adult populations and even more so for the pediatric population. Use of the indwelling catheter should be discontinued as soon as appropriate. If there is still an indication for an indwelling catheter, some evidence supports the practice of changing a long-term catheter prior to initiating therapy for a CAUTI especially if it has been in place greater than 2 weeks [8]. Most recommendations for the duration of antibiotics to treat CAUTI are based on expert opinion and range from 5 to 14 days and depend upon resolution of symptoms [8, 17].

Special Pediatric Populations and Complications of Urinary Tract Procedures

Congenital abnormalities of the genitourinary tract are relatively common among hospitalized children on a surgical service who may have had recent complex surgical repair, have reconstruction of congenital abnormalities of the urogenital system, or have a chronic indwelling catheter (urethral or suprapubic). Adult CAUTI prevention bundles utilize a closed drainage system, but many children with complex urologic problems and neonates may have an open drainage system. Despite a potential increased risk of urinary tract infection with an open system, there is insufficient data to determine whether there are specific patients that would benefit more from an open vs. closed drainage system.

Catheter-associated bacteriuria (CAB) which is defined as the presence of $\geq 10^5$ CFU/mL of one or more bacterial species in a single catheter urine specimen is almost universal in patients with long-term indwelling bladder catheters such as suprapubic catheters and is detected in most patients who have been catheterized for >1 week [18, 42]. In patients with long-term catheters, antimicrobial therapy for asymptomatic bacteriuria does not change the prevalence of bacteriuria or decrease progression to symptomatic UTI [43] and thus should be avoided.

A vast majority of patients with spina bifida suffer from neurogenic bladder and are prone to renal deterioration secondary to recurrent UTIs or deleterious bladder pressure. Over half of children with spina bifida will have their first urinary tract infection by 15 months of age, and 44% will have greater than five episodes by age 15 years. The introduction of clean intermittent catheterization (CIC), performed by over 70% of children with spina bifida, and antimuscarinic pharmacotherapy has resulted in improved renal protection and urinary continence in this patient population. Best practices for CIC include using a clean catheterization technique and ensuring complete drainage of the bladder to decrease the inherent risk of urinary tract infections in this population [44].

Definitions for diagnosis of UTI in patients with spina bifida/neurogenic bladder are heterogeneous and interpreted by various providers differently [45]. Frequent high bacterial counts in the urine, polymicrobial urine cultures, and colonization with multidrug-resistant organisms provide challenges for clinicians to differentiate between asymptomatic bacteriuria or urinary tract infection in patients performing clean intermittent catheterization. UTIs may contribute to renal deterioration when the infection involves the upper tract. Multiple reports have demonstrated preserved renal function in patients with asymptomatic bacteriuria and absence of vesicoureteral reflux (VUR). Low-dose antimicrobial prophylaxis is common in patients with spina bifida who perform CIC. Zegers et al. in a randomized clinical trial of 176 patients found that stopping low-dose antimicrobial prophylaxis in a subset of patients, males with low rates of UTI and patients without vesicoureteral reflux, did not increase the number of febrile urinary tract infections [46]. In those undergoing intermittent catheterization, treatment of asymptomatic bacteriuria in addition to antimicrobial prophylaxis may contribute to increased frequency of resistant organisms in subsequent symptomatic UTI episodes [43]. Madden-Fuentes et al. propose the definition of UTI in spina bifida patients to include (1) ≥ 2 signs/symptoms (fever >38 °C, abdominal pain, new back pain, new or worse incontinence, pain with catheterization or urination, or malodorous/cloudy urine), (2) $>100,000$ CFU/mL of a single organism, and (3) >10 WBC/HPF on urine microscopy [45]. Adoption of this more stringent definition of UTIs that require antimicrobial treatment may decrease antibiotic exposure in these patients and ultimately lead to a decrease in resistant organisms.

In the early 1980s, Mitrofanoff developed a surgical technique to use the appendix to create a catheterizable channel to empty the bladder increasing the continence of patients requiring use of CIC [47]. Known complications of this procedure are mainly related to poor emptying and include UTI, bladder stone formation, stomal problems, metabolic complications, and renal damage [48]. Rates of urinary tract infection in this population range from 19% to 63% in retrospective reviews of up to 10 years of follow-up. The variable rates of infection were primarily influenced by adherence to CIC best practices and the degree of patient compliance with the catheterizing regimen [48, 49].

References

1. Magill SS, Edwards JR, Bamberg W, et al. Emerging infections program healthcare-associated infections and antimicrobial use prevalence survey team. Multistate point-prevalence survey of health care-associated infections. N Engl J Med. 2014;370:1198–208. https://doi.org/10.1056/NEJMoa1306801.
2. Weber DJ, Sickbert-Bennett EE, Gould CV, et al. Incidence of catheter-associated and non-catheter-associated urinary tract infections in a healthcare system. Infect Control Hosp Epidemiol. 2011;32:822–3. https://doi.org/10.1086/661107.
3. Lo E, Nicolle LE, Coffin SE, et al. Strategies to prevent catheter-associated urinary tract infections in acute care hospitals: 2014 update. Infect Control Hosp Epidemiol. 2014;35:464–79.
4. Davis KF, Colebaugh AM, Eithun BL, et al. Reducing catheter-associated urinary tract infections: a quality-improvement initiative. Pediatrics. 2014;134:e857–64. https://doi.org/10.1542/peds.2013-3470.
5. Tambyah PA, Halvorson KT, Maki DG. A prospective study of pathogenesis of catheter-associated urinary tract infections. Mayo Clin Proc. 1999;74:131–6. https://doi.org/10.4065/74.2.131.
6. Stamm WE. Catheter-associated urinary tract infections: epidemiology, pathogenesis, and prevention. Am J Med. 1991;91:65S–71S.

7. Kabbani MS, Ismail SR, Fatima A, et al. Urinary tract infection in children after cardiac surgery: incidence, causes, risk factors and outcomes in a single-center study. J Infect Public Health. 2016;9:600–10.
8. Lake JG, Weiner LM, Milstone AM, Saiman L, Magill SS, See I. Pathogen distribution and antimicrobial resistance among pediatric healthcare-associated infections reported to the National Healthcare Safety Network. Infect Control Hosp Epidemiol. 2011-2014;2017:1–11. https://doi.org/10.1017/ice.2017.236.
9. Langley JM, Hanakowski M, Leblanc JC. Unique epidemiology of nosocomial urinary tract infection in children. Am J Infect Control. 2001;29:94–8.
10. Davies HD, Jones EL, Sheng RY, et al. Nosocomial urinary tract infections at a pediatric hospital. Pediatr Infect Dis J. 1992;11:349.
11. Zimlichman E, Henderson D, Tamir O, et al. Health care-associated infections: a meta-analysis of costs and financial impact on the US health care system. JAMA Intern Med. 2013;173:2039–46. https://doi.org/10.1001/jamainternmed.2013.9763.
12. Dudeck MA, Edwards J, Allen-Bridson K, et al. National Healthcare Safety Network report, data summary for 2013. Device-associated module. Am J Infect Control. 2015;43:206–21. https://doi.org/10.1016/j.ajic.2014.11.014.
13. Patrick S, Kawai A, Kleinman K, et al. Health care-associated infections among critically ill children in the US, 2000–2012. Pediatrics. 2014;134:705–12. https://doi.org/10.1542/peds.2014-0613.
14. Chenoweth CE, Saint S. Urinary tract infections. Infect Dis Clin N Am. 2016;30:869–85. https://doi.org/10.1016/j.idc.2016.07.007.
15. Lee NG, Marchalik D, Lipsky A, Rushton HG, Pohl HG, Song X. Risk factors for catheter associated urinary tract infections in a pediatric institution. J Urol. 2016;195:1306–11. https://doi.org/10.1016/j.juro.2015.03.121.
16. Kizilbash Q, Petersen N, Chen G, et al. Bacteremia and mortality with urinary catheter-associated bacteriuria. Infect Control Hosp Epidemiol. 2013;34:1153–9. https://doi.org/10.1086/673456.
17. AAP Subcommittee on Urinary Tract Infection, Steering Committee on Quality Improvement and Management. Clinical Practice Guideline. Urinary tract infection: clinical practice guideline for the diagnosis and management of the initial UTI in febrile infants and children 2–24 months. Pediatrics. 2011;128:595–610.
18. Hooton TM, Bradley SF, Cardenas DD, et al. Diagnosis, prevention, and treatment of catheter-associated urinary tract infection in adults: 2009 international clinical practice guidelines from the Infectious Diseases Society of America. Clin Infect Dis. 2010;50:625–63. https://doi.org/10.1086/650482.
19. Al-Qas Hanna F, Sambirska O, Iyer S, Szpunar S, Fakih MG. Clinician practice and the National Healthcare Safety Network definition for the diagnosis of catheter-associated urinary tract infection. Am J Infect Control. 2013;41:1173–7. https://doi.org/10.1016/j.ajic.2013.05.024.
20. O'Grady NP, Barie PS, Bartlett JG, et al. Guidelines for evaluation of new fever in critically ill adult patients: 2008 update from the American College of Critical Care Medicine and the Infectious Diseases Society of America. Crit Care Med. 2008;36:1330–49. https://doi.org/10.1097/CCM.0b013e318169eda9.
21. Tedja R, Wentink J, O'Horo JC, Thompson R, Sampathkumar P. Catheter-associated urinary tract infections in intensive care unit patients. Infect Control Hosp Epidemiol. 2015;36:1330–4. https://doi.org/10.1017/ice.2015/172.
22. Laupland KB, Shahpori R, Kirkpatrick AW, Ross T, Gregson DB, Stelfox HT. Occurrence and outcome of fever in critically ill adults. Crit Care Med. 2008;36:1531–5. https://doi.org/10.1097/CCM.0b013e318170efd3.
23. Mullin KM, Kovacs CS, Fatica C, et al. A multifaceted approach to reduction of catheter-associated urinary tract infections in the intensive care unit with an emphasis on "stewardship of culturing". Infect Control Hosp Epidemiol. 2017;38:186–8. https://doi.org/10.1017/ice.2016.266.

24. Carlson AL, Munigala S, Russo AJ, et al. Inpatient urine cultures are frequently performed without urinalysis or microscopy: findings from a large academic medical center. Infect Control Hosp Epidemiol. 2017;38:455–60. https://doi.org/10.1017/ice.2016.311.

25. CDC NHSN Website. https://www.cdc.gov/nhsn/index.html. Accessed 21 Jan 2018.

26. The Joint Commission National Patient Safety Goals. https://www.jointcommission.org/standards_information/npsgs.aspx. Accessed 21 Jan 2018.

27. Fakih MG, Gould CV, Trautner BW, et al. Beyond infection: device utilization ratio as a performance measure for urinary catheter harm. Infect Control Hosp Epidemiol. 2016;37:327–33. https://doi.org/10.1017/ice.2015.287.

28. Bardossy AC, Jayaprakash R, Alangaden AC, et al. Impact and limitations of the 2015 national health and safety network case definition on catheter-associated urinary tract infection rates. Infect Control Hosp Epidemiol. 2017;38:239–41. https://doi.org/10.1017/ice.2016.278.

29. Livorsi DJ, Perencevich EN. CAUTI surveillance: opportunity or opportunity cost? Infect Control Hosp Epidemiol. 2015;36:1335–6. https://doi.org/10.1017/ice.2015.174.

30. Wright MO, Kharasch M, Beaumont JL, Peterson LR, Robicsek A. Reporting catheter-associated urinary tract infections: denominator matters. Infect Control Hosp Epidemiol. 2011;32:635–40. https://doi.org/10.1086/660765.

31. Sen AI, Balzer K, Mangino D, et al. Electronic surveillance for catheter-associated urinary tract infections at a university-affiliated children's hospital. Am J Infect Control. 2016;44:599–601. https://doi.org/10.1016/j.ajic.2015.12.006.

32. Gould CV, Umscheid CA, Agarwal RK, et al. Guideline for prevention of catheter-associated urinary tract infections 2009. Infect Control Hosp Epidemiol 2010;31:319–326. https://www.cdc.gov/infectioncontrol/pdf/guidelines/cauti-guidelines.pdf. Accessed 28 Jan 2018.

33. APIC Implementation Guides: Guide to preventing catheter-associated urinary tract infections. http://www.apic.org/implementationguides. Accessed 21 Jan 2018.

34. Saint S, Greene MT, Krein SL, et al. A program to prevent catheter-associated urinary tract infection in acute care. N Engl J Med. 2016;374:2111–9. https://doi.org/10.1056/NEJMoa1504906.

35. Solutions for Patient Safety Website: http://www.solutionsforpatientsafety.org/. Accessed 21 Jan 2018.

36. Brilli RJ, McClead RE Jr, Crandall WV, et al. A comprehensive patient safety program can significantly reduce preventable harm, associated costs, and hospital mortality. J Pediatr. 2013;163:1638–45. https://doi.org/10.1016/j.jpeds.2013.06.031.

37. Esteban E, Ferrer R, Urrea M, et al. The importance of a quality improvement intervention to reduce nosocomial infections in a PICU. Pediatr Crit Care Med. 2013;14:525–32. https://doi.org/10.1097/PCC.0b013e31828a87cc.

38. Zavalkoff S, Korah N, Quach C. Presence of a physician safety champion is associated with a reduction in urinary catheter utilization in the pediatric Intensive care unit. Plos One. 10:e0144222. https://doi.org/10.1371/journal.pone.0144222.

39. Siddiq DM, Darouiche RO. New strategies to prevent catheter-associated urinary tract infections. Nat Rev Urol. 2012;9:305–14. https://doi.org/10.1038/nrurol.2012.68.

40. Meddings J, Rogers MAM, Macy M, Saint S. Systematic review and meta-analysis: reminder systems to reduce catheter-associated urinary tract infections and urinary catheter use in hospitalized patients. Clin Infect Dis. 2010;51:550–60. https://doi.org/10.1086/655133.

41. Maki DG, Tambyah PA. Engineering out the risk for infection with urinary catheters. Emerg Infect Dis. 2001;7:342–7.

42. Warren JW, Tenney JH, Hoopes JM, Muncie HL, Anthony WC. A prospective microbiologic study of bacteriuria in patients with chronic indwelling urethral catheters. J Infect Dis. 1982;146:719–23.

43. Nicolle LE. Urinary catheter-associated infections. Infect Dis Clin N Am. 2012;26:13–27. https://doi.org/10.1016/j.idc.2011.09.009.

44. Newman DK, Willson MM. Review of intermittent catheterization and current best practices. Urol Nurs. 2011;31:12–48.

45. Madden-Fuentes RJ, McNamara ER, Lloyd JC, et al. Variation in definitions of urinary tract infections in spina bifida patients: a systemic review. Pediatrics. 2013;132:132–9. https://doi.org/10.1542/peds.2013-0557.
46. Zegers B, Uiterwaal C, Kimpen J, et al. Antibiotic prophylaxis for urinary tract infections in children with spina bifida on intermittent catheterization. J Urol. 2011;186:2365–71. https://doi.org/10.1016/j.juro.2011.07.108.
47. Berkowitz J, North AC, Tripp R, Gearhart JP, Lakshmana Y. Mitrofanoff continent catheterizable conduits: top down or bottom up? J Pediatr Urol. 2009;5:122–5. https://doi.org/10.1016/j.jpurol.2008.11.003.
48. Clark T, Pope JC, Adams MC, Wells N, Brock JW. Factors that influence outcomes of the Mitrofanoff and Malone antegrade continence enema reconstructive procedures in children. J Urol. 2002;168:1537–40. https://doi.org/10.1097/01.ju.0000028619.08733.7f.
49. Bertschy C, Bawab F, Liard A, Valioulis I, Mitrofanoff P. Enterocystoplasty complications in children: a study of 30 cases. Eur J Pediatr Surg. 2000;10:30–4.

Healthcare-Associated Viral Infections: Considerations for Nosocomial Transmission and Infection Control

14

Gail J. Demmler-Harrison

Introduction

Viral infections are extremely common in children. Given the frequency with which they occur in the general pediatric population, as well as the prolonged period of shedding associated with many viruses, it is not surprising that these agents may pose a risk for transmission within the healthcare environment. This chapter will briefly review common and clinically significant viral pathogens with the potential for healthcare-associated transmission as well as infection control considerations related to these infections. In addition, isolation and containment procedures related to rare but highly virulent viral pathogens will be discussed.

Respiratory Viruses

Respiratory viruses are common healthcare-associated viral infections, especially in pediatric hospitals or health centers where children are seen, evaluated, and treated [1–6]. Respiratory virus nucleic acids were detected in 42% of samples taken from environmental surfaces in a children's hospital waiting room in one study [7]. The respiratory viruses of major importance to healthcare-associated infections are usually considered to include the paramyxoviruses (such as respiratory syncytial virus (RSV); parainfluenza viruses types 1, 2, 3, and 4; and human metapneumovirus); the orthomyxoviruses, including influenza A and B; the picornaviruses, some of which can be transmitted from the respiratory tract, such as rhinoviruses and respiratory enteroviruses; and the respiratory adenoviruses, of which

G. J. Demmler-Harrison
Department of Pediatrics, Baylor College of Medicine, Houston, TX, USA

Infectious Diseases Service, Texas Children's Hospital, Houston, TX, USA
e-mail: gdemmler@bcm.edu

© Springer Nature Switzerland AG 2019
J. C. McNeil et al. (eds.), *Healthcare-Associated Infections in Children*,
https://doi.org/10.1007/978-3-319-98122-2_14

there are many serotypes. Mimiviruses also may cause nosocomial pneumonia, especially in patients who are being mechanically ventilated in intensive care units. Respiratory virus infections may have potentially fatal consequences in children with hematologic malignancies or who have received bone marrow transplants. Therefore prompt isolation upon admission of patients with suspected respiratory viral infections, prior to confirmatory diagnosis, should be routine in healthcare centers to reduce nosocomial spread. In addition to contact precautions that have been traditionally recommended for many respiratory virus infections, enhanced isolation precautions (adding droplet precautions to contact precautions) have recently been shown to reduce the rate of nosocomial respiratory virus infections in pediatric hospitals and have now been adopted by many centers, especially bone marrow transplant units [1]. In such scenarios, caretakers wear gowns, gloves, and surgical masks during patient care encounters to reduce nosocomial spread of respiratory viruses. Therapy for the vast majority of respiratory viral infections in children, even in cases of hospital-acquired disease, is supportive with supplemental fluid and oxygen administered as needed and mechanical ventilation in cases of respiratory failure. Considerations related to specific viruses will be discussed below along with appropriate antiviral therapy when relevant.

Respiratory Syncytial Virus

Respiratory syncytial virus (RSV), an enveloped, RNA, paramyxovirus, causes acute respiratory tract infections and is probably the most common healthcare-associated viral infection in the pediatric setting [8–10]. Infection with RSV may occur at any age, although it is most frequently diagnosed in the first 2 years of life. Reinfections with RSV may occur. It causes upper respiratory tract symptoms, such as rhinorrhea (often copious in nature), cough, and otitis media, as well as lower respiratory tract disease, such as bronchiolitis and pneumonia. In newborns or premature infants, apnea may be a presenting symptom. Most infections with RSV occur during the fall and early winter, but there are annual and regional differences to the start and finish of each RSV season. Most RSV infections are self-limited; however, infection may cause serious, even life-threatening disease in medically fragile patients, such as those with congenital heart disease, neuromuscular disease, and/or immunocompromised hosts. RSV is a common cause for medical visits in clinics, urgent care centers, and emergency centers, as well as hospitalization in acute care and intensive care units, providing ample opportunity for nosocomial transmission. Nosocomial outbreaks in pediatric wards, pediatric intensive care units, bone marrow transplant units, and neonatal intensive care units have been reported [8, 10, 11] and are associated with prolonged hospitalizations, prolonged time receiving mechanical ventilation, and even increased mortality.

The diagnosis of RSV can be suspected clinically with reasonable reliability in an infant or child with bronchiolitis occurring during local "RSV season" and established definitively by point-of-care rapid diagnostic tests (POCT) frequently used in clinics and urgent care centers. Traditional viral culture or respiratory viral panels utilizing molecular diagnostics are alternative means of virologic diagnosis.

The treatment of RSV infection is usually supportive in normal hosts, with fluid and respiratory support and suctioning of the nose and airways as needed. Antiviral treatment with inhaled ribavirin may help reduce viral load and shedding and hasten recovery, especially in seriously ill infants and children and those who are immuno-compromised [12]. Additionally, there is growing interest in the use of oral ribavirin for the treatment of RSV and other respiratory viral illnesses in immunocompro-mised hosts; however, this is still under investigation [13].

The transmission of RSV is person-to-person or through direct or close contact with contaminated respiratory secretions. It also may aerosolize via large particle droplets and has been detected through molecular techniques in the air surrounding RSV-infected patients [14], although droplet transmission is not felt to be as impor-tant a mode of transmission as contact transmission. It also can persist on environ-mental surfaces and hands. Healthcare-associated transmission from patient to healthcare worker often occurs via hand to nose or hand to eye self-inoculation after contact with contaminated secretions. Patients hospitalized with suspected or proven RSV infection should be cared for under standard and contact precautions (Table 14.1), using gown and gloves, and rigorous hand hygiene. Some centers, especially bone marrow transplant units, will also use enhanced isolation precau-tions, and add droplet precautions, with healthcare workers wearing surgical masks during patient encounters [15–17]. In a quasi-experimental study in a children's hospital, the use of contact and droplet precautions was associated with a 39% reduction in nosocomial respiratory viral infections (including RSV) [1]. The use of eye goggles or face masks is not routinely recommended to reduce nosocomial transmission of RSV from patient to healthcare worker. Additional measures found to be helpful in some centers to minimize nosocomial spread of RSV include cohort-ing infants with suspected or proven RSV infection and excluding visitors with respiratory tract infections.

Parainfluenza Viruses

Parainfluenza viruses types 1, 2, 3, and 4 (PIVs) are enveloped RNA viruses belong-ing to the family *Paramyxoviridae*. They are common and an important cause of upper respiratory infections, as well as lower tract respiratory infections, such as laryngotracheobronchitis (croup), bronchiolitis, and pneumonia. The PIVs are also seasonal viruses, and usually circulate in early fall and late spring/early summer, with different serotypes having distinct seasonal patterns. Most children are infected with PIVs prior to 5 years of age. Infection with PIVs is usually self-limited; how-ever, prolonged viral shedding, often associated with severe lower respiratory tract disease which may be fatal, may occur in immunocompromised patients. In chil-dren who have received bone marrow transplants, PIV infections commonly result in serious lower respiratory tract infections, especially if they occur before

Table 14.1 Summary of infection control recommendations for common childhood viral infections

Virus	Isolation precautions				Comments
	Standard	Contact	Droplet	Airborne	
Respiratory viruses					
RSV	X	X			Droplet precautions may be used for immunocompromised patients in some centers
Parainfluenza viruses	X	X			Droplet precautions may be used for immunocompromised patients in some centers
Human metapneumoviruses	X	X			Droplet precautions may be used for immunocompromised patients in some centers; Single-room or cohorting
Influenza	X		X		
Rhinovirus	X	X	X		
Respiratory adenoviruses	X	X	X		
Childhood exanthems					
Measles	X	X		X	Airborne precautions recommended for 4 days after the onset of rash in immunocompetent hosts
Mumps	X	X	X		Droplet precautions recommended until 5 days after onset of parotid swelling
Rubella (postnatal)	X	X	X		Recommended for 7 days after onset of rash
Congenital rubella syndrome	X	X			Consultation with local public health authorities is recommended
Roseola	X				
Chicken pox	X	X		X	Should be continued for a minimum of 5 days after onset of rash and until all lesions are crusted; see text for recommendations in neonates and immunocompromised hosts
Zoster	X	X			Airborne precautions recommended for immunocompromised patients or those with disseminated zoster
Parvovirus B19	X	X	X		Droplet precautions recommended for patients with aplastic crises and PPGSS or immunocompromised patients with chronic infection; otherwise standard precautions are sufficient
Gastrointestinal viruses					
Rotavirus	X	X			
Norovirus	X	X			Soap and water preferred over alcohol-based rubs for hand hygiene

				Comments
Non-polio enteroviruses	X	X		
Enteric adenovirus	X	X		
Mucocutaneous viral infections				
Human papillomavirus	X			N95 respirators are recommended during photoangiolytic/laser therapy
Herpes simplex virus	X	X		
Other common viruses				
Cytomegalovirus	X			

engraftment [18]. In such patients, ribavirin may be administered in efforts to shorten the duration and lessen the severity of disease [19].

Diagnosis of PIV infection can be suspected with reasonable certainty if a pediatric patient presents with a croup-like illness during the appropriate seasonal time period. It can be confirmed using traditional viral culture, direct immunofluorescence, or utilizing molecular diagnostics available in larger hospitals and reference laboratories.

Parainfluenza viruses are transmitted from person to person, primarily by direct contact with infected secretions, and also by droplet spread, when an infected person coughs or sneezes. Environmental surfaces may also harbor PIVs for several hours. Patients admitted to the hospital with croup or a suspected or proven PIV infection should be isolated under contact precautions, although some centers will also use droplet precautions.

Human Metapneumovirus

Human metapneumovirus (HMPV) was discovered in 2001 and is an enveloped, RNA, paramyxovirus. It causes acute respiratory tract illnesses in all ages. Most HMPV infections occur during late winter or early spring. Hospital outbreaks of HMPV have been reported and may have fatal consequences in patients with malignancies or who are immunocompromised from transplants [20, 21].

Diagnosis of HMPVs may be suspected in children presenting with upper or lower respiratory tract symptoms during late winter or early spring; however, it may mimic RSV or PIV infection, making precise clinical diagnosis with any certainty difficult. Therefore, HMPV infection is usually diagnosed definitively by viral respiratory panels utilizing molecular diagnostic techniques. Direct immunofluorescence may also be used to detect HMPV antigens in infected respiratory secretions.

Transmission of HMPVs is from person to person via contact with infected secretions, close personal contact, and from objects and surfaces that have been in contact with infected secretions. Contact precautions are recommended for patients hospitalized with suspected or proven HMPV infection. Some centers, especially bone marrow transplant units, will also add droplet precautions as described above.

Influenza Viruses

Influenza is caused by influenza A, B, or C virus, which are RNA viruses in the orthomyxovirus family. Influenza A virus can be further classified into subtypes based on two surface antigens (hemagglutinin (HA) and neuraminidase (NA)) and subtyped even further by the type of HA and NA (e.g., influenza A H1N1 or H3N2). Most infections with influenza virus in the Northern Hemisphere occur during the late fall and throughout winter into early spring, but there are annual and regional differences to the start and finish of each influenza season around the world. Pandemics with new and novel influenza viruses may also occur with periodicity of approximately every 20–30 years, most recently during the 2009 influenza A H1N1 pandemic. This then novel influenza A virus appeared to have enhanced transmissibility compared to previous seasonal influenza viruses, resulting in large numbers of patients presenting for medical treatment, a large number of critically ill patients requiring hospitalization for prolonged periods of time, and subsequently greater nosocomial transmission risk [22–27]. This particular influenza season was also associated with a large number of healthcare workers becoming ill, with up to 40% experiencing an influenza like illness (ILI) [28].

Influenza virus causes a febrile respiratory illness associated with fever, chills, malaise, myalgia, and cough in all age groups. Pediatric patients also commonly have vomiting and diarrhea. Newborns may present with apnea. Some children present with acute myositis, myocarditis, a sepsis-like syndrome, or neurological disease. Secondary bacterial pneumonia with *Staphylococcus aureus*, *Streptococcus pyogenes*, or *S. pneumoniae* can occur after influenza, sometimes resulting in serious, life-threatening disease.

Treatment of influenza virus infection and disease includes a variety of available antiviral medications, such as oseltamivir, peramivir, and zanamivir for influenza A and B virus infections. Influenza A and B viruses are also susceptible to inhaled ribavirin. Influenza B is never susceptible to amantadine or rimantadine; currently circulating influenza A virus subtypes are also not susceptible to amantadine/rimantadine, limiting the utility of these agents

In addition to standard precautions with strict hand hygiene procedures, droplet precautions are recommended for children hospitalized with influenza. Many hospitals will enforce droplet precautions at the time of admission, for all patients presenting with ILI, until the cause can be established through appropriate diagnostic testing. During the 2009 influenza A (H1N1) pandemic, infection control recommendations from the Centers for Disease Control and Prevention included the use of N95 respirators for healthcare workers caring for patients with suspected pandemic influenza, in addition to contact and droplet precautions. Realistically, however, many institutions had difficulty complying with these enhanced isolation precautions, either due to unavailability of N95 respirators, poor tolerability, work flow concerns, or patient volume, among other reasons. In addition, to their impact on individual patient symptoms, antiviral agents have a role in the prevention of spread of influenza within a hospital unit. Prompt antiviral therapy with oseltamivir or zanamivir for children hospitalized with ILI or confirmed influenza virus infections has been shown to reduce nosocomial spread of influenza by reducing viral shedding in infected patients [24]. Oseltamivir resistance may emerge during prolonged antiviral treatment of hospitalized immunocompromised hosts who have persistent and prolonged viral shedding while receiving antiviral therapy. Routine immunization of all healthcare workers with the seasonal influenza vaccine, prior to the beginning of the influenza season, is also recommended (and even mandatory in many hospitals) to reduce healthcare worker-to-patient transmission of infection.

Rhinoviruses and Respiratory Enteroviruses

Rhinoviruses and the respiratory enteroviruses are small, non-enveloped, RNA, picornaviruses with over 100 serotypes. They are very common causes of upper respiratory tract infections, such as the "common cold," pharyngitis, and lower respiratory tract infections, such as bronchiolitis and pneumonia. Rhinoviruses also may exacerbate acute asthma. Most infections are mild and self-limited; however, severe and even fatal respiratory infections in premature infants and in immunocompromised hosts have been linked to rhinovirus and enterovirus infections [29–31]. Patients with hypogammaglobulinemia may be particularly susceptible to persistent or severe infections. Rhinoviruses may occur year round and in all parts of the world. Nosocomial outbreaks of rhinovirus infection and disease in pediatric hospitals and neonatal intensive care units have been documented. A notable emerging pathogen included in this group is Enterovirus D68 (EV-D68); EV-D68 can cause respiratory illness or asthma exacerbation in children, as well as acute flaccid paralysis similar to poliomyelitis [32].

Transmission of rhinoviruses is predominantly person-to-person through prolonged and close contact with infected secretions, with subsequent autoinoculation by touching hands to the face, eyes, mouth, or nose. However, there is also experimental evidence to support indirect contact with contaminated fomites and surfaces as modes of transmission [33], as well as large droplet contact transmission. Nosocomial outbreaks of rhinovirus infection have been documented, especially in preterm infants hospitalized in neonatal intensive care units [30]. Patients in the healthcare setting with suspected or proven rhinovirus or respiratory enterovirus infections should be cared for under standard, contact, and droplet precautions. Rigorous hand hygiene should also be encouraged.

Respiratory Adenoviruses

Adenoviruses (ADV) are non-enveloped, DNA viruses with over 50 distinct serotypes. Some adenoviruses are associated primarily with respiratory tract disease (usually serotypes 1–5, 7, 14 [recently shown to be a potentially severe, fatal serotype], and 21). The respiratory adenoviruses infect pediatric patients of all ages. They may cause upper respiratory tract disease, such as rhinorrhea, pharyngitis, exudative tonsillitis, a pertussis-like syndrome, conjunctivitis, and epidemic keratoconjunctivitis, as well as lower respiratory tract disease, such as croup, bronchiolitis, and pneumonia. They do not appear to have a distinct seasonality and may occur in all seasons of the year. Most infections are self-limited in healthy hosts, but severe and fatal disease may occur in newborns and the immunocompromised.

Transmission of ADV in the healthcare setting is primarily through person-to-person spread via contact with infected secretions, as well as by fomites, contaminated environmental surfaces (where ADV may remain for extended periods of time due to their non-enveloped nature), and by droplet spread. In one study, 37% of environmental samples taken from a children's hospital waiting room in the winter had evidence of adenovirus [7], highlighting the potential for this virus to persist in the environment. Nosocomial outbreaks in pediatric wards, bone marrow transplant units, intensive care units, ophthalmology clinics, and neonatal intensive care units have been documented [34, 35]. Medical devices, such as eye specula (blepharostat) used to examine the eyes of newborns and preterm infants at risk for retinopathy of prematurity in the nurseries and neonatal intensive care units, have also been linked to nosocomial outbreaks [34]. In addition, tonometer prisms used in ophthalmology clinics may be a source of ADV infection after eye exams [36]. Given this notable risk of infection transmission, single-use eye specula and tonometers are preferred if available. Autoclave sterilization is the preferred method of sterilization of reusable eyelid specula between neonate examinations. However, if autoclave use is not available or will damage the instrument, washing the specula with chlorhexidine gluconate or dilute bleach (sodium hypochlorite) in between examinations may be more effective than cleaning with an alcohol swab [37–39]. Patients in the healthcare setting with suspected or proven ADV infections should be cared for under standard, contact, and droplet precautions. In addition, rigorous hand hygiene with soap and water or an alcohol-based hand rub should be enforced and environmental surfaces should be disinfected frequently [40]. Notably, one laboratory-based study found that alcohol-based solutions in hand sanitizers may not be effective against some strains of adenovirus [36].

Treatment of routine ADV infections is supportive, as most infections are self-limited. Severe, life-threatening adenovirus infections in immunocompromised hosts or newborns have been treated with cidofovir or brincidofovir.

Mimiviruses

Mimiviruses ("mimicking microbes") are the largest known DNA viruses and are considered an emerging cause of pneumonia [41–43]. They are a member of the Mimiviridae order, Mimiviridae family of nucleocytoplasmic large DNA viruses, and *Mimivirus* genus, and can be found within the amoeba, *Acanthamoeba polyphaga*. They were originally discovered in amoeba in 1992 and were thought to be bacteria, but in 2003 they were confirmed to be giant viruses. They can be cultured using special isolation techniques involving amoebae as a eukaryotic co-host and detected by molecular techniques. Clinical diagnosis, however, remains a challenge since they are difficult to detect. However, serologic assays have suggested these viruses may play a role in community-acquired and healthcare-associated pneumonia in adults [44]. Knowledge of their role, if any, in healthcare-associated, pediatric pneumonia is evolving.

Childhood Viral Diseases and Exanthems

The childhood viral diseases and exanthems may contribute to healthcare viral infections though transmission in the hospital and include measles, mumps, rubella, roseola, varicella (or chicken pox), and parvovirus B19. Measles and chicken pox are considered among the most highly contagious infectious diseases and therefore pose a significant risk for nosocomial transmission.

Measles (Rubeola)

Measles, or rubeola, is a highly contagious febrile childhood exanthem, characterized by cough, coryza, and conjunctivitis. Complications such as otitis media, pneumonia, and meningoencephalitis also may occur. Fatalities may occur in immunocompromised hosts and patients who develop subacute sclerosing panencephalitis.

Measles is caused by the measles virus, an RNA paramyxovirus. Measles is transmitted person-to-person through direct contact with infected secretions or via droplet or airborne spread. Measles is considered one of the most highly contagious infectious diseases with an average of 12–18 secondary cases in a susceptible population following exposure to a primary case; however, variability exists in the exact degree of contagion depending on the specific population studied [45, 46]. Healthcare-associated transmission of measles is well documented [47, 48]. The pediatric emergency room has been reported as a particularly common healthcare venue for measles exposure and transmission [49]. Measles transmission in the healthcare setting has involved both patients and healthcare workers. Patients with suspected or proven measles admitted to the hospital or seen in clinics or emergency centers should be cared for under standard and airborne precautions. In addition, patients exposed to measles in the hospital should be placed on airborne precautions from day 5 to day 21 after the exposure and maintained in airborne precautions if they develop measles illness and require continued hospitalization. Postexposure immunoprophylaxis in nonimmune individuals through measles vaccine is effective if given within 72 h of exposure and through immune globulin if given within 6 days of exposure [50]. Healthcare workers should be immunized against measles or provide serologic evidence of immunity prior to caring for patients.

Diagnosis of measles can be suspected clinically in children exhibiting the classic signs and symptoms and confirmed by detection of measles IgM antibody in serum if obtained at least 72 h after the onset of the measles rash. Measles virus may also detected by viral culture and molecular assays, performed in reference or public health laboratories.

Treatment of measles is primarily supportive. The World Health Organization (WHO) recommends vitamin A treatment for all children, in all countries, diagnosed with measles. Ribavirin has been administered to severely ill, immunocompromised patients with measles with variable success.

Mumps

Mumps (epidemic parotitis) is a febrile, childhood respiratory disease uniquely characterized by parotitis and orchitis. Meningoencephalitis, myocarditis, and other systemic manifestations may also occur.

Mumps is caused by the mumps virus, an RNA paramyxovirus, and is a vaccine-preventable illness. Mumps occurs all over the world, and community outbreaks occur, even in areas where immunization is routine. Healthcare-associated transmission of mumps has also occasionally been reported [51–53]. The virus is spread by contact with infected saliva and respiratory secretions. Patients hospitalized with suspected or proven mumps should be isolated under standard and droplet precautions until 5 days after onset of parotitis. Healthcare workers should be immunized against mumps or provide serologic evidence of immunity prior to performing patient care duties

Rubella

Rubella is a febrile childhood exanthem, with a generalized erythematous maculo-papular rash and lymphadenopathy. It is caused by the RNA virus, rubella virus, a member of the *Togaviridae* family. Rubella virus also causes congenital rubella syndrome (CRS) in congenitally infected infants, which is associated with intrauterine growth restriction, petechiae, hepatosplenomegaly, microcephaly, eye findings (cataracts, pigmentary retinopathy, glaucoma), cardiac disease (patent ductus arteriosus), sensorineural hearing loss, and neurologic abnormalities [5].

Rubella and thus CRS are vaccine-preventable diseases in most developed countries. However, there are still resource-limited areas where rubella immunization is not routine and rubella/CRS occurs. Therefore, healthcare professionals should be vigilant about suspecting CRS in infants from resource-limited countries, especially if they present with one or more clinical symptoms associated with CRS.

Rubella and CRS may be diagnosed by serologic detection of rubella IgM. Isolation of rubella virus in cell culture and detection of rubella virus by molecular diagnostic techniques may also be done in specialized public health laboratories, such as the Centers for Disease Control and Prevention (CDC).

Patients admitted to the hospital or cared for in the outpatient setting with suspected or proven rubella should be cared for under standard and droplet precautions [50]. Infants with CRS should be cared for in the hospital and outpatient setting under contact precautions, until they are 1 year of age or until two samples of clinical specimens (saliva/throat and urine) obtained at least 1 month apart are negative for rubella virus in tests performed by a reliable public health laboratory.

Varicella Zoster Virus Infections (Chicken Pox and Zoster)

Varicella zoster virus (VZV) is a DNA herpesvirus and the cause of chicken pox, a highly contagious, febrile, papulovesicular childhood exanthem, and zoster (shingles), a localized dermatomal papulovesicular reactivation. Infection with VZV may be associated with severe infections, such as pneumonia, hepatitis with hepatic necrosis, encephalitis, or hemorrhagic varicella in immunocompromised children. Chicken pox and zoster are vaccine-preventable diseases, with currently no clear seasonable distribution in countries where routine vaccination is recommended. In countries without routine immunization, a late winter-early spring seasonal distribution may be observed.

Infection with VZV, in both normal and immunocompromised hosts, is commonly treated with antivirals, such as acyclovir and valacyclovir; antivirals are not typically required in otherwise healthy children given the self-limited nature of the illness. Consideration should be given to the treatment of VZV in immunocompetent children >12-years old, those with chronic pulmonary or skin disorders, and those taking salicylates or corticosteroids [50]. Intravenous acyclovir is recommended for immunocompromised patients. Other antivirals commonly used to treat cytomegalovirus (CMV), such as ganciclovir, valganciclovir, foscarnet, and cidofovir, also have activity against VZV. Administration of varicella immune globulin (VariZIG) or intravenous immune globulin (IVIG) may be used in select situations for postexposure immunoprophylaxis, in addition to antiviral therapy with acyclovir or valacyclovir [50].

Transmission of VZV is person-to-person through the airborne route and from direct contact with patients with VZV infection. Skin lesions from chicken pox and zoster contain high titers of infectious virus which may aerosolize or be deposited on fomites or surfaces and are the most likely sources of viral transmission. Molecular techniques have also detected VZV DNA in the air surrounding patients with varicella zoster infections (chicken pox and zoster) [54]. Transmission from respiratory droplets is thought to be much less common. Nosocomial transmission of VZV infections is well documented in the healthcare setting (especially pediatric wards), and healthcare-associated outbreaks, sometimes with fatal outcomes in immunocompromised hosts, may occur [55, 56]. Patients hospitalized with chicken pox or disseminated zoster (or immunocompromised patients with simple zoster who may be at risk for dissemination) should be isolated in a private room equipped with a separate exhaust system and negative pressure air relative to the hallway, if such rooms are available [50]. They should also, in addition to standard precautions, be cared for with contact and airborne precautions. Isolation should continue until no new lesions occur, and all lesions that have occurred are completely crusted over. In addition, nonimmune patients in the hospital setting who have been exposed to varicella should also be isolated under airborne and contact precautions for 8–21 days after exposure (and up to 28 days after exposure if VariZIG or IVIG were received as postexposure immunoprophylaxis) if they require ongoing hospitalization. Newborns born to mothers with varicella at the time of delivery should also be isolated and cared for under contact and airborne precautions while hospitalized (or until 21 days of age or 28 days if immunoglobulin is provided). Normal patients with localized zoster may not require special isolation with airborne and contact precautions if the zoster lesions are able to be completely covered. However, some hospital infection control officers may prefer to isolate even immunocompetent patients with localized zoster under airborne precautions and, if available, place them in a negative pressure room, especially if they are roomed near immunocompromised patients.

Healthcare workers should provide documentation of either immunization with two doses of varicella vaccine or immunity to varicella zoster virus infection (through serologic testing for the presence of VZV IgG from a previous infection) prior to assuming patient care responsibilities.

Parvovirus

Parvovirus B19 is a common, single-stranded DNA virus that causes erythema infectiosum or fifth disease in normal healthy children. It also may cause a polyarthropathy syndrome or papular purpuric gloves and socks syndrome (PPGSS). Chronic anemia and red cell aplasia may occur in immunocompromised hosts, and transient aplastic crisis in patients with sickle cell anemia accompanied by prolonged viral excretion; such severe manifestations are potentially contagious in the healthcare setting. Newborns may also present with hydrops fetalis or congenital anemia. Nosocomial transmission of parvovirus B19 infections can occur from person to person through droplet transmission and, rarely, through blood products [57]. Healthcare-associated outbreaks of parvovirus B19 affecting both patients and hospital personnel have been described [58].

Detection of parvovirus B19 infection is by serologic assays of virus-specific IgG and IgM and detection of viral DNA using molecular techniques. Most blood products used for transfusion do not contain parvovirus B19, and when they do, it is often present only at a very low level. Blood product transmission of parvovirus B19 rarely results in symptomatic illness [57].

Patients hospitalized with parvovirus B19 infections who have aplastic crises, PPGSS, or chronic infection, should be isolated with standard and droplet precautions, because they often shed virus in larger quantities for extended periods of time and are therefore potentially contagious in the healthcare setting. Pregnant healthcare providers should be informed about the risks for exposure to parvovirus B19 and strategies to mitigate this risk (i.e., strict adherence to infection control policies).

Gastrointestinal Viruses

The gastrointestinal viruses are a major cause of healthcare-associated viral infections, and the viruses of major nosocomial importance include rotavirus, caliciviruses (including norovirus), astrovirus, toroviruses, enteric adenoviruses (especially serotypes 40/41), enteric enteroviruses, parechoviruses, and hepatitis A virus. The treatment of such infections is largely supportive with fluid and electrolyte replacement as needed.

Rotavirus

Rotavirus is an RNA virus and is a common cause of febrile diarrhea in young infants, often resulting in dehydration and electrolyte and acid-base abnormalities. It is usually a seasonal virus, with peak transmission occurring in fall and winter. Rotavirus commonly infects young infants who are in diapers, is often shed in large quantities in the stool even for many days after diarrhea has resolved, and survives for long periods of time on environmental surfaces. These specific characteristics allow for the ready nosocomial spread of rotavirus. Since the advent of the rotavirus vaccine, the epidemiology of rotavirus diarrhea has changed in developed countries who employ routine immunization, with a substantial decrease in outpatient visits and hospitalizations for rotavirus diarrhea as well as reduced nosocomial acquisition of infection [59]. Rotavirus is discussed in more detail in Chap. 12.

Caliciviruses, Including Norovirus

Caliciviruses, including norovirus, are a diverse group of RNA viruses that cause a self-limited gastrointestinal illness characterized by nausea, vomiting, and crampy abdominal pain with diarrhea. In premature infants, as well as immunocompromised or medically fragile patients, norovirus can be a severe, protracted and even fatal diarrheal illness [60]. Norovirus also has been associated with necrotizing enterocolitis in neonatal intensive care units [61]. Since the advent of routine immunization with rotavirus vaccine, norovirus has now become a leading cause of gastroenteritis in the United States and other developed countries, and an important nosocomial viral pathogen. Norovirus is discussed in more detail in Chap. 12.

Non-polio Gastrointestinal Enteroviruses and Parechoviruses

The non-polio enteroviruses are small RNA viruses and include coxsackie viruses groups A and B, echoviruses, and a variety of other enteroviruses, comprising over 100 serotypes. Enteroviruses also are classified genetically as belonging to groups A, B, C, or D, while still retaining serotype designations. The parechoviruses were formerly known as echoviruses 22 and 23. These viruses are common and distributed worldwide, with a summer and fall seasonal pattern in most countries.

The non-polio enteroviruses and parechoviruses cause vomiting and diarrhea, hepatitis, hand-foot-mouth disease, and severe disease with an acute viral sepsis syndrome. An exanthem, myocarditis, and meningoencephalitis may also occur in neonates and immunocompromised patients, including transplant recipients, children with cancer, and those with hypogammaglobulinemia. Outbreaks of enterovirus and parechovirus infections, often with severe disease, have been documented in pediatric hospitals, especially neonatal intensive care units [62–65].

Patients with suspected or documented infections with enteroviruses or parechovirus should be under both standard and contact precautions. In nursery outbreaks, cohorting may be helpful to limit spread of the virus. Vigorous hand hygiene and decontamination of environmental surfaces are also recommended.

Enteric Adenoviruses

Many adenoviruses may cause gastrointestinal disease, but the serotypes 40/41 as well as serotypes 12, 18, 31, 52, and 61 are associated primarily with diarrhea. Most infections are self-limited in healthy hosts, but severe and fatal disease may occur in newborns and immunocompromised hosts [66].

Transmission of ADV in the healthcare setting is primarily person-to-person through contact with infected secretions, as well as by fomites, infected environmental surfaces, and by droplet spread. Nosocomial outbreaks in pediatric wards, intensive care units, and neonatal intensive care units have been documented [67]. All patients hospitalized with a suspected or proven gastrointestinal virus should be isolated under standard and contact precautions for duration of illness.

As discussed above, the treatment of routine ADV infections is supportive, as most infections are self-limited; severe infections in immunocompromised hosts may be managed with cidofovir or brincidofovir.

Mucocutaneous Viruses

Human Papillomaviruses

The human papillomaviruses (HPV) are DNA viruses which can be grouped by their ability to infect cutaneous or mucosal sites and their capacity (defined as high or low risk) to cause cancer. The HPVs of nosocomial transmission interest are primarily those low risk, cutaneous types 6 and 11, which cause oral or cutaneous warts, laryngeal papillomas, and juvenile respiratory papillomatosis. The latter is a chronic disease of the respiratory tract that often requires repeated surgical procedures or photoangiolytic laser treatments to alleviate long-term stenotic complications in the airways. Oral warts and oropharyngeal cancers caused by HPV types 16 and 18 also may require laser/electrosurgery procedures. These procedures may generate laser plumes, aerosols, or smoke that may contain HPV virus particles and therefore are a potential risk for healthcare workers. The risk of inhalation of potentially infectious aerosols that may be generated during the procedure can be mitigated by performing the procedures in a well-ventilated room, while using localized smoke evacuator exhaust ventilation, and wearing of N95 respirators during the procedure [68]. Reports also exist of HPV contamination of improperly sterilized gynecologic instruments and vaginal ultrasound probes [69, 70]. Patients with HPV infections, however, do not require special precautions during normal, routine medical encounters that are not associated with laser therapy.

Herpes Simplex Viruses

The herpes simplex viruses (HSV) types 1 and 2 are enveloped DNA viruses which commonly cause asymptomatic infections, as well as a variety of illnesses, including the following: neonatal HSV syndromes; skin, oral, and/or genital lesions; eczema herpeticum; keratoconjunctivitis; acute retinal necrosis; and disseminated disease, which may have a fatal outcome. Patients who are critically ill and intubated, have extensive burns, or are immunocompromised may experience a reactivation of HSV infection and may develop oropharyngeal or cutaneous herpetic lesions. As such, it is not uncommon for patients to experience HSV reactivation and recurrent disease while in the hospital. Alternatively, physiologic stress may induce laboratory detectable HSV reactivation without overt disease [71]. Up to 14% of patients with septic shock develop HSV reactivation with transient viremia, although the clinical significance of this is a bit unclear [72, 73]. Primary corneal graft failure has also been reported due to reactivation of latent corneal HSV in donor tissue following corneal transplantation [74]. Nosocomial outbreaks with HSV have been reported in eye clinics.

Antiviral treatment with acyclovir or valacyclovir is commonly used for active HSV disease, suppression of HSV infection after successful treatment, or prevention of reactivation HSV infection. The antivirals ganciclovir, valganciclovir, foscarnet, and cidofovir also have activity against HSV and are second-line antivirals for HSV treatment.

In addition to standard precautions, patients with HSV mucocutaneous or skin lesions should be placed on contact precautions. However if the HSV recurrence consists of a single lesion or small, localized lesions, standard precautions may be appropriate, with good hand hygiene technique. Single use eye instruments are preferred for routine eye exams and exams in neonates for retinopathy or prematurity. Sodium hypochlorite (dilute bleach) appears to effectively disinfect HSV on reusable tonometers and specula used for eye exams. In some studies 70% isopropyl alcohol was also an effective disinfectant against HSV on eye specula [37, 38, 75].

Blood-Borne and Tissue-Borne Viruses

Viruses that may be found in, and potentially transmitted by, blood product or tissue or organ donation include hepatitis B, hepatitis C, hepatitis E, cytomegalovirus (CMV), human herpes virus 8, parvovirus B19, HIV, HTLV-1 and HTLV-2, dengue virus, West Nile virus, and Colorado tick fever virus. In addition, prions may also be potentially transmitted in this manner. Of these, CMV is the most commonly transmitted through blood products in the United States [76]. Since an in-depth discussion on blood-borne pathogens is beyond the scope of this chapter, the reader seeking more details on blood product screening and safety and the management of these infections is asked to see reviews on potential transfusion-transmitted viruses [4, 50].

Breast Milk-Borne Infections

A variety of viruses may be detected and potentially transmitted through maternal breast milk, including CMV, hepatitis B, hepatitis C, HIV, HTLV-1 and HTLV-2, herpes simplex virus, rubella, varicella, and West Nile virus. Of these, CMV has the most relevance as a healthcare-associated virus [50]. Additional discussion of this topic is provided in Chap. 15.

Cytomegalovirus

CMV is a common herpes family DNA virus that most commonly causes asymptomatic infection but also may cause mononucleosis syndrome, hepatitis, pneumonitis, or a viral sepsis-like syndrome in premature infants. It can be transmitted via breast milk, blood product transfusions, and tissue or organ donation. Person-to-person transmission of CMV has not been documented to occur in the hospital setting, even though CMV transmission is common in the family and daycare settings, where close contact and the sharing of food, drink, and toys are common. CMV infections may also reactivate in immunocompromised patients, such as transplant recipients, burn patients, or patients in intensive care units, and cause serious disease [77, 78].

Postnatal CMV infection in the very low birth weight infant is an important healthcare-associated viral infection in the neonatal intensive care unit. Primary sources for postnatal CMV infection in these vulnerable neonates include blood transfusions and breast milk. Most neonatal intensive care units provide CMV-seronegative or CMV-"safe," leukocyte-depleted sources of blood products, reducing the risk of blood product transmission considerably. Recent studies have shown that maternal breast milk is a primary source of postnatal CMV infection and disease in preterm infants [79]. Fresh or refrigerated breast milk is more likely to transmit CMV than frozen-thawed breast milk, and pasteurized breast milk carries very little to nil risk of CMV transmission [79–81].

Infants with postnatal CMV infection from breast milk feedings typically become ill after the first month of life and may present with apnea and bradycardia, thrombocytopenia, neutropenia, hepatitis, viral sepsis syndrome, necrotizing enterocolitis, or pneumonitis. Postnatal CMV infection is best documented by a negative CMV urine or saliva culture or molecular detection test performed in the first 21 days of life (to exclude congenital CMV), followed by a subsequent positive CMV detection test on the same samples after 1 month of life. These infants are often viremic and CMV can be detected and quantified in blood by molecular techniques. Since severe illness and even death may occur in postnatal CMV infections in very low birth weight infants, antiviral therapy with ganciclovir or valganciclovir may be indicated in infants who present with serious symptoms and/or demonstrate significant viremia. Antiviral treatment is often administered for 3–6 weeks, depending on clinical and virologic response.

Infants with postnatal CMV infection do not require special isolation procedures and standard precautions are recommended.

Viruses that Require Special Containment and Special Circumstances

Recent worldwide outbreaks of emerging/re-emerging highly virulent viral infections have highlighted the importance of continued vigilance in infection control and prevention in an increasingly "global world." The following section will highlight infection control considerations for highly virulent viral pathogens.

Severe Acute Respiratory Syndrome Coronavirus (SARS-CoV) and Middle East Respiratory Syndrome Coronavirus (MERS-CoV)

The severe acute respiratory syndromes (SARS) include SARS-coronavirus (CoV) and Middle East respiratory syndrome coronavirus (MERS-CoV) [82, 83]. These syndromes are acute viral respiratory and gastrointestinal illnesses caused by novel coronaviruses and are spread from person to person through close contact. MERS-CoV may also be transmitted through contact with infected camels. Infection with SARS-CoV was first reported in Asia in 2003 and becomes a global epidemic, affecting over 20 countries in North and South America, Europe, and Asia. Since 2004, there have been no reported cases of SARS-CoV anywhere in the world. Infection with MERS-CoV was first reported in Jordan and Saudi Arabia in 2012 and has spread in the Arabian Peninsula and to the Republic of Korea. The WHO and CDC monitor SARS-CoV and MERS-CoV activity globally.

Both SARS-CoV and MERS-CoV infections in children can be suspected if patients have had contact with a known case of SARS-CoV (hypothetically) or MERS-CoV, recent travel to areas of the world with active SARS-CoV or MERS-CoV transmission, or close contact with someone ill who had such travel. Usually infants and young children have milder illness, such as fever, rhinorrhea, and slight cough. However, older children and adolescents may have severe illness with fever, cough rhinorrhea, headache, chills, lymphopenia, dyspnea, hypoxemia, and/or respiratory failure requiring mechanical ventilation. Unilateral or bilateral pneumonia on chest radiographs also are typically present in severe illness. While the illness is primarily respiratory, diarrhea also may occur. Both SARS-CoV and MERS-CoV infections have a high reported mortality rate (a mortality rate ranging from 20% to 50% has been reported for MERS-CoV in some series) [84, 85]. There are no specific antiviral medications available proven to be effective against coronaviruses. Treatment is therefore primarily symptomatic, with fluid management and mechanical ventilation administered as needed.

Importantly, a number of cases of transmission of these viruses from patients or family members to other patients or hospital staff with serious consequences have been documented [86]. Given the potential severity of these illnesses, attention to appropriate isolation and infection control measures is essential. While most coronaviruses require only routine and contact precautions, patients suspected to have infection with (often referred to as a person under investigation or PUI) or proven to be infected with SARS-CoV or MERS-CoV require airborne, droplet, and contact precautions. Patients should be given a mask to wear over their nose and mouth and isolated in an airborne infection isolation room (AIIR) or a special isolation unit (SIU), if available. Only specially trained, essential personnel should enter the hospital room to care for the patient, and a log of all persons should be maintained, and their symptoms monitored for fever, cough, or other acute illnesses for 14 days after contact with the patient. Personnel should be trained in both standard hand hygiene and personal protective equipment (PPE), such as gloves, gowns, and eye protection, as well as use of fit-tested, N95 filtering facepiece respirators in AIIRs or powered air-purifying respirators (PAPRs) used in SIUs (Figs. 14.1 and 14.2) [82, 83]. Caution should be used when performing aerosol-generating procedures, such as suctioning, intubation, linen changing, and toilet flushing [87]. Patients suspected or proven to be infected with either SARS-CoV or MERS-CoV should be reported to the healthcare facility infection control officer and the local public health authorities immediately.

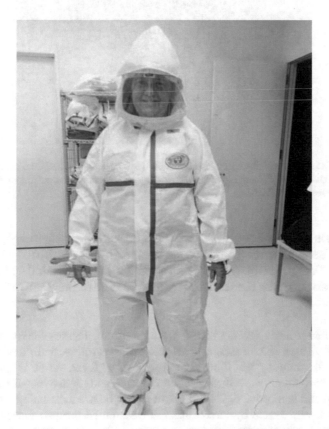

Fig. 14.1 The author, wearing special isolation unit (SIU) personal protective equipment (PPE) – inner layer – consisting of a liquid impervious jump suit with powered air-purifying respirator (PAPR)

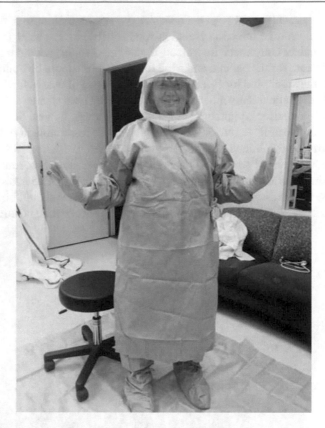

Fig. 14.2 The author, wearing special isolation unit (SIU) personal protective equipment (PPE) – outer layer – consisting of liquid impervious gown, three layers of gloves, and boots, with powered air-purifying respirator (PAPR)

Viral Hemorrhagic Fevers: Filoviruses (Ebola and Marburg), Bunyaviruses (Hemorrhagic Fever with Renal Syndrome (HFRS), Crimean-Congo Hemorrhagic Fever (CCHF) and Rift Valley Fever (RVF), Arenaviruses (Lassa Fever), and Flaviviruses (Dengue Fever)

The viral hemorrhagic fevers (VHFs) are a group of illnesses caused by different families of viruses (filoviruses, bunyaviruses, arenaviruses, and flaviviruses) that cause a similar multisystem illness characterized by fever, vomiting and diarrhea, respiratory symptoms, as well as vascular damage, with disseminated intravascular coagulation and hemorrhage. These infections can be life threatening.

Dengue fever, caused by flaviviruses, is transmitted through mosquito vectors and is not transmitted through person-to-person contact (with the exception of rare cases of transfusion-associated transmission). Therefore standard precautions are usually recommended, since the healthcare-associated risks of this VHF is low.

Similarly, the VHF caused by bunyaviruses (HFRS, CCHF, and RVF) require standard precautions, with the addition of contact, droplet, or airborne precautions for some cases of CCHF, with isolation in an AAIR or SIU required in certain circumstances which should be individualized. Consultation with public health authorities is recommended in suspected cases of CCHF.

Of the VHFs, Ebola virus disease (EVD) poses the greatest healthcare-associated transmission risk and therefore will be the focus of this section [88]. Ebola virus disease (EVD) is caused by infection with one of the five known Ebola viruses. Ebola virus was first discovered in 1976 near the Ebola River in the Democratic Republic of Congo. It has caused many severe outbreaks in Africa, and in 2014–2016, an Ebola virus outbreak in West Africa spread to urban areas in Africa. Subsequently, through commercial air travel, the outbreak became a global epidemic with spread to the United States and Europe and also involving infection in healthcare workers. Ebola virus transmission should always be considered to be potentially occurring in sub-Saharan Africa, and with global air travel common, the potential spread outside of Africa remains an ongoing concern for healthcare workers. The CDC and WHO constantly monitor EVD activity.

Ebola virus is spread from person to person through direct contact with bodily fluids or contaminated linens, trash, medical equipment, and instruments in contact with a person who is sick or who has died from EVD. Ebola virus may also be transmitted through needle sticks or sexual contact. Vertical transmission from mother to fetus/newborn has been documented. It is also been spread through direct contact with infected fruit bats or primates, especially if eaten as "bushmeat."

Ebola virus infection usually causes fever, headache, myalgias, and weakness early in the course of illness. It may mimic a flu-like illness. A rash is often present, and vomiting and diarrhea are common, as well. Respiratory symptoms may also occur, especially in children. Infection with Ebola virus should be suspected in patients with these symptoms who have had recent travel in an area where Ebola virus transmission is reported to be occurring; furthermore, such suspected cases should be reported to public health authorities at once. In the latter stages of the illness, disseminated intravascular coagulation occurs, followed by hemorrhage and death in up to 50% of patients. All bodily fluids should be considered to be highly infectious and handled with extreme care [88].

The diagnosis of Ebola virus can be established by detection of Ebola virus in the blood by PCR. The PCR test must be performed at first suspicion of EVD and also at least 3 days after the onset of febrile symptoms, at which time significant viremia may be present. Consultation with public health officials (such as the CDC) is highly recommended regarding the handling and processing of specimens from patients with suspected or proven EVD.

Treatment of EVD is primarily symptomatic, with fluid resuscitation and, if needed and determined to be medically beneficial on an individual basis, mechanical ventilation and other critical care support. Currently, there are no antiviral medications licensed for treatment of EVD. However, experimental antiviral clinical trial protocols are available. In addition, immunotherapeutics, using convalescent plasma or blood transfusions from EVD survivors, has been administered with some promise of benefit. Finally, a variety of monoclonal antibodies and vaccine strategies are under development or in clinical trials.

PUIs or those proven to be infected with Ebola virus should be given a mask to wear over their nose and mouth if they are coughing and not vomiting; isolated in an AIIR or SIU, if available; and transferred, if possible, to a designated Ebola treatment center for children, which is available in developed countries [88]. In resource-limited healthcare facilities, mobile Ebola treatment units (ETUs) are typically set up, with "cold zone" and "hot zone" designations to minimize the risk of healthcare-associated transmission between patients, from patients to healthcare workers, and to the community [88]. Only specially trained, essential personnel should enter the SIU, ETU, or hospital room to care for the patient with suspected or proven EVD, and a log of all persons should be maintained, and their symptoms monitored for fever, cough, or other acute illnesses for 14 days after contact with the patient. Personnel should be trained in both standard hand hygiene and PPE, such as gloves, gowns, and eye and face shield protection, as well as use of fit-tested, N95 filtering facepiece respirators and face shields in AIIRs or PAPRs used in SIUs [89]. Caution should be used when performing all aerosol-generating procedures. All procedures, such as blood drawing or central line access, should be minimized, carefully planned, and performed with extreme care. All trash contaminated with bodily fluids requires special handling and should be double-bagged, taped closed, and autoclaved or incinerated prior to leaving the SIU or ETU. Toilets should be flushed with the lid closed, or with a covering over the bowl during the flush, to minimize aerosols of potentially infectious material [87]. All surfaces in contact with the patient, or near the patient, should be frequently cleaned and decontaminated, and special handling is required after a spill or body fluid contamination. PUIs or those proven to be infected with Ebola virus should be reported to the healthcare facility infection control officer and the local public health authorities at once. If the patient dies, special precautions are recommended for autopsy and handling of the human remains.

Smallpox (Variola) and Monkeypox

Smallpox is an ancient and serious illness caused by variola virus, a large DNA virus in the *Orthopoxvirus* genus and *Poxviridae* family, and is primarily of historical significance, although the risk of a bioterrorism event involving smallpox remains a real concern. While many patients infected with smallpox survived, often with scars on their body or blindness, the mortality rate historically was approximately 30%. The last known case of naturally occurring smallpox in the United States was documented in 1949 and globally occurred in 1977 [90].

Monkeypox is a member of the same virus genus and family as smallpox, and was discovered in 1958 in monkey colonies [91]. The first human case was reported in 1970 in Africa, in the Democratic Republic of Congo, and in 2003 an outbreak spread to the United States. Given this relatively recent emergence, clinicians should be vigilant for new cases of monkeypox.

Smallpox is spread from human-to-human through respiratory droplets during coughing and sneezing in the early stage, and via their sores in the mouth and on the skin, once the disease has become established. Patients are contagious until the last smallpox lesion scab crusts over and falls off. It is also possible for smallpox to be transmitted via the airborne route and on fomites such as linens that were in contact with smallpox lesions. There is no known animal or insect vector for smallpox.

Monkeypox is transmitted from person to person through close contact with bodily fluids or large respiratory droplets; contact with fomites or animals, such as African rodents or prairie dogs, infected with monkeypox may also lead to human disease.

Smallpox can be suspected in children with known contact with someone who had smallpox (e.g., in the event of a bioterrorism event); however, healthcare personnel should be vigilant for a possible first or sentinel case of this highly contagious disease and suspect it in any acutely ill patient with an acute, generalized pustular rash. The illness may have several stages, first starting with high fever, myalgias, and vomiting. The first stage is followed by the early rash stage, with lesions on the tongue, in the mouth, and then on the skin, which spread rapidly to all parts of the body, in the same stage or time frame. The pustular rash stage then occurs, and within 2–3 weeks, the lesions crust into scabs and then fall off. Once all scabs have fallen off, the patient is no longer contagious. Smallpox rarely if ever causes significant lymphadenopathy.

Monkeypox illness may cause fever, headache, myalgias, and significant lymphadenopathy. The rash associated with monkeypox begins within 1–3 days after the constitutional symptoms and usually progresses, similar to smallpox, through the stages of macules, papules, vesicles, pustules, and scabs. The pustular rash stage lasts 2–3 weeks; the lesions crust into scabs and then fall off. Similar to small pox, the patient is no longer contagious once all scabs have fallen off. Monkeypox can be a severe illness, with a mortality rate of approximately 10%.

Smallpox or monkeypox infection may be confirmed using special virus isolation techniques or PCR identification of specific viral DNA in a clinical specimen at a public health laboratory. Electron microscopy of a lesion may provide presumptive identification if orthopoxvirus virions are detected.

Treatment of smallpox or monkeypox includes antiviral treatment with antivirals such as tecovirimat, cidofovir, or brincidofovir, as well as supportive care with fluids and respiratory support, as needed. It is not recommended to give vaccinia immune globulin (VIG) for treatment of established disease caused by smallpox. It is not known if VIG can be beneficial in the treatment of monkeypox disease. Prior immunization or postexposure prophylaxis with the smallpox vaccine given within 3–7 days of exposure may provide protection against smallpox and monkeypox infection or severe disease. In patients with severe immune deficiency who cannot receive smallpox vaccine, use of VIG may be beneficial for postexposure prophylaxis.

Patients suspected or proven to be infected with smallpox virus or monkeypox virus should be isolated with standard, contact, and droplet precautions, preferably in an AIIR or SIU, if available. The patient should wear a mask placed over the nose and mouth, and their exposed skin with lesions covered with a sheet or gown or linens. Only specially trained, essential personnel should enter the hospital room to care for the patient, and a log of all persons should be maintained, and their symptoms monitored for fever, cough or other acute illnesses for 14 days after contact with the patient. Similar care regarding use of PPE, the generation of aerosols, the disposal of waste, and care of deceased patients used for patients with EVD apply to those with known or proven smallpox/monkeypox. Patients suspected or proven to be infected with either smallpox or monkeypox should be reported to the healthcare facility infection control officer and the local public health authorities immediately.

Prions

Human prion diseases, also called the transmissible spongiform encephalopathies, are very rare, uniformly fatal neurodegenerative disorders. These naturally occurring diseases include Creutzfeldt-Jakob disease (CJD), fatal insomnia, and Gerstmann-Straussler-Scheinker syndrome. Iatrogenic CJD may occur by nosocomial prion transmission after contaminated growth hormone injections, cadaveric dura mater graft, stereotactic EEG electrodes and other neurosurgical procedures, ophthalmologic procedures such as corneal transplants, or blood product transfusions [92]. Prions are small, highly resilient proteins which are capable of self-propagation via autocatalytic templating and are highly resistant to conventional methods of decontamination. The presence of prion-contaminated instruments in the operating room, especially when neurosurgical and ophthalmologic procedures are performed, poses a rare but potentially serious risk of healthcare-associated transmission.

The diagnosis of CJD, and other prion disorders, is most reliably established by examination of brain tissue obtained by brain biopsy or at autopsy. Noninvasive diagnostic tests are under investigation. The prion disorders are uniformly fatal and no treatment is available except supportive therapies.

Patients suspected to have or diagnosed with a prion disease, such as CJD, do not require special isolation, and standard precautions are indicated for routine, noninvasive, patient care encounters. However, if patients require invasive procedures, tissues such as the brain, eye, and spinal cord, as well as the surgical instruments in contact with these tissues, should be considered to be highly infectious. During procedures in patients with known or suspected prion disease, protective measures should include a minimum of healthcare workers in the operating room, covering all non-disposable, multiple-use instruments, employing single-use equipment whenever possible, unidirectional flow of instruments, disposal of all single-use items by incineration, and thorough cleaning of all work surfaces.

Prions are highly resistant to chemical disinfectants such as alcohol, ammonia, and formalin, as well as boiling, dry heating, and ultraviolet or microwave exposure. Incineration is probably the most effective means of decontamination; however, some experts feel thorough cleaning with concentrated bleach or sodium hydroxide for an hour, followed by prolonged autoclaving, may be sufficient to decrease infectivity of prion-contaminated surgical instruments. Special handling for autopsy and body remains should also be followed. The WHO has detailed infection control guidelines and practices for prion infection [93].

References

1. Rubin LG, Kohn N, Nullet S, Hill M. Reduction in rate of nosocomial respiratory virus infections in a children's hospital associated with enhanced isolation precautions. Infect Control Hosp Epidemiol. 2018;39(2):152–6.
2. Goldmann DA. Epidemiology and prevention of pediatric viral respiratory infections in healthcare institutions. Emerg Infect Dis. 2001;7(2):249–53.
3. Hutspardol S, Essa M, Richardson S, Schechter T, Ali M, Krueger J, et al. Significant transplantation-related mortality from respiratory virus infections within the first one hundred days in children after hematopoietic stem cell transplantation. Biol Blood Marrow Transplant. 2015;21(10):1802–7.
4. Huskins C, Shaklee-Sammons J, Coffin S. Health-care associated infections. In: Cherry J, Harrison G, Kaplan S, Steinbach W, Hotez P, editors. Feigin and Cherry's textbook of pediatric infectious diseases. Philadelphia: Elsevier; 2018. p. 2514–42.
5. Quach C, Shah R, Rubin LG. Burden of healthcare-associated viral respiratory infections in children's hospitals. J Pediatric Infect Dis Soc. 2018;7(1):18–24.
6. Verboon-Maciolek MA, Krediet TG, Gerards LJ, Fleer A, van Loon TM. Clinical and epidemiologic characteristics of viral infections in a neonatal intensive care unit during a 12-year period. Pediatr Infect Dis J. 2005;24(10):901–4.
7. D'Arcy N, Cloutman-Green E, Klein N, Spratt DA. Environmental viral contamination in a pediatric hospital outpatient waiting area: implications for infection control. Am J Infect Control. 2014;42(8):856–60.
8. Halasa NB, Williams JV, Wilson GJ, Walsh WF, Schaffner W, Wright PF. Medical and economic impact of a respiratory syncytial virus outbreak in a neonatal intensive care unit. Pediatr Infect Dis J. 2005;24(12):1040–4.
9. Thorburn K, Eisenhut M, Riordan A. Mortality and morbidity of nosocomial respiratory syncytial virus (RSV) infection in ventilated children--a ten year perspective. Minerva Anestesiol. 2012;78(7):782.
10. Thorburn K, Kerr S, Taylor N, van Saene HK. RSV outbreak in a paediatric intensive care unit. J Hosp Infect. 2004;57(3):194–201.
11. Taylor GS, Vipond IB, Caul EO. Molecular epidemiology of outbreak of respiratory syncytial virus within bone marrow transplantation unit. J Clin Microbiol. 2001;39(2):801–3.
12. Shah DP, Ghantoji SS, Shah JN, El Taoum KK, Jiang Y, Popat U, et al. Impact of aerosolized ribavirin on mortality in 280 allogeneic haematopoietic stem cell transplant recipients with respiratory syncytial virus infections. J Antimicrob Chemother. 2013;68(8):1872–80.
13. Burrows FS, Carlos LM, Benzimra M, Marriott DJ, Havryk AP, Plit ML, et al. Oral ribavirin for respiratory syncytial virus infection after lung transplantation: efficacy and cost-efficiency. J Heart Lung Transplant. 2015;34(7):958–62.
14. Kulkarni H, Smith CM, Lee Ddo H, Hirst RA, Easton AJ, O'Callaghan C. Evidence of respiratory syncytial virus spread by aerosol. Time to revisit infection control strategies? Am J Respir Crit Care Med. 2016;194(3):308–16.
15. Sung AD, Sung JAM, Thomas S, Hyslop T, Gasparetto C, Long G, et al. Universal mask usage for reduction of respiratory viral infections after stem cell transplant: a prospective trial. Clin Infect Dis. 2016;63(8):999–1006.
16. Sokol KA, De la Vega-Diaz I, Edmondson-Martin K, Kim S, Tindle S, Wallach F, et al. Masks for prevention of respiratory viruses on the BMT unit: results of a quality initiative. Transpl Infect Dis. 2016;18(6):965–7.

17. Sim SA, Leung VKY, Ritchie D, Slavin MA, Sullivan SG, Teh BW. Viral respiratory tract infections in allogeneic hematopoietic stem cell transplantation recipients in the era of molecular testing. Biol Blood Marrow Transplant. 2018;24(7):1490–6.
18. Kakiuchi S, Tsuji M, Nishimura H, Wang L, Takayama-Ito M, Kinoshita H, et al. Human parainfluenza virus type 3 infections in patients with hematopoietic stem cell transplants: the mode of nosocomial infections and prognosis. Jpn J Infect Dis. 2018;71(2):109–15.
19. Casey J, Morris K, Narayana M, Nakagaki M, Kennedy GA. Oral ribavirin for treatment of respiratory syncitial virus and parainfluenza 3 virus infections post allogeneic haematopoietic stem cell transplantation. Bone Marrow Transplant. 2013;48(12):1558–61.
20. Kim S, Sung H, Im HJ, Hong SJ, Kim MN. Molecular epidemiological investigation of a nosocomial outbreak of human metapneumovirus infection in a pediatric hemato-oncology patient population. J Clin Microbiol. 2009;47(4):1221–4.
21. Hoellein A, Hecker J, Hoffmann D, Gottle F, Protzer U, Peschel C, et al. Serious outbreak of human metapneumovirus in patients with hematologic malignancies. Leuk Lymphoma. 2016;57(3):623–7.
22. Houlihan C, Frampton D, Ferns RB, Raffle J, Grant P, Reidy M, et al. The use of whole genome sequencing in the investigation of a nosocomial influenza virus outbreak. J Infect Dis. 2018 [E pub ahead of print].
23. Bearden A, Friedrich TC, Goldberg TL, Byrne B, Spiegel C, Schult P, et al. An outbreak of the 2009 influenza a (H1N1) virus in a children's hospital. Influenza Other Respir Viruses. 2012;6(5):374–9.
24. Fanella ST, Pinto MA, Bridger NA, Bullard JM, Coombs JM, Crockett ME, et al. Pandemic (H1N1) 2009 influenza in hospitalized children in Manitoba: nosocomial transmission and lessons learned from the first wave. Infect Control Hosp Epidemiol. 2011;32(5):435–43.
25. Pollara CP, Piccinelli G, Rossi G, Cattaneo C, Perandin F, Corbellini S, et al. Nosocomial outbreak of the pandemic Influenza A (H1N1) 2009 in critical hematologic patients during seasonal influenza 2010-2011: detection of oseltamivir resistant variant viruses. BMC Infect Dis. 2013;13:127.
26. Xiao S, Tang JW, Hui DS, Lei H, Yu H, Li Y. Probable transmission routes of the influenza virus in a nosocomial outbreak. Epidemiol Infect. 2018;146(9):1114–22.
27. Feemster K, Localio R, Grundmeier R, Metlay JP, Coffin SE. Incidence of healthcare-associated influenza-like illness after a primary care encounter among young children. J Pediatric Infect Dis Soc. 2018 [E pub ahead of print].
28. Bhadelia N, Sonti R, McCarthy JW, Vorenkamp J, Jia H, Saiman L, et al. Impact of the 2009 influenza A (H1N1) pandemic on healthcare workers at a tertiary care center in New York City. Infect Control Hosp Epidemiol. 2013;34(8):825–31.
29. Steiner M, Strassl R, Straub J, Bohm J, Popow-Kraupp T, Berger A. Nosocomial rhinovirus infection in preterm infants. Pediatr Infect Dis J. 2012;31(12):1302–4.
30. Reid AB, Anderson TL, Cooley L, Williamson J, McGregor AR. An outbreak of human rhinovirus species C infections in a neonatal intensive care unit. Pediatr Infect Dis J. 2011;30(12):1096–5.
31. Reese SM, Thompson M, Price CS, Young HL. Evidence of nosocomial transmission of human rhinovirus in a neonatal intensive care unit. Am J Infect Control. 2016;44(3):355–7.
32. Centers for Disease Control and Prevention. Enterovirus D68. https://www.cdc.gov/non-polio-enterovirus/about/EV-D68.html. Published 2018. Accessed 13 June 2018.
33. Gralton J, McLaws ML, Rawlinson WD. Personal clothing as a potential vector of respiratory virus transmission in childcare settings. J Med Virol. 2015;87(6):925–30.
34. Ersoy Y, Otlu B, Turkcuoglu P, Yetkin F, Aker S, Kuzucu C. Outbreak of adenovirus serotype 8 conjunctivitis in preterm infants in a neonatal intensive care unit. J Hosp Infect. 2012;80(2):144–9.
35. Palomino MA, Larranaga C, Avendano LF. Hospital-acquired adenovirus 7h infantile respiratory infection in Chile. Pediatr Infect Dis J. 2000;19(6):527–31.

36. Uzuner H, Karadenizli A, Kadir Er D, Osmani A. Investigation of the efficacy of alcohol-based solutions on adenovirus serotypes 8, 19 and 37, the common cause of epidemic keratoconjunctivitis, after an adenovirus outbreak occurred in the hospital. J Hosp Infect. 2018 [E pub ahead of print].

37. Woodman TJ, Coats DK, Paysse EA, Demmler GJ, Rossmann SN. Disinfection of eyelid speculums for retinopathy of prematurity examination. Arch Ophthalmol. 1998;116(9):1195–8.

38. Junk AK, Chen PP, Lin SC, Nouri-Mahdavi K, Radhakrishnan S, Singh K, et al. Disinfection of Tonometers: a report by the American academy of ophthalmology. Ophthalmology. 2017;124(12):1867–75.

39. Cloutman-Green E, Canales M, Pankhurst L, Evenor T, Malone D, Klein N, et al. Development and implementation of a cleaning standard algorithm to monitor the efficiency of terminal cleaning in removing adenovirus within a pediatric hematopoietic stem cell transplantation unit. Am J Infect Control. 2015;43(9):997–9.

40. Weber DJ, Anderson D, Rutala WA. The role of the surface environment in healthcare-associated infections. Curr Opin Infect Dis. 2013;26(4):338–44.

41. Saadi H, Pagnier I, Colson P, Cherif JK, Beji M, Boughalmi M, et al. First isolation of Mimivirus in a patient with pneumonia. Clin Infect Dis. 2013;57(4):e127–34.

42. Vincent A, La Scola B, Papazian L. Advances in Mimivirus pathogenicity. Intervirology. 2010;53(5):304–9.

43. dos Santos Silva LK, Arantes TS, Andrade KR, Lima Rodrigues RA, Miranda Boratto PV, de Freitas Almeida GM, et al. High positivity of mimivirus in inanimate surfaces of a hospital respiratory-isolation facility, Brazil. J Clin Virol. 2015;66:62–5.

44. Bousbia S, Papazian L, Saux P, Forel JM, Auffray JP, Martin C, et al. Serologic prevalence of amoeba-associated microorganisms in intensive care unit pneumonia patients. PLoS One. 2013;8(3):e58111.

45. Anderson RM, May RM. Directly transmitted infections diseases: control by vaccination. Science. 1982;215(4536):1053–60.

46. Guerra FM, Bolotin S, Lim G, Heffernan J, Deeks SL, Li Y, et al. The basic reproduction number (R0) of measles: a systematic review. Lancet Infect Dis. 2017;17(12):e420–8.

47. Botelho-Nevers E, Gautret P, Biellik R, Brouqui P. Nosocomial transmission of measles: an updated review. Vaccine. 2012;30(27):3996–4001.

48. Farizo KM, Stehr-Green PA, Simpson DM, Markowitz LE. Pediatric emergency room visits: a risk factor for acquiring measles. Pediatrics. 1991;87(1):74–9.

49. Centers for Disease Control and Prevention. Hospital-associated measles outbreak – Pennsylvania, March–April 2009. MMWR Morb Mortal Wkly Rep. 2012;61(2):30–2.

50. American Academy of Pediatrics. Red book report of the committee on infectious diseases. 31st ed. Itasca: American Academy of Pediatrics; 2018.

51. Kutty PK, Kyaw MH, Dayan GH, Brady MT, Bocchini JA, Reef SE, et al. Guidance for isolation precautions for mumps in the United States: a review of the scientific basis for policy change. Clin Infect Dis. 2010;50(12):1619–28.

52. Fischer PR, Brunetti C, Welch V, Christenson JC. Nosocomial mumps: report of an outbreak and its control. Am J Infect Control. 1996;24(1):13–8.

53. Gilroy SA, Domachowske JB, Johnson L, Martin D, Gross S, Bode M, et al. Mumps exposure of a health care provider working in a neonatal intensive care unit leads to a hospital-wide effort that prevented an outbreak. Am J Infect Control. 2011;39(8):697–700.

54. Sawyer MH, Chamberlin CJ, Wu YN, Aintablian N, Wallace MR. Detection of varicella-zoster virus DNA in air samples from hospital rooms. J Infect Dis. 1994;169(1):91–4.

55. Yoshikawa T, Ihira M, Suzuki K, Suga S, Tomitaka A, Ueda H, et al. Rapid contamination of the environments with varicella-zoster virus DNA from a patient with herpes zoster. J Med Virol. 2001;63(1):64–6.

56. Depledge DP, Brown J, Macanovic J, Underhill G, Breuer J. Viral genome sequencing proves nosocomial transmission of fatal varicella. J Infect Dis. 2016;214(9):1399–402.

57. Juhl D, Ozdemir M, Dreier J, Gorg S, Hennig H. Look-back study on recipients of parvovirus B19 (B19V) DNA-positive blood components. Vox Sang. 2015;109(4):305–11.
58. Sungkate S, Phongsamart W, Rungmaitree S, Lapphra K, Wittawatmongkol O, Pumsuwan V, et al. Human parvovirus B19 nosocomial outbreak in healthcare personnel in a paediatric ward at a national tertiary referral centre in Thailand. J Hosp Infect. 2017;96(2):163–7.
59. Standaert B, Strens D, Li X, Schecroun N, Raes M. The sustained rotavirus vaccination impact on nosocomial infection, duration of hospital stay, and age: the RotaBIS study (2005-2012). Infect Dis Ther. 2016;5(4):509–24.
60. Fraenkel CJ, Inghammar M, Johansson PJ, Bottiger B. Incidence of hospital norovirus outbreaks and infections using 2 surveillance methods in Sweden. Infect Control Hosp Epidemiol. 2017;38(1):96–102.
61. Turcios-Ruiz RM, Axelrod P, St John K, Bullitt E, Donahue J, Robinson N, et al. Outbreak of necrotizing enterocolitis caused by norovirus in a neonatal intensive care unit. J Pediatr. 2008;153(3):339–44.
62. de Jong EP, van den Beuken MGA, van Elzakker EPM, Wolthers KC, Sprij AJ, Lopriore E, et al. Epidemiology of Sepsis-like illness in young infants: major role of enterovirus and human parechovirus. Pediatr Infect Dis J. 2018;37(2):113–8.
63. Ferreras Antolin L, Kadambari S, Braccio S, Tang JW, Xerry J, Allen DJ, et al. Increased detection of human parechovirus infection in infants in England during 2016: epidemiology and clinical characteristics. Arch Dis Child. 2018 [E pub ahead of print].
64. Abedi GR, Watson JT, Nix WA, Oberste MS, Gerber SI. Enterovirus and Parechovirus surveillance - United States, 2014–2016. MMWR Morb Mortal Wkly Rep. 2018;67(18):515–8.
65. Strenger V, Diedrich S, Boettcher S, Richter S, Maritschnegg P, Gangl D, et al. Nosocomial outbreak of Parechovirus 3 infection among newborns, Austria, 2014. Emerg Infect Dis. 2016;22(9):1631–4.
66. Pankhurst L, Cloutman-Green E, Canales M, D'Arcy N, Hartley JC. Routine monitoring of adenovirus and norovirus within the health care environment. Am J Infect Control. 2014;42(11):1229–32.
67. Rodriguez-Baez N, O'Brien R, Qiu SQ, Bass DM. Astrovirus, adenovirus, and rotavirus in hospitalized children: prevalence and association with gastroenteritis. J Pediatr Gastroenterol Nutr. 2002;35(1):64–8.
68. Dodhia S, Baxter PC, Ye F, Pitman MJ. Investigation of the presence of HPV on KTP laser fibers following KTP laser treatment of papilloma. Laryngoscope. 2018;128(4):926–8.
69. Casalegno JS, Le Bail CK, Eibach D, Valdeyron ML, Lamblin G, Jacquemoud H, et al. High risk HPV contamination of endocavity vaginal ultrasound probes: an underestimated route of nosocomial infection? PLoS One. 2012;7(10):e48137.
70. Gallay C, Miranda E, Schaefer S, Catarino R, Jacot-Guillarmod M, Menoud PA, et al. Human papillomavirus (HPV) contamination of gynaecological equipment. Sex Transm Infect. 2016;92(1):19–23.
71. Saugel B, Jakobus J, Huber W, Hoffmann D, Holzapfel K, Protzer U, et al. Herpes simplex virus in bronchoalveolar lavage fluid of medical intensive care unit patients: association with lung injury and outcome. J Crit Care. 2016;32:138–44.
72. Walton AH, Muenzer JT, Rasche D, Boomer JS, Sato B, Brownstein BH, et al. Reactivation of multiple viruses in patients with sepsis. PLoS One. 2014;9(2):e98819.
73. Lepiller Q, Sueur C, Solis M, Barth H, Glady L, Lefebvre F, et al. Clinical relevance of herpes simplex virus viremia in intensive care unit patients. J Infect. 2015;71(1):93–100.
74. Farooq AV, Shukla D. Corneal latency and transmission of herpes simplex virus-1. Future Virol. 2011;6(1):101–8.
75. Hutchinson AK, Coats DK, Langdale LM, Steed LL, Demmler G, Saunders RA. Disinfection of eyelid specula with chlorhexidine gluconate (Hibiclens) after examinations for retinopathy of prematurity. Arch Ophthalmol. 2000;118(6):786–9.
76. Drew WL, Tegtmeier G, Alter HJ, Laycock ME, Miner RC, Busch MP. Frequency and duration of plasma CMV viremia in seroconverting blood donors and recipients. Transfusion. 2003;43(3):309–13.

77. Lachance P, Chen J, Featherstone R, Sligl WI. Association between cytomegalovirus reactivation and clinical outcomes in immunocompetent critically ill patients: a systematic review and meta-analysis. Open Forum Infect Dis. 2017;4(2):ofx029.
78. Limaye AP, Kirby KA, Rubenfeld GD, Leisenring WM, Bulger EM, Neff MJ, et al. Cytomegalovirus reactivation in critically ill immunocompetent patients. JAMA. 2008;300(4):413–22.
79. Josephson CD, Caliendo AM, Easley KA, Knezevic A, Shenvi N, Hinkes MT, et al. Blood transfusion and breast milk transmission of cytomegalovirus in very low-birth-weight infants: a prospective cohort study. JAMA Pediatr. 2014;168(11):1054–62.
80. Lanzieri TM, Dollard SC, Josephson CD, Schmid DS, Bialek SR. Breast milk-acquired cytomegalovirus infection and disease in VLBW and premature infants. Pediatrics. 2013;131(6):e1937–45.
81. Civardi E, Tzialla C, Baldanti F, Strocchio L, Manzoni P, Stronati M. Viral outbreaks in neonatal intensive care units: what we do not know. Am J Infect Control. 2013;41(10):854–6.
82. Centers for Disease Control and Prevention. Guidance for persons who may have been exposed to SARS. https://www.cdc.gov/sars/infection/exposure.html. Published 2005. Accessed 13 June 2018.
83. Centers for Disease Control and Prevention. Interim infection prevention and control recommendations for hospitalized patients with Middle East respiratory syndrome coronavirus (MERS-CoV). https://www.cdc.gov/coronavirus/mers/infection-prevention-control.html. Published 2015. Accessed 13 June 2018.
84. Assiri A, Al-Tawfiq JA, Al-Rabeeah AA, Al-Rabiah FA, Al-Hajjar S, Al-Barrak A, et al. Epidemiological, demographic, and clinical characteristics of 47 cases of Middle East respiratory syndrome coronavirus disease from Saudi Arabia: a descriptive study. Lancet Infect Dis. 2013;13(9):752–61.
85. Ahmed AE. Estimating survival rates in MERS-CoV patients 14 and 45 days after experiencing symptoms and determining the differences in survival rates by demographic data, disease characteristics and regions: a worldwide study. Epidemiol Infect. 2018;146(4):489–95.
86. Hastings DL, Tokars JI, Abdel Aziz IZ, Alkhaldi KZ, Bensadek AT, Alraddadi BM, et al. Outbreak of Middle East respiratory syndrome at tertiary care hospital, Jeddah, Saudi Arabia, 2014. Emerg Infect Dis. 2016;22(5):794–801.
87. Sassi HP, Reynolds KA, Pepper IL, Gerba CP. Evaluation of hospital-grade disinfectants on viral deposition on surfaces after toilet flushing. Am J Infect Control. 2018;46(5):507–11.
88. Arrington A, Hilmers D, Campbell J, Harrison G. Filoviral hemorrhagic fever: Marburg and Ebola virus fevers. In: Cherry J, Harrison G, Kaplan S, Steinbach W, Hotez P, editors. Feigin and Cherry's textbook of pediatric infectious diseases. 8th ed. Philadelphia: Elsevier; 2018. p. 1839–41.
89. Centers for Disease Control and Prevention. Guidance on personal protective equipment (PPE) to be used by healthcare workers during management of patients with confirmed ebola or persons under investigation (PUIs) for ebola who are clinically unstable or have bleeding, vomiting or diarrhea in US hospitals, including procedures for donning and doffing PPE. https://www.cdc.gov/vhf/ebola/healthcare-us/ppe/guidance.html. Published 2015. Accessed 13 June 2018.
90. Centers for Disease Control and Prevention. Smallpox. https://www.cdc.gov/smallpox/clinicians/index.html. Published 2017. Accessed 13 June 2018.
91. Centers for Disease Control and Prevention. Monkeypox. https://www.cdc.gov/poxvirus/monkeypox/clinicians/infection-control-hospital.html. Published 2015. Accessed 13 June 2018.
92. Bonda DJ, Manjila S, Mehndiratta P, Khan F, Miller BR, Onwuzulike K, et al. Human prion diseases: surgical lessons learned from iatrogenic prion transmission. Neurosurg Focus. 2016;41(1):E10.
93. World Health Organization. WHO infection control guidelines for transmissible spongiform encephalopathies. Geneva: World Health Organization (WHO); 1999.

Part III

Infections in Vulnerable Hosts

Healthcare-Associated Infections in the NICU: A Brief Review

15

J. B. Cantey

Special Considerations in the Nursery Setting

Neonatal Intensive Care Unit

The neonatal intensive care unit (NICU) is a unique setting within acute care hospitals. NICUs are first and foremost intensive care units, for preterm infants on the cusp of viability to the term infant with critical illness. However, a meaningful proportion of NICU infants are moderately preterm infants – colloquially called "feeder/growers" – who require long-term but not particularly intensive care. Finally, many NICUs admit slightly older infants from the community, often for infectious concerns such as fever in the neonate or viral bronchiolitis. As such, NICUs must incorporate aspects of intensive care units, long-term care facilities, and medical/surgical wards to provide appropriate care for a relatively heterogeneous population of infants.

NICU layout and staffing also introduce specific challenges. Many NICUs utilize an open-unit style (i.e., "bays"), while the trend for newer NICUs is to include single-patient rooms or even combined maternal/infant rooms. The bay-style NICU has less physical barriers between patients and often greater density of patients. Approximately 150 ft^2 per intensive care infant is recommended, and overcrowding has been associated with increased nosocomial infections [1, 2]. Finally, nursing understaffing has been linked to increased risk for healthcare-associated infection [2, 3]. Presumably, higher infant-to-nurse ratios mean more work and less attention to routine control practices such as hand hygiene; higher density of infants in a fixed space means closer "jumps" for horizontal transmission of pathogens. This wide

J. B. Cantey
Department of Pediatrics, University of Texas Health San Antonio, San Antonio, TX, USA
e-mail: cantey@uthscsa.edu

© Springer Nature Switzerland AG 2019
J. C. McNeil et al. (eds.), *Healthcare-Associated Infections in Children*,
https://doi.org/10.1007/978-3-319-98122-2_15

range of NICU structure and function means that infection control and prevention in the nursery setting must incorporate a broad variety of methods to be successful.

Infants

The immune system of infants, particularly those born preterm, are functionally immature compared with older children and adults. Virtually all aspects of innate immunity, including granulocyte chemotaxis, complement, and opsonization, are markedly reduced [4, 5]. Among preterm infants, the skin is thinner and has less desmosomes which make it an imperfect barrier to pathogens. In addition, the skin is frequently breached for blood draws and catheter placement. Adaptive immunity is similarly deficient. The concentration and function of T cells, B cells, and natural killer cells are reduced relative to older children. The only antibody available to newborns is transplacentally derived maternal immunoglobulin G (IgG). Preterm infants, especially those born before 28 weeks of gestation, have minimal serum IgG concentrations at birth. Therefore, while preterm infants are not immunodeficient in the usual sense of the word, they are at substantially increased risk for infection due to the physiologic immaturity of their immune system.

Late-Onset Sepsis

Late-onset sepsis (LOS) is defined as infection of a sterile site such as blood, urine, or cerebrospinal fluid that occurs >72 h after delivery [6]. In contrast to early-onset sepsis, in which the source of infection is perinatal exposure to organisms in the amniotic fluid or genital tract, the etiology of LOS is secondary to the postnatal (e.g., nursery) environment [7]. Over the past two decades, the incidence of LOS has slowly decreased, but LOS remains a major cause of morbidity and mortality among preterm infants [8].

Like all healthcare-associated infections in the NICU, risk for LOS increases with decreasing gestational age and birth weight. Approximately 20% of all very-low-birth-weight infants (VLBW, <1500 g) have at least one episode of LOS, and the risk increases to 35–40% for extremely-low-birth-weight infants (ELBW, <1000 g) [6, 8]. Indwelling hardware such as central venous catheters, bladder catheters, or endotracheal tubes are major risk factors as well; specific clinical conditions associated with these are described below. Finally, medications may increase the risk for LOS by interfering with innate immunity (e.g., postnatal corticosteroids, gastric acid blockers) or by disrupting the normal microbiome (e.g., antibiotics).

Gram-positive organisms account for the majority of LOS cases, with coagulase-negative staphylococci (CoNS, 50–60%) and *Staphylococcus aureus* (~10%) predominating. Gram-negative organisms collectively account for approximately 20% of all LOS, with *Candida* species rounding out the remainder (~5–10%). Specific clinical scenarios are described below.

Central Line-Associated Bloodstream Infections

Central line-associated bloodstream infections (CLABSIs) are the most common hospital-acquired infection in the NICU and represent a large proportion of all late-onset sepsis episodes [9]. In addition to prolonged length of stay, increased costs, and higher risk of mortality, CLABSIs in neonates are also associated with adverse neurodevelopmental outcomes such as cerebral palsy and intellectual disability [10–12]. However, central lines are used extensively in the NICU and often necessary to administer medications, fluid, and nutrition; furthermore, average dwell time is significantly longer in the NICU than in other pediatric settings [9]. Therefore, strategies to minimize CLABSIs are critically important.

Epidemiology and Risk Factors

As discussed above, the major risk factors for CLABSIs in the NICU setting include birth weight, degree of prematurity, and catheter dwell time. Birth weight and gestational age are highly correlated in most cases; at present the National Healthcare Safety Network (NHSN) uses birth weight rather than gestational age in their summary reporting [13]. Not only do the most preterm infants have the most impaired defenses against infection, but they also have the greatest central line requirements. The more total days that a central line remains in place (i.e., greater dwell time), the higher the risk for CLABSI. Each manipulation of the central line (including – but not limited to – opening and recapping the hub, infusing medications or flushes, changing tubing or dressings, and insertion and removal) carries a small risk of infection if proper technique is not adhered to; it is estimated that preterm infants average >1 of these catheter manipulations per hour [14]. Unsurprisingly, the incidence of CLABSI remains the highest among the smallest infants (Fig. 15.1) despite significant reduction in the overall incidence of CLABSI.

Another risk factor for CLABSI is the presence of intra-abdominal pathology (e.g., necrotizing enterocolitis, congenital malformation, spontaneous intestinal perforation) [22]. Infants with intra-abdominal pathology generally require a period of bowel rest and total parenteral nutrition through a central line, which markedly increases the absolute number of line-days and therefore the infant's risk for CLABSI. The use of histamine-2 receptor blockers or proton pump inhibitors has been associated with increased risk for necrotizing enterocolitis, sepsis, and CLABSIs [23, 24]. Presumably, this increased risk for CLABSI is the result of both direct impairment of innate immunity by lowering gastric acidity and increased need for central lines if necrotizing enterocolitis develops.

The majority of organisms responsible for CLABSI are gram-positive. CoNS are the most commonly implicated organisms for CLABSI and the most common cause of late-onset sepsis overall in the NICU (50–70% of cases) [9, 25]. The burden of CoNS on the skin combined with their ability to form biofilms on catheters makes them particularly effective colonizers of central lines. S. aureus (methicillin-susceptible and methicillin-resistant) is the second most common cause of CLABSI

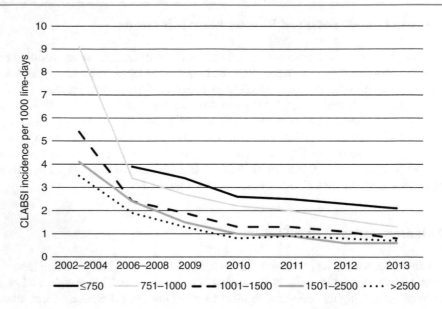

Fig. 15.1 Central line-associated bloodstream infection (CLABSI) incidence among preterm infants in the NHSN, 2002–2013, stratified by birth weight (in grams). (Adapted from Refs. [15–21])

(10–15%), and some studies have suggested that the proportion of CLABSIs due to *S. aureus* is increasing as effective prevention techniques have decreased infections due to CoNS [25]. Gram-negative pathogens are less common, but the risk for gram-negative CLABSI seems to increase with significant intestinal pathology and dwell times >50 days [26]. Finally, *Candida* species also contribute to CLABSI and are associated with high risk for morbidity and mortality (see section "Candidiasis in the NICU", below).

CLABSI Prevention

Several large, well-done quality improvement studies have demonstrated that CLABSI reduction in the NICU setting is possible; selected studies and their areas of focus are shown in Table 15.1. Evidence-based strategies to prevent CLABSIs in the NICU (Table 15.2) are similar to CLABSI prevention in other hospital settings, with a few exceptions:

1. Unlike in adults, catheter insertion in the lower extremity is not associated with increased risk for CLABSI among infants or young children [31]. Therefore, femoral or other lower-extremity central line placement sites are acceptable.
2. Skin disinfection with 2% chlorhexidine solution is recommended prior to line insertion in adults. However, chlorhexidine has been associated with low-level systemic absorption and contact dermatitis, particularly among ELBW infants

Table 15.1 Features of selected central line-associated bloodstream infection bundles in the neonatal intensive care unit. All bundles included insertion and maintenance checklists, attention to hand hygiene, and addressing the ongoing need for central access on a daily basis

Study	Population	Notable features	Impact
Fisher et al. [27]	13 North Carolina NICUs	Assessing need for line placement – "If there was no line in place today, would we place one?" Prompt removal at 120 cc/kg/day of enteral feeds	71% reduction in CLABSIs in 3.5-year period (3.94 → 1.16 per 1000 line-days)
Piazza et al. [28]	17 children's hospital NICUs participating in the Children's Hospital Neonatal Database	Specifically evaluated 4 practices: 1. Clean versus sterile tubing change technique 2. Hub care compliance monitoring 3. Catheter entry limitations 4. Catheter removal tracking	19% reduction in CLABSIs in a 2-year period(1.33 → 1.08 per 1000 line-days) Sterile tubing change and hub care compliance associated with greater decreases in CLABSI
Shepherd et al. [29]	6 level II, III, and IV nurseries within the Nationwide Children's Hospital system	For infants >2 months chronologic age, chlorhexidine-ethanol skin antisepsis For infants ≥28 weeks and ≥1000 g birth weight, chlorhexidine-impregnated disks used for insertion of central lines	89% reduction in CLABSIs in a 7-year period (6 → 0.7 per 1000 line-days)
Wilder et al. [30]	Single-center level IV NICU	Daily line rounds; nurse-led team would review need for line or dressing change	92% reduction in CLABSIs in a 3-year period (3.9 → 0.3 per 1000 line-days)

[32, 33]. Therefore, there is no recommendation for or against the use of chlorhexidine in neonates. NICU surveys report a fairly even split between centers using povidone-iodine solution and those using 2% chlorhexidine [34].

3. Dressing changes for central lines in neonates are performed only as needed when the dressing is displaced, wet, or soiled. There is no recommendation to change the dressing every 7 days if the dressing is in good condition, as constant removal of adhesive dressings can cause significant irritation or breakdown.

Insertion of central lines must be an area of focus to prevent CLABSIs. Efforts should be made to avoid placing unnecessary lines, and quality improvement programs that institute patient criteria for umbilical catheters or peripherally inserted central catheters (PICCs) have been successful in reducing both line-days and CLABSI incidence [35]. Although not currently included in the formal recommendations, facilities are increasingly using a dedicated team of providers who receive specialized training in the insertion and maintenance of central lines (e.g., PICC teams).

Table 15.2 Evidence-based strategies to prevent central line-associated bloodstream infections and neonatal intensive care unit-specific differences

General recommendation for non-NICU settings	NICU recommendations
1. Hand hygiene before catheter insertion	Same
2. Maximal sterile barrier precautions for catheter insertion	Same
3. Use of 2% chlorhexidine before insertion	No specific recommendation for neonates given concern for systemic absorption or skin irritation. Many centers use chlorhexidine for older infants; povidone-iodine may be used for younger or more preterm infants
4. Avoid femoral site for insertion	Femoral or other lower-extremity sites may be used
5. Disinfect catheter hubs and connectors before accessing catheter	Same
6. Perform dressing changes every 7 days or more frequently if dressing loose or soiled	Perform dressing changes only if loose or soiled (i.e., no dressing change at 7 days if dressing clean and intact)
7. Remove catheter promptly once no longer required	Same

Such teams have been associated with increased compliance with proper insertion techniques and decreased risk for CLABSI [36, 37].

In addition to proper insertion and maintenance, providers should strive to minimize dwell times. For infants in the NICU, this equates to a focus on establishing enteral feeding and switching intravenous medications to oral medications as soon as feasible. The general practice for the most preterm infants is to begin low-volume enteral feeds and advance steadily in order to reduce the risk for feeding intolerance or necrotizing enterocolitis. In some cases, minimal enteric feeding ("trophic feeds") is given for several days before feeding advancement begins. Therefore, among the smallest preterm infants, even those with no signs of feeding intolerance, typically require 7–14 days to reach full enteral feeds. However, slow feeding advancement (15–20 cc/kg/day) does not reduce the risk of necrotizing enterocolitis compared with more rapid advancement (30–40 cc/kg/day), and slower regimens have been associated with increased central line requirements and increased risk for CLABSI [38]. Prevention bundles that focus on reaching 120 cc/kg/day of enteral feeds and prompt removal of the central lines when this goal has been achieved have been successful in reducing CLABSIs [27].

The type of catheter may play a role in risk for CLABSI in preterm infants. Central venous catheters in the NICU commonly include umbilical venous catheters (UVCs), PICCs, or tunneled catheters. UVCs are often placed shortly after birth in order to administer fluid, nutrition, and medications to critically ill infants. The convenience of using the umbilical vein and the relative simplicity of insertion make UVCs a popular initial choice. However, studies suggest that the CLABSI risk per line-day is higher with UVCs than with other catheters and increases with UVC dwell times beyond 7–14 days [39]. In contrast, the CLABSI risk per line-day for

PICC lines is more constant. Therefore, nursery providers will generally exchange UVCs for PICC lines at some point for infants who require ongoing central access. The optimal time for exchange has not been determined. Butler-O'Hara et al. [40] investigated CLABSI risk with two central line strategies in a single-center cohort of neonates. One group of infants had a UVC placed initially which was exchanged for a PICC at age 7 days; another group had a UVC placed initially and had no mandate for exchange. The relative risk for CLABSI was similar through age 10 days in both groups; after 10 days, risk increased significantly for infants whose UVCs had not been exchanged for PICC lines. Similarly, Sanderson et al. [39] found an increased risk for CLABSI among infants whose UVCs were exchanged for PICCs after age 3 days compared with infants whose UVC was exchanged before age 3 days. Similar to Butler-O'Hara et al., this difference became apparent after 10–14 total line-days. The same study showed a decreased CLABSI rate when UVC placement was bypassed and infants instead received a PICC as their first central line, but no clear differences were seen once confounders such as birth weight were controlled for. Finally, a case-control study of infants <30 weeks of gestation in the Canadian Neonatal Network showed no reduction in line-days or CLABSI incidence among infants who had PICC lines placed on day of life 1 [41]. However, a randomized controlled trial of immediate PICC placement versus traditional UVC-to-PICC practice would provide valuable information. In the interim, the most evidence-based practice is to begin with UVC placement, exchange for a PICC line within 7–10 days, and remove the central line promptly once no longer needed.

Ventilator-Associated Pneumonia

Ventilator-associated pneumonia (VAP) is pneumonia in mechanically ventilated patients occurring >48 h after intubation [42]. Although less common than CLABSI, VAP accounts for a substantial portion of healthcare-associated infections in the NICU [43]. VAP is a challenging diagnosis under the best of circumstances due to the criteria's reliance on radiographic findings and subjective clinical features [44]. For preterm infants, many of whom have myriad reasons for abnormal respiratory physiology and imaging (e.g., surfactant deficiency, bronchopulmonary dysplasia, apnea of prematurity, etc.) neonatal VAP is even more difficult to objectively measure. Therefore, in 2014 the NHSN discontinued reporting of neonatal VAP, limiting our understanding of the contemporary epidemiology of this entity. VAP remains, however, an important cause of morbidity and mortality among mechanically ventilated neonates [45].

Epidemiology and Risk Factors

Obviously, the primary risk factor for VAP is the need for endotracheal intubation. The presence of an endotracheal tube allows bacteria to bypass much of the innate

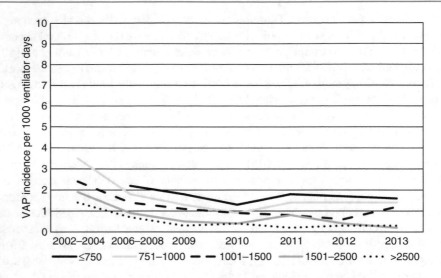

Fig. 15.2 Ventilator-associated pneumonia (VAP) incidence among preterm infants in the NHSN, 2002–2013, stratified by birth weight (in grams). (Adapted from Refs. [15–21])

defense of the airway on their way to the distal airways and alveoli [46]. In addition, endotracheal tubes for neonates are generally uncuffed or microcuffed rather than cuffed, as the cricoid bone is the narrowest aspect of the upper airway and serves as a natural cuff [47]. In the absence of a perfect seal, however, uncuffed tubes may allow gastric and oral secretions a route to the lower airway. The other primary risk factor for neonatal VAP is prematurity, which is directly related to the degree of lung immaturity. Compared with larger infants, ELBW infants are more likely to be intubated and require longer durations of mechanical ventilation. Consequently, ELBW infants have the highest incidence of VAP per 1000 ventilator days (Fig. 15.2). Gestational age, birth weight, and length of mechanical ventilation account for the majority of VAP risk in neonates.

By controlling for prematurity and length of mechanical ventilation, other risk factors have been identified. Frequency of reintubation has been associated with increased risk for VAP [48, 49]. These reintubations may be due to unplanned extubation or due to medical necessity (e.g., if the infant develops significant air leak or fails a planned trial of extubation). The underlying condition that necessitates intubation does not seem to impact VAP rates; odds ratios for VAP among patients with respiratory distress syndrome, meconium aspiration, perinatal asphyxia, and congenital anomalies are not significantly different [49]. Finally, pharmacologic acid suppression in neonates has been repeatedly linked to infection in general, including pneumonia [50–52].

The organisms responsible for VAP in neonates are predominantly gram-negative, although a wide variety of organisms have been associated with VAP. Epidemiologic studies are limited by a dearth of bronchoscopy-based cultures; instead, many studies rely on sputum or tracheal aspirate culture, making it difficult to distinguish between pathogens and colonizing flora. Enteric (*Klebsiella, Escherichia coli, Enterobacter, Serratia*) and environmental (*Pseudomonas, Stenotrophomonas, Chryseobacterium*) gram-negatives have been identified in neonatal VAP cases [53, 54]. Gram-positive organisms such as *S. aureus* and *Enterococcus* are less commonly identified. CoNS or *Candida* from the upper airway are not generally considered pathogens and should typically not be treated.

VAP Prevention

There are limited prospective data regarding VAP prevention in neonates. Most of the successful efforts reported in the literature have used an approach modified from VAP bundles designed for other settings (Table 15.3) [54, 55]. The common themes of successful neonatal bundles include:

1. Endotracheal tube care: A sterile tube should be used whenever possible for each intubation attempt. Suctioning should be performed during oral care as well as before maneuvers that may result in endotracheal tube movement (e.g., repositioning or retaping the tube). Closed suctioning systems are favored as the catheters are less likely to be contaminated with pathogenic bacteria [56]. Finally, efforts to minimize unplanned extubations should be prioritized [57].
2. Patient positioning: Neonatal VAP bundles have generally incorporated the recommendation that mechanically ventilated patients should have their heads elevated 30–45°.
3. Oral care: Oral care is an important aspect of VAP prevention at all ages. Most neonatal VAP bundles have used sterile water every 3–4 h to maintain the oral cavity. However, there is increasing interest in using colostrum for infants who

Table 15.3 Evidence-based strategies to prevent ventilator-associated pneumonia and neonatal intensive care unit-specific differences

General recommendation for Non-NICU settings	NICU recommendations
Head of bed elevation to ≥30°	In addition, lateral positioning after feeding has been associated with decreased aspiration
Oral care with 2% chlorhexidine or other antiseptic solution	No formal recommendation for chlorhexidine in neonates due to safety concerns (skin irritation, systemic absorption)
Daily evaluation for readiness to extubate	Same
Daily spontaneous awakening and breathing trials	Not directly applicable, but sedation should be kept to minimum amount necessary
Change breathing circuit only when malfunctioning or visibly soiled	Same
Peptic ulcer disease prophylaxis	Risks may outweigh benefits for neonates
Deep venous thrombosis prophylaxis	Not indicated in neonates

are otherwise not receiving enteral feeds. Early colostrum oral care results in increased detection of IgA, lactoferrin, and other antibacterial substances [58]. Whether this early colostrum exposure is associated with decreased risk for pneumonia has not been determined.

4. Minimizing sedation: VAP bundles for older patients generally include a "sedation vacation" at least once daily. Neonates are less likely to be paralyzed or heavily sedated, but the importance of limiting sedation to the minimum amount necessary cannot be overstated.

5. Assessing readiness for extubation: As with central lines, the daily need for the endotracheal tube and mechanical ventilation should be continually assessed.

Finally, nursery providers should strive to avoid culturing the endotracheal tube unless absolutely necessary. The upper airway is not sterile, and endotracheal tubes are rapidly colonized within days or even hours of intubation [59, 60]. As a result, providers in the nursery are often tasked with determining whether a positive endotracheal tube culture represents colonization or infection. When cultures are obtained in low-pretest-probability settings (e.g., when another source of infection is likely or in the absence of radiographic or clinical changes), the already poor positive predictive value of endotracheal tube cultures declines even further. Therefore, endotracheal tube cultures should only be considered when pneumonia is suspected based on both clinical and radiographic findings and alternative sources of infection have also been evaluated [61].

Ventricular Shunt Infection

The majority of children requiring ventricular shunting have their initial surgical intervention during the first few months of life. Common indications for ventricular shunts include congenital anomalies that involve obstruction of cerebrospinal fluid drainage (e.g., myelomeningocele, congenital aqueductal stenosis, Dandy-Walker malformation) or acquired conditions that lead to impaired cerebrospinal fluid reabsorption (e.g., post-hemorrhagic hydrocephalus following intraventricular hemorrhage, meningitis). For children with an indication for ventricular shunt, the long-term approach is placement of a ventriculoperitoneal shunt (VPS) or ventriculoatrial shunt. However, the usual size requirement for an infant to receive a definitive VPS is approximately 1500–2000 g. Therefore, smaller infants who require diversion generally undergo a temporizing measure until they achieve the required weight. These temporizing approaches include ventricular reservoirs, subgaleal shunts, or serial lumbar punctures. Such temporizing measures not only provide time for the infant to grow but in some cases may preclude the need for permanent shunting down the road if cerebrospinal fluid reabsorption improves in the interim [62]. Both definitive and temporizing shunts carry an increased risk for introduction of infection (meningitis, ventriculitis). A thorough discussion of CSF shunt infections in older children is provided in Chap. 10.

Epidemiology and Risk Factors

One of the primary risk factors for shunt infection is earlier placement. The risk of infection following shunting increases with decreasing weight at the time of placement [63]. For older children with a VPS, approximately 10% will have at least one shunt infection. The risk per shunt-year is approximately 6–8% [64, 65]. However, temporizing diversion measures have greater risk for infection than VPS; approximately 15–20% of subgaleal shunts or ventricular reservoirs may become infected despite relatively short dwell times, generally only a few months [66, 67]. Regardless of the type of shunt, the majority of infections occur within a few weeks of initial placement; infection risk then decreases markedly with increasing dwell time but never reaches zero [68]. Shunt revisions are associated with increased risk for infection – up to fourfold increase after a first revision and > tenfold increase after two revisions [69]. The need for shunt revision decreases as age at placement, birth weight, and gestational age increase, which is another reason that many neurosurgeons favor early temporizing measures for preterm infants [70].

Organisms responsible for shunt-associated infections are most commonly gram-positive. *Staphylococcus* spp. (CoNS and *S. aureus*) account for the majority of shunt infections in infants, as in older children [71, 72]. *Enterococcus* species are also commonly identified; gram-negative organisms including *Pseudomonas* represent a clinically significant minority of shunt infections [73].

Shunt Infection Prevention

Prevention of shunt infection among NICU infants is predicated on careful management of the temporizing shunts and minimizing the risk for VPS infection or dysfunction. This requires a careful balance between allowing the infant to grow while avoiding prolonged dwell times of the relatively higher-risk temporizing shunt.

Temporizing measures There does not appear to be a difference in the incidence of infection depending on the approach to temporization whether that is ventricular reservoirs, subgaleal shunts, or serial lumbar punctures. Meta-analysis of temporization measures showed a nonsignificant trend toward increased risk of infection when cerebrospinal fluid was obtained on a regular schedule compared to a conservative approach in which fluid was only obtained when signs of increased intracranial pressure were evident (relative risk 1.73 [95% confidence interval 0.53, 5.67]) [74]. However, other studies have found that the number of taps is not associated with increased risk for infection when there is strict adherence to sterile technique [75]. In the absence of clear evidence, the optimal strategy likely involves a standardized approach to ventricular diversion at a given center, with input from pediatric neurosurgery, neonatology, infectious diseases, and infection prevention.

Definitive shunting Once the infant has reached the preferred weight and corrected gestational age for neurosurgical intervention and still requires ongoing cerebrospinal fluid diversion, placement of a VPS will lower the risk of ventricular infection compared to continuing temporizing measures. Centers that have implemented a standardized surgical approach to VPS placement have reported lower postoperative infection rates [76]. Protocols that include antibiotic-impregnated shunt catheters or injection of antibiotics into the shunt after placement have been associated with a reduction in shunt infection risk [76–78]. Double-gloving, in which the neurosurgeon removes the first pair of gloves intraoperatively before handling the shunt catheter, has also been associated with decreased risk for infection [79].

Candidiasis in the NICU

Candida infection is a major cause of morbidity and mortality in the NICU, particularly among ELBW infants. Although *Candida* is a less common cause of LOS relative to bacteria, it accounts for a disproportionate amount of mortality with a case fatality rate of approximately 30–40%. In contrast, gram-positive LOS is associated with <10% mortality, and specifically CoNS sepsis is not associated with any increased risk for mortality [6, 80]. This may be due in part to the association between *Candida* and ELBW infants, however, as the case fatality rate for LOS increases with decreasing gestational age [81]. One of the most striking features of neonatal candidiasis is the wide variation in epidemiology seen among different NICUs due to differences in care practices. The incidence of candidiasis among ELBW infants ranged from 0% to 28% in one study of NICUs participating in the National Institute of Child Health and Human Development Neonatal Research Network [82].

Epidemiology and Risk Factors

Candida spp. may colonize the skin and gastrointestinal tract of infants following environmental exposure. *Candida* may be transmitted horizontally following contact with the skin (including during breastfeeding) or, less commonly, vertically from the maternal genital tract during labor and delivery [83]. *Candida* colonization is a major risk factor for subsequent candidiasis, and infection is most often caused by the colonizing strain. Risk for colonization and subsequent infection increases with decreasing gestational age and birth weight. Postnatal risk factors also mimic CLABSI risk factors, such as prolonged central line requirements, intra-abdominal pathology, and acid blocking medication. One risk factor that is highly specific for *Candida* colonization and infection is exposure to broad-spectrum antibiotic therapy, particularly third-generation cephalosporins or carbapenems. Indeed, a given NICU's rate of third-generation cephalosporin utilization correlates directly with the risk for invasive candidiasis within that NICU [84, 85]. Interestingly, this increased risk for candidiasis following cephalosporin exposure can be seen among term infants as well; while the absolute risk is drastically lower, the odds ratio (~1.6x increased risk) following cephalosporin exposure is unchanged [86].

Prevention of Candidiasis

In addition to CLABSI bundles, close attention to minimizing exposure to third-generation cephalosporins and carbapenems is critical to reduce the risk for invasive candidiasis. Prophylaxis with fluconazole given twice weekly either orally or intravenously reduces the risk for death or invasive candidiasis by approximately 50%. Fluconazole is generally well tolerated and has not been associated with subsequent increases in azole resistance within the NICU [87]. However, fluconazole prophylaxis is not a substitute for standard precautions, CLABSI reduction efforts, or vigilant antimicrobial stewardship. With these caveats being stated, fluconazole prophylaxis should be considered for NICUs who have ongoing candidiasis despite other efforts. Studies suggest that fluconazole prophylaxis is cost-effective if the incidence of candidiasis among ELBW infants exceeds 2.8% [88]. Finally, prophylaxis with probiotic therapy is receiving increased attention, and preliminary studies are promising. However, to date there has not been a large randomized controlled trial of probiotic prophylaxis in the NICU setting evaluating invasive candidiasis as a primary outcome.

Infections Associated with Human Milk

Human milk is an important aspect of NICU care. Numerous studies support the nutritional, immunological, and developmental benefits of human milk. As a result, NICUs are increasingly promoting exclusive human milk diets, either with mother's milk (direct breastfeeding or, more commonly, expressed breast milk) or with donor milk. However, there are several potential infectious contraindications to human milk use (Table 15.4). The only infection that is an absolute contraindication to breast milk use in the United States is maternal human immunodeficiency virus (HIV). In addition, although hepatitis C infection is not transmitted via breast milk, it can be transmitted by ingestion of maternal blood, and therefore maternal hepatitis C infection is a contraindication to breast milk if there is cracking or bleeding of the nipples, which may introduce maternal blood into the milk [89]. Several other conditions may preclude direct latching on the breast due to breast infection; in these cases, expressed milk is still safe to use. Untreated, active maternal tuberculosis is a contraindication to close proximity to the infant and therefore serves as a barrier to direct breastfeeding, but again expressed breast milk is safe to use.

Notably, Cytomegalovirus (CMV) can also be transmitted via human milk. In the era of CMV-safe blood transfusion practices (e.g., CMV-seronegative donors and irradiation to reduce leukocytes), breast milk is the predominant source of postnatally acquired CMV disease in the NICU setting [90]. Freezing of breast milk reduces but does not eliminate the CMV viral load; pasteurization inactivates CMV

Table 15.4 Maternal infectious contraindications to breastfeeding or breast milk use

Breast milk contraindicated	Human immunodeficiency virus (HIV)[a]
	Human T-cell lymphotropic virus
	Untreated brucellosis
	Hepatitis C and cracked or bleeding nipples
Direct breastfeeding contraindicated but expressed breast milk safe	Breast infection: Acute mastitis (bacterial or candida) Breast abscess Herpetic outbreak Active maternal tuberculosis Maternal varicella from up to 5 days prior to through up to 2 days following delivery
Direct breastfeeding safe	All other common infectious diseases
	Maternal hepatitis B infection
	Maternal hepatitis C infection if no nipple bleeding

Note: Noninfectious contraindications to breastfeeding include maternal use of certain medications, including but not limited to chemotherapy or radioactive agents, certain antipsychotics, and illicit substances such as cocaine or amphetamines
[a]Unless in a country where benefits of breastfeeding outweigh risk of HIV exposure

but also removes the majority of the nutritional benefit of breast milk [91, 92]. Therefore, the use of human milk must be weighed against the risk of CMV transmission. Postnatal CMV infection among preterm infants may be asymptomatic in the majority of cases; a minority of infants present with findings consistent with LOS such as pneumonitis, hepatitis, colitis, or disseminated intravascular coagulopathy [93]. However, in virtually all settings, the benefits of human milk over formula outweigh the risks of postnatal CMV acquisition. The one exception may be for the infant with proven or suspected severe combined immunodeficiency (SCID), which can be identified via newborn screening programs [94]. CMV is capable both of causing severe disease among infants with SCID and reducing the survival of hematopoietic stem cell transplantation. Therefore, if suspicion for SCID is high, some experts recommend a temporary cessation of breastfeeding until SCID can be definitely diagnosed and treated. However, the rate of false-positive SCID screening is not insignificant especially among preterm infants, for whom the benefits of human milk are greatest [95]. Therefore, providers must weigh the likelihood of real T cell dysfunction against the risks of temporarily withholding breast milk.

References

1. Kilpatrick SJ, Papile L, Macones GA, Watteberg KL, editors. Guidelines for perinatal care. 8th ed. Elk Grove: American Academy of Pediatrics; 2017.
2. Andersen BM, Lindemann R, Bergh K, et al. Spread of methicillin-resistant Staphylococcus aureus in a neonatal intensive care unit associated with understaffing, overcrowding and mixing of patients. J Hosp Infect. 2002;50:18–24.
3. Rogowski JA, Staiger D, Patrick T, et al. Nurse staffing and NICU infection rates. JAMA Pediatr. 2013;167:444–50.

4. Strunk T, Currie A, Richmond P, Simmer K, Burgner D. Innate immunity in human newborn infants: prematurity means more than immaturity. J Matern Fetal Neonatal Med. 2011;24:25–31.
5. Cuenca AG, Wynn JL, Moldawer LL, Levy O. Role of innate immunity in neonatal infection. Am J Perinatol. 2013;30:105–12.
6. Stoll BJ, Hansen N, Fanaroff AA, et al. Late-onset sepsis in very low birth weight neonates: the experience of the NICHD neonatal research network. Pediatrics. 2002;110:285–91.
7. Stoll BJ, Hansen NI, Sanchez PJ, et al. Early onset neonatal sepsis: the burden of group B Streptococcal and E. coli disease continues. Pediatrics. 2011;127:817–26.
8. Greenberg RG, Kandefer S, Do BT, et al. Late-onset sepsis in extremely premature infants: 2000-2011. Pediatr Infect Dis J. 2017;36:774–9.
9. Cantey JB, Milstone AM. Bloodstream infections: epidemiology and resistance. Clin Perinatol. 2015;42:1–16.
10. Hsu JF, Chu SM, Lee CW, et al. Incidence, clinical characteristics and attributable mortality of persistent bloodstream infection in the neonatal intensive care unit. PLoS One. 2015;10:e0124567.
11. Patel AL, Johnson TJ, Engstrom JL, et al. Impact of early human milk on sepsis and healthcare costs in very low birth weight infants. J Perinatol. 2013;33:514–9.
12. Johnson TJ, Patel AL, Jegier BJ, Engstrom JL, Meier PP. Cost of morbidities in very low birth weight infants. J Pediatr. 2013;162:243–9.
13. Centers for Disease Control and Prevention. Instructions for completion of denominators for neonatal intensive care unit (NICU, CDC 57.116). Available at https://www.cdc.gov/nhsn/forms/instr/57_116.pdf. Accessed 4 Dec 2017.
14. Mahieu LM, De Muynck AO, Ieven MM, et al. Risk factors for central vascular catheter-associated bloodstream infections among patients in a neonatal intensive care unit. J Hosp Infect. 2001;48:108–16.
15. Dudeck MA, Edwards JR, Allen-Bridson K, et al. National healthcare safety network report, data summary for 2013, device-associated module. Am J Infect Control. 2015;43:206–21.
16. Dudeck MA, Weiner LM, Allen-Bridson K, et al. National healthcare safety network report, data summary for 2012, device-associated module. Am J Infect Control. 2013;41:1148–66.
17. Dudeck MA, Horan TC, Peterson KD, et al. National healthcare safety network report, data summary for 2011, device-associated module. Am J Infect Control. 2013;41:286–300.
18. Dudeck MA, Horan TC, Peterson KD, et al. National healthcare safety network report, data summary for 2010, device-associated module. Am J Infect Control. 2011;39:798–816.
19. Dudeck MA, Horan TC, Peterson KD, et al. National healthcare safety network report, data summary for 2009, device-associated module. Am J Infect Control. 2011;39:349–67.
20. Edwards JR, Peterson KD, Mu Y, et al. National healthcare safety network report: data summary for 2006 through 2008, issued December 2009. Am J Infect Control. 2009;37:783–805.
21. National nosocomial infections surveillance system. National nosocomial infections surveillance system report, data summary from January 1992 through June 2004, issued October 2004. Am J Infect Control. 2004;32:470–85.
22. Dahan M, O'Donnell S, Hebert J, et al. CLABSI risk factors in the NICU: potential for prevention: a PICNIC study. Infect Control Hosp Epidemiol. 2016;37:1446–52.
23. Romaine A, Ye D, Ao Z, et al. Safety of histamine-2 receptor blockers in hospitalized VLBW infants. Early Hum Dev. 2016;99:27–30.
24. More K, Athalye-Jape G, Rao S, Patole S. Association of inhibitors of gastric acid secretion and higher incidence of necrotizing enterocolitis in preterm very low-birth-weight infants. Am J Perinatol. 2013;30:849–56.
25. Steiner M, Langgartner M, Cardona F, et al. Significant reduction of catheter-associated blood stream infections in preterm neonates after implementation of a care bundle focusing on simulation training of central line insertion. Pediatr Infect Dis J. 2015;34:1193–6.
26. Milstone AM, Reich NG, Advani S, et al. Catheter dwell time and CLABSIs in neonates with PICCs: a multicenter cohort study. Pediatrics. 2013;132:e1609–15.

27. Fisher D, Cochran KM, Provost LP, et al. Reducing central line-associated bloodstream infections in North Carolina NICUs. Pediatrics. 2013;132:e1664–71.
28. Piazza AJ, Brozanski B, Provost L, et al. SLUG bug: quality improvement with orchestrated testing leads to NICU CLABSI reduction. Pediatrics. 2016;137:1–12.
29. Shepherd EG, Kelly TJ, Vinsel JA, et al. Significant reduction of central-line associated bloodstream infections in a network of diverse neonatal nurseries. J Pediatr. 2015;167: 41–6.
30. Wilder KA, Wall B, Haggard D, Epperson T. CLABSI reduction strategy: a systematic central line quality improvement initiative integrating line-rounding principles and a team approach. Adv Neonatal Care. 2016;16:170–7.
31. Wrightson DD. Peripherally inserted central catheter complications in neonates with upper versus lower extremity insertion sites. Adv Neonatal Care. 2013;13:198–204.
32. Garland JS, Alex CP, Uhing MR, et al. Pilot trial to compare tolerance of chlorhexidine gluconate to povidone-iodine antisepsis for central venous catheter placement in neonates. J Perinatol. 2009;29:808–13.
33. Garland JS, Alex CP, Mueller CD, et al. A randomized trial comparing povidone-iodine to a chlorhexidine gluconate-impregnated dressing for prevention of central venous catheter infections in neonates. Pediatrics. 2001;107:1431–6.
34. Sharpe E, Kuhn L, Ratz D, Krein SL, Chopra V. Neonatal peripherally inserted central catheter practices and providers: results from the neonatal PICC1 survey. Adv Neonatal Care. 2017;17:209–21.
35. Shahid S, Dutta S, Symington A, Shivananda S. Standardizing umbilical catheter usage in preterm infants. Pediatrics. 2014;133:e1742–52.
36. Sharpe E, Kuhn L, Ratz D, Krein SL, Chopra V. Neonatal peripherally inserted cetnral catheter practices and providers: results from the neonatal PICC1 survey. Adv Neonatal Care. 2017; 17(3):209–21.
37. Taylor T, Massaro A, Williams L, et al. Effect of a dedicated percutaneously inserted central catheter team on neonatal catheter-related bloodstream infection. Adv Neonatal Care. 2011;11:122–8.
38. Oddie SJ, Young L, McGuire W. Slow advancement of enteral feed volumes to prevent necrotising enterocolits in very low birth weight infants. Cochrane Database Syst Rev. 2017;8:CD001241.
39. Sanderson E, Yeo KT, Wang AY, et al. Dwell time and risk of central-line associated bloodstream infection in neonates. J Hosp Infect. 2017;97:267–74.
40. Butler-O'Hara M, D'Angio CT, Hoey H, Stevens TP. An evidence-based catheter bundle alters central venous catheter strategy in newborn infants. J Pediatr. 2012;160:972–7.
41. Shalabi M, Adel M, Yoon E, et al. Risk of infection using peripherally inserted central and umbilical catheters in preterm neonates. Pediatrics. 2015;136:1073–9.
42. Mourani PM, Sonag MK. Ventilator-associated pneumonia in critically ill children: a new paradigm. Pediatr Clin N Am. 2017;64:1039–56.
43. Gaynes RP, Edwards JR, Jarvis WR, et al. Nosocomial infections among neonates in high-risk nurseries in the United States: national nosocomial infections surveillance system. Pediatrics. 1996;98:357–61.
44. Centers for Disease Control and Prevention. Pneumonia (ventilator-associated [VAP] and non-ventilator-associated pneumonia [PNEU]) event. Available at https://www.cdc.gov/nhsn/pdfs/pscmanual/6pscvapcurrent.pdf. Accessed 4 Dec 2017.
45. Apisarnthanarak A, Holzmann-Pazgal G, Hamvas A, Olsen MA, Fraser VJ. Ventilator-associated pneumonia in extremely preterm neonates in a neonatal intensive care unit: characteristics, risk factors, and outcomes. Pediatrics. 2003;112:1283–9.
46. Rouze A, Jaillette E, Poissy J, Preau S, Nseir S. Tracheal tube design and ventilator-associated pneumonia. Respir Care. 2017;62:1316–23.
47. De Orange FA, Andrade RG, Lemos A, et al. Cuffed versus uncuffed endotracheal tubes for general anesthesia in children aged eight years and under. Cochrane Database Syst Rev. 2017;11:CD011954.

48. Kawanishi F, Yoshinaga M, Morita M, et al. Risk factors for ventilator-associated pneumonia in neonatal intensive care unit patients. J Infect Chemother. 2014;20:627–30.
49. Tan B, Xian-Yang X, Zhang X, et al. Epidemiology of pathogens and drug resistance of ventilator-associated pneumonia in Chinese neonatal intensive care units: a meta-analysis. Am J Infect Control. 2014;42:902–10.
50. Santana RNS, Santos VS, Ribeiro-Junior RF, et al. Use of ranitidine is associated with infections in newborns hospitalized in a neonatal intensive care unit: a cohort study. BMC Infect Dis. 2017;17:375.
51. Bianconi S, Gudavalli M, Sutija VG, et al. Ranitidine and late-onset sepsis in the neonatal intensive care unit. J Perinat Med. 2007;35:147–50.
52. Terrin G, Passariello A, De Curtis M, et al. Ranitidine is associated with infections, necrotizing enterocolitis, and fatal outcome in newborns. Pediatrics. 2012;129:e40–5.
53. Lee PL, Lee WT, Chen HL. Ventilator-associated pneumonia in low birth weight neonates at a neonatal intensive care unit: a retrospective observational study. Pediatr Neonataol. 2017;58:16–21.
54. Azab SF, Sherbiny HS, Saleh SH, et al. Reducing ventilator-associated pneumonia in neonatal intensive care unit using "VAP prevention bundle": a cohort study. BMC Infect Dis. 2015;15:314.
55. Weber CD. Applying adult ventilator-associated pneumonia bundle evidence to the ventilated neonate. Adv Neonatal Care. 2016;16:178–90.
56. Akerman E, Larsson C, Ersson A. Clinical experience and incidence of ventilator-associated pneumonia using closed versus open suction-system. Nurs Crit Care. 2014;19:34–41.
57. Merkel L, Beers K, Lewis MM, et al. Reducing unplanned extubations in the NICU. Pediatrics. 2014;133:e1367–72.
58. Zhang Y, Ji F, Hu X, Cao Y, Latour JM. Oropharyngeal colostrum administration in very low birth weight infants: a randomized controlled trial. Pediatr Crit Care Med. 2017;18:869–75.
59. Willson DF, Conaway M, Kelly R, Hendley JO. The lack of specificity of tracheal aspirates in the diagnosis of pulmonary infection in intubated children. Pediatr Crit Care Med. 2014;15:299–305.
60. Gibbs K, Holzman IR. Endotracheal tube: friend or foe? Bacteria, the endotracheal tube, and the impact of colonization and infection. Semin Perinatol. 2012;36:454–61.
61. Cantey JB. Optimizing the use of antibacterial agents in the neonatal period. Paediatr Drugs. 2016;18:109–22.
62. Wellons JC, Shannon CN, Kulkarni AV, et al. A multicenter retrospective comparison of conversion from temporary to permanent cerebrospinal fluid diversion in very low birth weight infants with posthemorrhagic hydrocephalus. J Neurosurg Pediatr. 2009;4:50–5.
63. Pople IK, Bayston R, Hayward RD. Infection of cerebrospinal fluid shunts in infants: a study of etiological factors. J Neurosurg. 1992;77:29–36.
64. Lee JK, Seok JY, Lee JH, et al. Incidence and risk factors of venticuloperitoneal shunt infections in children: a study of 333 consecutive shunts in 6 years. J Korean Med Sci. 2012;27:1563–8.
65. Simon TD, Hall M, Riva-Cambrin J, et al. Infection rates following initial cerebrospinal fluid shunt placement across pediatric hospitals in the United States. J Neurosurg Pediatr. 2009;4:156–65.
66. Wellons JC, Shannon CN, Holubkov R, et al. Shunting outcomes in posthemorrhagic hydrocephalus: results of a hydrocephalus clinical research network prospective cohort study. J Neurosurg Pediatr. 2017;20:19–29.
67. Wang JY, Amin AG, Jallo GI, Ahn ES. Ventricular reservoir versus ventriculoperitoneal shunt for posthemorrhagic hydrocephalus in preterm infants: infection risks and ventriculoperitoneal shunt rate. J Neurosurg Pediatr. 2014;14:447–54.
68. Conen A, Walti LN, Merlo A, et al. Characteristics and treatment outcome of cerebrospinal fluid shunt-associated infections in adults: a retrospective analysis over an 11-year period. Clin Infect Dis. 2008;47:73–82.
69. Simon TD, Butler J, Whitlock KB, et al. Risk factors for first cerebrospinal fluid shunt infection: findings from a multi-center prospective cohort study. J Pediatr. 2014;164:1462–8.

70. Bir SC, Konar S, Maiti TK, et al. Outcome of ventriculoperitoneal shunt and predictors of shunt revision in infants with posthemorrhagic hydrocephalus. Childs Nerv Syst. 2016;32:1405–14.
71. McGirt MJ, Zaas A, Fuchs HE, et al. Risk factors for pediatric ventriculoperitoneal shunt infection and predictors of infectious pathogens. Clin Infect Dis. 2003;36:858–62.
72. Arnell K, Cesarini K, Lagerqvist-Widh A, Wester T, Sjolin J. Cerebrospinal fluid shunt infections in children over a 13-year period: anaerobic cultures and comparison of clinical signs of infection with Propionibacterium acnes and with other bacteria. J Neurosurg Pediatr. 2008;5:366–72.
73. Kebriaei MA, Shoja MM, Salinas SM, et al. Shunt infection in the first year of life. J Neurosurg Pediatr. 2013;12:44–8.
74. Whitelaw A, Lee-Kelland R. Repeated lumbar or ventricular punctures in newborns with intraventricular haemorrhage. Cochrane Database Syst Rev. 2017;4:CD000216.
75. Kormanik K, Praca J, Garton HJ, Sarkar S. Repeated tapping of ventricular reservoir in preterm infants with post-hemorrhagic ventricular dilatation does not increase the risk of reservoir infection. J Perinatol. 2010;30:218–21.
76. Kestle JR, Riva-Cambrin J, Wellons JC, et al. A standardized protocol to reduce cerebrospinal fluid shunt infection: the hydrocephalus clinical research network quality improvement initiative. J Neurosurg Pediatr. 2011;8:22–9.
77. Konstantelias AA, Vardakas KZ, Polyzos KA, Tansarli GS, Falagas ME. Antimicrobial-impregnated and -coated shunt catheters for prevention of infections in patients with hydrocephalus: a systematic review and meta-analysis. J Neurosurg. 2015;122:1096–112.
78. Klimo P, Thompson CJ, Baird LC, et al. Pediatric hydrocephalus: systematic literature review and evidence-based guidelines. Part 7: antibiotic-impregnated shunt systems versus conventional shunts in children: a systematic review and meta-analysis. J Neurosurg Pediatr. 2014;14(S1):53–9.
79. Rehman AU, Rehman TU, Bashir HH, Gupta V. A simple method to reduce infection of ventriculoperitoneal shunts. J Neurosurg Pediatr. 2010;5:569–72.
80. Cantey JB, Anderson KR, Kalagiri RR, Mallet LH. Morbidity and mortality of coagulase-negative staphylococcal sepsis in very-low-birth-weight infants. World J Pediatr. 2018;14(3):269–73.
81. Piening BC, Geffers C, Gastmeier P, Schwab F. Pathogen-specific mortality in very low birth weight infants with primary bloodstream infection. PLoS One. 2017;12:e0180134.
82. Benjamin DK, Stoll BJ, Gantz MG, et al. Neonatal candidiasis: epidemiology, risk factors, and clinical judgement. Pediatrics. 2010;126:e865–73.
83. Bliss JM, Basavegowda KP, Watson WJ, Sheikh AU, Ryan RM. Vertical and horizontal transmission of Candida albicans in very low birth weight infants using DNA fingerprinting techniques. Pediatr Infect Dis J. 2008;27:231–5.
84. Saiman L, Ludington E, Dawson JD, et al. Risk factors for Candida species colonization of neonatal intensive care unit patients. Pediatr Infect Dis J. 2001;20:1119–24.
85. Cotton CM, McDonald S, Stoll B, et al. The association of third-generation cephalosporin use and invasive candidiasis in extremely low birth-weight infants. Pediatrics. 2006;118:717–22.
86. Lee JH, Hornik CP, Benjamin DK, et al. Risk factors for invasive candidiasis in infants ≥1500 g birth weight. Pediatr Infect Dis J. 2013;32:222–6.
87. Ericson JE, Kaufman DA, Kicklighter SD, et al. Fluconazole propylaxis for the prevention of candidiasis in premature infants: a meta-analysis using patient-level data. Clin Infect Dis. 2016;63:604–10.
88. Swanson JR, Vergales J, Kaufman DA, Sinkin RA. Cost analysis of fluconazole prophylaxis for prevention of neonatal invasive candidiasis. Pediatr Infect Dis J. 2016;35:519–23.
89. Centers for Disease Control and Prevention. Breastfeeding: Hepatitis B and C infections. Available at https://www.cdc.gov/breastfeeding/disease/hepatitis.htm. Accessed 4 Dec 2017.
90. Josephson CD, Caliendo AM, Easley KA, et al. Blood transfusion and breast milk transmission of cytomegalovirus in very-low-birth-weight infants: a prospective cohort study. JAMA Pediatr. 2014;168:1054–62.

91. Omarsdottir S, Casper C, Naver L, et al. Cytomegalovirus infection and neonatal outcome in extremely preterm infants after freezing of maternal milk. Pediatr Infect Dis J. 2015;34:482–289.
92. Hamprecht K, Maschmann J, Muller D, et al. Cytomegalovirus inactivation in breast milk: reassessment of pasteurization and freeze-thawing. Pediatr Res. 2004;56:529–35.
93. Kelly MS, Benjamin DK, Puopolo KM, et al. Postnatal cytomegalovirus infection and the risk for bronchopulmonary dysplasia. JAMA Pediatr. 2015;169:e153785.
94. Kwan A, Abraham RS, Currier R, et al. Newborn screening for severe combined immunodeficiency in 11 screening programs in the United States. JAMA. 2014;312:729–38.
95. Ward CE, Baptist AP. Challenges of newborn severe combined immunodeficiency screening among premature infants. Pediatrics. 2013;131:e1298–302.

Infection Prevention in Pediatric Oncology and Hematopoietic Stem Cell Transplant Recipients

16

Ankhi Dutta and Ricardo Flores

Children with malignancies or those who are hematopoietic stem cell transplant (HSCT) recipients are at increased risk for healthcare-associated infections (HAI) due to their underlying diagnoses as well as the receipt of immunosuppressive medications that are part of their treatment. In addition, frequent visits to healthcare settings increase the risk for exposure to resistant organisms. Thus, while adherence to infection control and prevention measures recommended for all hospitalized children is essential, additional interventions to reduce the inherent risk of morbidity associated with HAIs are warranted in this special population.

Infection Prevention in Pediatric Oncology Patients and Hematopoietic Stem Cell Transplant Recipients

There are various factors which contribute to the increased susceptibility to infections in pediatric hematology/oncology (PHO) and HSCT patients, most prominent of them being disruption of cutaneous and mucosal barriers (oral, gastrointestinal, etc.), microbial gastrointestinal translocation, defects in cell-mediated immunity, and insufficient quantities and inadequate function of phagocytes. Goals of infection control and prevention in this population are based on mitigating the risk inherent with the underlying malignancy and associated treatments (i.e., chemotherapy,

A. Dutta (✉)
Department of Pediatrics, Section of Pediatric Infectious Diseases, Texas Children's Hospital and Baylor College of Medicine, Houston, TX, USA
e-mail: adutta@bcm.edu

R. Flores
Department of Pediatrics, Texas Children's Cancer and Hematology Centers and Baylor College of Medicine, Houston, TX, USA
e-mail: rjflores@txch.edu

© Springer Nature Switzerland AG 2019
J. C. McNeil et al. (eds.), *Healthcare-Associated Infections in Children*,
https://doi.org/10.1007/978-3-319-98122-2_16

radiation). This chapter discusses infection control and prevention measures specifically in patients with hematological malignancies as well as HSCT recipients.

General Measures

Hand hygiene and standard precautions during the care of PHO and HSCT patients are key components in reducing the risk of infections. Additional isolation precautions may also be undertaken depending on the pathogen isolated and/or symptoms that the patient is experiencing (e.g., contact precautions would be appropriate in patients experiencing diarrhea). Further information on general infection prevention measures can be found in Chap. 1.

Skin Care and Hygiene

Minimizing injury to mucosal surfaces and decreasing heavy colonization of the skin reduce the likelihood of microbial invasion through these sites. Thus, the importance of meticulous skin care and daily inspection in PHO and HSCT patients is paramount and provides opportunities to identify areas of inflammation or breakdown early. Skin inspection should be done routinely, with special attention to high-risk areas like intravascular catheter insertion sites and the perineum. Rectal thermometers, digital rectal examinations, and suppositories should be avoided to prevent mucosal breakdown. As part of an effort to reduce colonization of cutaneous surfaces, daily chlorhexidine baths have been shown to reduce HAIs and transmission of multidrug-resistant organisms (MDRO) in oncology patients [1, 2]. Chlorhexidine gluconate (CHG) is a cationic bisbiguanide that serves as a topical antiseptic. CHG binds to negatively charged bacterial cell wall proteins altering the bacterial cell wall equilibrium and helps in reducing bacterial colonization of the skin [1]. Education of patients, families, and staff on the importance of these practices is key to compliance with this preventative strategy and should be made a priority.

Oral Hygiene

Many experts recommend a complete periodontal examination be performed prior to initiation of chemotherapy with reevaluations throughout the treatment course and after completion [3, 4]. Oral mucositis, which can be considered an acute inflammation and/or ulceration of the oral/oropharyngeal mucus membranes, is a common adverse effect of chemotherapeutic agents. It can cause oral pain/discomfort as well as difficulties in eating, swallowing, and speech. Mucositis is most commonly caused by chemotherapeutic agents which prevent DNA synthesis such as methotrexate, 5-fluorouracil, and cytarabine, particularly in HSCT recipients. Oral rinses with normal saline or CHG-containing products are recommended 4–6 times per day to prevent oral mucositis [2, 3]. Patients with painful mucositis might not comply with oral care regimens, however, putting them at increased risk for infections from oral flora such as bacteremia due to viridans streptococci. Mouth rinses containing alcohol should be avoided because they can aggravate mucositis. Neutropenic patients should also be instructed to brush their teeth carefully in order to prevent gingival injury [3]. A regular soft toothbrush or an electric brush can be used to minimize trauma [3].

Any elective dental procedure should be ideally performed prior to starting chemotherapy and after discussion with the primary medical team. The absolute neutrophil count, platelet count, and stage of treatment should be considered before performing any dental procedures in this vulnerable population [2, 3].

Central Line-Associated Bloodstream Infection (CLABSI) Prevention

The presence of central venous catheters (CVC) in this population puts them at risk for central line-associated bloodstream infection (CLABSI) and its related complications. CLABSI is the most commonly reported HAI in most pediatric series. Among all the pediatric HAI reported to National Healthcare Surveillance Network (NHSN), 15% were from oncology units; *Streptococcus viridans* (15%) and *Klebsiella pneumoniae/oxytoca* (12%) were the two most common pathogens in this study [5]. In the NHSN report, antibiotic resistance was noted to be high in oncology units, including ampicillin and/or vancomycin resistance for *Enterococcus faecium* and fluoroquinolone resistance for *Escherichia coli* [5]. Although less than 4% of *Enterobacteriaceae* were reported to have carbapenem resistance, the emergence of such organisms in this population is of significant concern [6]. Among *Candida* infections in this population, fluconazole resistance among non-*C. albicans* and non-*C. parapsilosis* isolates was up to 41%, whereas fluconazole resistance in *C. albicans* and *C. parapsilosis* was <4% [5].

Mucosal barrier injury (MBI)-associated laboratory-confirmed bloodstream infections (MBI-LCBI) have gained attention in recent years [7, 8]. These are CLABSIs related primarily to mucosal barrier injury (i.e., mucositis) and not due to the direct presence of the CVC per se. In the NHSN definition, a positive blood culture would qualify as a MBI-LCBI if it results from one or more groups of selected commensal organisms of the oral cavity or gastrointestinal tract and occurred in the presence of signs and symptoms consistent with mucosal barrier injury (MBI) in PHO or HSCT patients [7]. Eligible organisms for MBI-LCBI include *Candida* species, *Enterococcus*, *Enterobacteriaceae*, viridans group streptococci, other *Streptococcus* species, and anaerobes [7].

Specific guidelines for central line insertion and maintenance bundles have been proposed by the Centers for Disease Control and Prevention (CDC) and the Infectious Diseases Society of America (IDSA) to reduce the CLABSI rates and healthcare costs [9, 10]. Several studies have demonstrated that a multifaceted approach reduces CLABSI rates in this population [11, 12] and includes standardizing CVC insertion practices and maintenance bundles, tracking CVC infections using standardized definitions, and using dedicated nursing staff or "CVC champions" specifically trained in CVC maintenance and tracking in conjunction with other infection control methods (including oral and hand hygiene, optimizing nurse/patient ratio, etc.). CLABSI is discussed in greater detail in Chap. 6.

Environmental and Dietary Considerations

The American Society for Blood and Marrow Transplantation recommends a low microbial diet for HSCT recipients [13]. There is little evidence, however, to suggest that this helps in PHO patients. Routine safety in handling and preparing food should be practiced by patients and parents. In general, eating unpasteurized milk/cheese, undercooked meat, and raw fruits and vegetables is discouraged during periods of neutropenia to reduce incidence of infection. The need to minimize risk of infection, however, should be balanced with the nutritional needs and quality of life of the patient [2, 13].

Pet Ownership

Pets can be a great source of companionship and comfort to children; however, there are several diseases that can be transmitted by pets to these immunosuppressed hosts [14–16]. Certain animals like reptiles, birds, rodents, or other exotic animals that cannot be immunized and could carry unusual human pathogens should not be kept as pets in households with PHO or HSCT patients. Immunosuppressed patients should avoid petting zoos due to the risk of diseases secondary to enteric pathogens (such as *Salmonella* or *Campylobacter*) [13–16].

Dogs and cats, preferably more than 1 year old, are generally considered safe for PHO and HSCT patients. They should be routinely evaluated by veterinarians for diseases and their immunizations kept up-to-date. Extreme care should be taken to maintain hand hygiene during and after handling the pets [13–16]. Further information regarding pet therapy is available in Chap. 4.

Prevention of Bacterial Infections: Antibiotic Prophylaxis in Neutropenic Patients Without Fever

Studies performed in adult oncology patients have consistently shown the benefit of using prophylactic antibiotics in reducing the incidence of bacterial infections [17]. Levofloxacin prophylaxis in adults has been shown to reduce the incidence of fever, bacterial infection, hospitalization rates, and all-cause mortality [18, 19]. Based upon such data in adults, the IDSA Guidelines for the Use of Antimicrobial Agents in Neutropenic Patients with Cancer state that fluoroquinolone prophylaxis should be considered for high-risk patients with prolonged severe neutropenia [20].

Pediatric studies on antibiotic prophylaxis are limited. A pediatric pilot study on the use of ciprofloxacin prophylaxis for pediatric patients receiving delayed intensification therapy for acute lymphoblastic leukemia (ALL) showed a reduction in hospitalization, intensive care admission, and bacteremia when compared to controls [21]. In another study, levofloxacin prophylaxis in patients with ALL reduced the odds of febrile neutropenia, possible bacterial infection, and confirmed bloodstream infection by $\geq 70\%$. It also reduced the use of other broad-spectrum antibiotics and the incidence of *C. difficile* infections [22]. In other studies, however, ciprofloxacin prophylaxis did not decrease the incidence of overall bacteremia or duration of fever or mortality in pediatric acute myelogenous leukemia (AML) patients [23]. Furthermore, increasing quinolone resistance among gram-negative organisms is a concern recently observed in the NHSN database of pediatric oncology patients with CLABSI [5]. In addition, the use of antimicrobial prophylaxis in PHO could increase the possibility of developing other MDROs, invasive fungal infections, or drug-related toxicities. Though some authors suggest that antibiotic prophylaxis should be considered in children undergoing induction chemotherapy for ALL, there is currently insufficient data to inform definitive guidelines for antibiotic prophylaxis to prevent bacterial infections in pediatric oncology patients [19–21]. Notably, an open-label randomized clinical trial was recently conducted of levofloxacin prophylaxis vs. no prophylaxis in children with AML, relapsed ALL, and HSCT recipients. Among patients with AML and relapsed ALL, prophylaxis was associated with a reduction in rates of bacteremia; there was a numeric reduction in bacteremia in the HSCT recipients, but this did not achieve statistical significance. It is unclear at this time how these new findings will influence practice and future guidelines [24].

Prevention of Viral Infections

Infections with common respiratory and gastrointestinal viruses can result in significant morbidity and mortality in PHO and HSCT patients. The most common respiratory viruses encountered include rhinovirus, coronavirus, adenovirus, RSV, parainfluenza, human metapneumovirus, and influenza. Common gastrointestinal viruses affecting both healthy and immunocompromised children include norovirus, rotavirus, enteric adenoviruses, and enteroviruses among others. Infection prevention strategies should include education provided to the patient and the family about hand hygiene, prevention techniques, avoidance of ill visitors, disease surveillance in the community and hospital, vaccination against influenza and prompt identification, and testing and treatment (if possible) of any respiratory viral illness. Implementation of routine infection control prevention policies on oncology wards should reduce transmission of common respiratory and gastrointestinal viruses. All visitors should be screened for any signs and symptoms of acute viral illness and restricted from visitation on the unit or contact with any immunocompromised hosts. Chapter 4 outlines infection control guidance for hospital visitors in greater detail.

Immunization of Healthcare Workers and Household Contacts

Immunization of healthcare workers and household contacts needs special consideration in settings with PHO and HSCT patients. Given the immunosuppressed status of children with malignancy and/or HSCT, immunization of those closest to them at home and those caring for them in the hospital is critically important in preventing infections. Live attenuated vaccines contain a theoretical risk of being transmitted to an immunocompromised host. Live oral polio vaccine, which is no longer administered in the United States, is an absolute contraindication for people taking care of this high-risk population. However, data suggests that measles, mumps, and rubella (MMR), varicella zoster, and herpes zoster vaccines can be safely provided to healthcare workers and household contacts [25]. If healthcare personnel develop a rash that cannot be covered within the first 42 days following receipt of the varicella vaccine, they should avoid any contact with immunocompromised patients until all rash has crusted to avoid the potential risk of transmitting vaccine strain varicella to patients [25]. Infants living in households with persons who are immunocompromised including PHO and HSCT patients may be safely immunized against rotavirus; it is recommended, however, that immunocompromised persons avoid contact with the infant's diapers/stool for 4 weeks following vaccination to minimize risk of acquiring vaccine strain rotavirus infection [26]. An inactivated influenza vaccine is preferred for personnel taking care of immunocompromised children as opposed to live attenuated influenza vaccine [25]. Vaccination against other non-viral pathogens (such as pneumococcus or pertussis) by family members is another important method to minimize the risk of serious infection in PHO patients.

Physical Measures to Prevent Fungal Infections

Hospital environments are designed to minimize the potential for fungal disease in the highest-risk patients. High efficiency particulate air (HEPA) filters have been shown to reduce nosocomial infection in HSCT patients, and the CDC recommends HEPA filters in HSCT recipient's rooms. The rooms should also have directed airflow and positive air pressure and be properly ventilated (≥ 12 air changes per hour) [2]. Avoidance of carpets and upholstery is also recommended. Since outbreaks secondary to *Aspergillus* have been reported during hospital renovation or construction, appropriate containment should be in place, and strict precautions should be taken to prevent exposure to patients during such periods [2]. Infection control and prevention departments should be involved in risk assessment, planning, and approval of all construction or renovation projects in healthcare facilities including inpatient units, clinics, and infusion centers caring for these patients [27].

Fever and Neutropenia

Cytotoxic chemotherapies and radiation therapy used in the treatment of malignancies are myelosuppressive and result in variable duration and severity of neutropenia. In addition, certain malignancies that originate from bone marrow precursors (i.e., leukemia) or metastasize to the bone marrow (e.g., lymphoma, neuroblastoma, and sarcomas) can result in a decreased number of normal blood cell precursors and consequent neutropenia. Hence, pediatric cancer and HSCT patients are frequently immunosuppressed and at risk for a wide range of pathogens.

Febrile neutropenia is a common condition in the PHO/HSCT population. With regard to this entity, fever is defined as a single temperature >38.3 °C (101 °F) or a temperature ≥38.0 °C (100.4 °F) on two occasions 1 hour apart. Neutropenia is classified as mild (absolute neutrophil count [ANC] >500–1000/mm^3), moderate (ANC ≥200–500/mm^3), or severe (ANC <200/mm^3). Febrile neutropenia (also known as fever and neutropenia) is the combination of these two events in the patient with malignancy or HSCT and is a common complication of cancer treatment. It has been estimated that 10–50% of patients with solid tumors and up to 80% of patients with hematologic malignancies will develop fever during at least one chemotherapy cycle associated with neutropenia [28]. Moreover, fever may be the only indication of a severe underlying infection as other signs and symptoms are often absent or minimized due to an inadequate inflammatory response. Therefore, physicians must be particularly aware of the infection risks, diagnostic methods, and antimicrobial therapies required for the management of febrile neutropenia in cancer patients.

In the majority of febrile episodes, a pathogen is not identified, with a clinically documented infection occurring in only 20–47% of cases. Of these patients, bacteremia occurs in 10–25%, with most episodes seen in the setting of prolonged and/or profound neutropenia (ANC < 100 neutrophils/mm^3) [29, 30]. On the other hand, the most common sites of focal infection include the gastrointestinal tract, lung, and skin [31].

Common Organisms

Over the past five decades, the rates, antibiotic resistance, and epidemiologic spectrum of bloodstream pathogens isolated from febrile neutropenic patients have changed substantially under the selective pressure of broad-spectrum antimicrobial therapy and/or prophylaxis [32, 33]. Early in the development of cytotoxic chemotherapies, during the 1960s and 1970s, gram-negative pathogens predominated in febrile neutropenia. Subsequently, during the 1980s and 1990s, gram-positive organisms became more common as use of indwelling plastic venous catheters became more prevalent, which can allow for colonization and subsequent infection by gram-positive skin flora [31, 34]. Gram-positive bacteria currently account for 60–70% of culture-positive infections in pediatric cancer patients [5].

Importantly, a recent systematic review of the epidemiology and antibiotic resistance of pathogens causing bacteremia in cancer patients since 2008 showed a recent shift from gram-positive to gram-negative organisms [35]. The main causes for this new trend are to be determined, but the use and duration of antibiotic prophylaxis are an important factor to consider as the incidence of gram-negative bacteria was significantly higher in groups who did not receive antibiotic prophylaxis. The use of antibiotic prophylaxis, however, may conceivably select for resistant organisms; increasing rates of antibiotic resistance in both gram-negative and

Table 16.1 Common bacterial pathogens in neutropenic patients

Gram-positive bacteria
Staphylococci (coagulase-negative staphylococci and *Staphylococcus aureus*)
Enterococci (*E. faecium* and *E. faecalis*)
Streptococci (viridans group streptococci, *S. pneumoniae*, and *S. pyogenes*)
Bacillus species
Gram-negative bacteria
Enterobacteriaceae (*Escherichia coli*, *Enterobacter* species, *Klebsiella* species, *Citrobacter* species, etc.)
Non-fermenting gram-negative rods (*Pseudomonas aeruginosa* and *Stenotrophomonas* species)
Acinetobacter species

Modified from [20, 29, 30]

gram-positive bacteria have been reported in the global community as well as the cancer population and are of significant concern [5, 31, 35].

Overall, the most common blood isolate in the setting of febrile neutropenia is coagulase-negative staphylococci. Other less common blood isolates include *Enterobacteriaceae*, non-fermenting gram-negative bacteria (such as *Pseudomonas*), *S. aureus*, and streptococci (see Table 16.1). Providers should review the local data at their institution for prevalent blood isolates and antimicrobial susceptibility profiles.

Stratification and Management of Neutropenic Patients

Management of febrile neutropenia continues to evolve given the awareness that interventions previously considered standard of care (such as inpatient treatment with intravenous broad-spectrum antibiotics) may not be necessary nor appropriate for all patients [36]. It has become increasingly important to identify patients at high risk of infectious complications requiring more aggressive management and monitoring (i.e., inpatient setting with intravenous antibiotics). In addition, clinicians may be able to identify low-risk patient populations who may be managed in a less aggressive and more cost-effective manner (i.e., outpatient setting and/or with oral antibiotics). In order to address these issues, algorithmic approaches to neutropenic fever, infection prophylaxis, diagnosis, and treatment have been developed [20, 37–39].

It is well established that stratification of patients to determine the risk for complications of severe infection should be undertaken at presentation of fever [20, 37]. This determines the type of empiric antibiotic therapy (oral vs. intravenous), venue of treatment (inpatient vs. outpatient), and duration of antibiotic therapy.

Generally, the risk for serious infection is directly related to the degree and duration of neutropenia. Pediatric patients with mild (ANC ≥500) and brief periods of neutropenia (<7 days) are less likely to have infectious complications than those with moderate to severe neutropenia (ANC ≤500) lasting more than 7 days. Similarly, the risk for bacteremia and septicemia increases dramatically when the ANC is <200. Infectious complications that are more common with severe and prolonged neutropenia include bacteremia, pneumonitis, cellulitis, and abscess formation.

Risk Stratification

It is important to consider individual patient risk incorporating the latest recommendations for the management of neutropenic fever in children with cancer and HSCT [37, 38]. Patients are generally stratified as either high or low risk as follows:

1. High-risk patients – anticipated prolonged (>7 days duration) and profound neutropenia (ANC <100 cells/mm^3 following cytotoxic chemotherapy) and/or significant medical comorbid conditions, including hypotension, pneumonia, new-onset abdominal pain, or neurologic changes [20]
2. Low-risk patients – anticipated brief (<7 days duration) neutropenic periods in those with no or few comorbidities [20]

In addition, risk classification may be based on the Multinational Association for Supportive Care in Cancer (MASCC) score (Table 16.2) [40]. A MASCC risk score of ≥21 is recommended as the threshold for definition of low risk, with 6% of such patients developing serious medical complications compared to 39% of those scoring <21 [40]. However the MASCC score was developed and validated in adults and has not been validated in a pediatric population.

Table 16.2 MASCC risk-index score

Patient characteristic	Assigned weight
Burden of illness: no or mild symptoms[a]	5
Absence of hypotension	5
No chronic obstructive pulmonary disease	4
Solid tumor or no previous fungal infection	4
No dehydration	3
Burden of illness: moderate symptoms[a]	3
Outpatient status	3
Age < 60 years	2

Legend: The MASCC index score is calculated as the sum of the above variables. For patients meeting any given criteria, they are assigned weighted points specific to that individual criteria
[a]Represent mutually exclusive categories

Evaluation

Upon presentation of the neutropenic fever patient, blood cultures should be obtained from all lumens of central venous catheters and consideration given to concomitant cultures from peripheral blood. Urinalysis and urine culture should be considered in patients with a readily available midstream specimen. Chest radiography should only be obtained in patients with signs or symptoms of respiratory infection. Other diagnostic tests should be performed based upon the presenting signs and symptoms. In children with upper respiratory symptoms, several viruses should be considered in the differential diagnosis as discussed above with the inclusion of molecular diagnostic studies as appropriate. Patients with gastrointestinal symptoms might be evaluated for gastrointestinal pathogens including *Clostridium difficile*, particularly if they have recently been treated with antibiotics (see Chap. 12).

Treatment

The consensus in the field is for all patients considered to be at high risk by MASCC or by clinical criteria to be treated as inpatients with empiric IV antibiotic therapy. Carefully selected low-risk patients may be candidates for oral and/or outpatient empiric antibiotic therapy. Table 16.3 summarizes the recommendation for the management of febrile neutropenia based on recommendations of the IDSA and the International Pediatric Fever and Neutropenia Guideline Panel. Importantly, in neutropenic febrile patients with an obvious source of infection on clinical exam, management should be tailored to that source.

Of note, adequate antibiotic stewardship is of utmost importance during the treatment of neutropenic patients in order to decrease the incidence of antibiotic-related

Table 16.3 Summary of recommendations for management of fever and neutropenia (FN) in pediatric hematology/oncology and HSCT patients

Recommendation	Strength of recommendation Quality of evidence
Initial management	
Risk stratification	
Adopt a validated risk stratification strategy and incorporate it into routine clinical management	Strong recommendation Low-quality evidence
Evaluation	
Obtain blood cultures at the onset of FN from all lumens of central venous catheters	Strong recommendation Low-quality evidence
Consider obtaining peripheral blood cultures concurrent with central venous catheter cultures	Weak recommendation Moderate-quality evidence
Consider urinalysis and urine culture in patients in whom a clean-catch, midstream specimen is readily available	Weak recommendation Low-quality evidence
Obtain chest radiography only in patients with respiratory signs or symptoms	Strong recommendation Moderate-quality evidence

Table 16.3 (continued)

Recommendation	Strength of recommendation Quality of evidence
Treatment	
High-risk patients	
Use monotherapy with an antipseudomonal β-lactam, a fourth generation cephalosporin, or a carbapenem as empirical therapy in pediatric high-risk FN depending on the local prevalence of multidrug-resistant gram-negative rods	Strong recommendation High-quality evidence
Reserve addition of a second gram-negative agent or a glycopeptide for patients who are clinically unstable, when a resistant infection is suspected, or for centers with a high rate of resistant pathogens	Strong recommendation Moderate-quality evidence
Low-risk patients	
Consider initial or step-down outpatient management if the infrastructure is in place to ensure careful monitoring and follow-up	Weak recommendation Moderate-quality evidence
Consider oral antibiotic administration if the child is able to tolerate this route of administration reliably	Weak recommendation Moderate-quality evidence

Adapted from [20, 37, 41]

adverse drug events, prevalence of antibiotic resistance, and decrease treatment costs. Blood cultures must be closely monitored, and once a microorganism has been identified, an appropriate plan for antibiotic de-escalation and/or treatment duration should be promptly instituted.

Invasive Fungal Infections

Invasive fungal diseases (IFD) are one of the leading causes of morbidity and mortality in PHO and HSCT patients and present many diagnostic and therapeutic challenges.

Risk Factors

One of the principal risk factors contributing to the development of IFD relates to the patient's oncologic diagnosis. Patients with AML and high-risk and relapsed ALL, recipients of allogenic HSCT, and those with chronic or severe acute graft-versus-host disease (GVHD) are at the highest risk of IFD [42, 43]. Often a combination of other risk factors is present in these patients which may include prolonged neutropenia, high-dose corticosteroid use, immunosuppressive therapy, parenteral nutrition, presence of a CVC, preceding antibiotic therapy, presence of bacterial coinfection, oral mucositis, and admission to an intensive care unit [44, 45]. The highest risk of IFD is during periods of profound neutropenia which for HSCT recipients occurs during the first 30 days posttransplant and during neutrophil engraftment [46]; for PHO patients, the highest risk period is during induction chemotherapy [46].

In an era of growing prophylactic antifungal use, children receiving mold-active agents have been shown to be at higher risk of non-*Aspergillus* species fungal infection [43]. Voriconazole prophylaxis in adults has been shown to be an independent risk factor for mucormycoses [47]. Likewise, breakthrough trichosporonosis has also been reported in patients receiving micafungin as prophylaxis [48]. These phenomena are likely in part related to the selection of fungi with reduced intrinsic susceptibility to the prophylactic agent.

Species Distribution

The most common IFD are invasive aspergillosis (IA) and invasive candidiasis (IC), with a recent upward trend seen in non-*Aspergillus* mold infections [43–45]. Among *Aspergillus* species, *A. fumigatus* is the most common, followed by *A. flavus* and *A.niger* [45]. Among non-*Aspergillus* molds, mucormycoses (*Rhizopus*, *Mucor*, *Absidia*) are most frequently reported followed by a number of other species (e.g., *Fusarium*, *Scedosporium*, *Curvularia*, *Exserohilum*, etc.) [45].

Among IC, *C. albicans* is the single most common *Candida* species, but non-*albicans Candida* species (especially *C. parapsilosis* and *C. tropicalis*) have been increasingly reported among this population [49].

Clinical Presentation

IFD should be suspected in patients with fever and neutropenia lasting for more than 4 days without any identifiable cause [20]. IC can present as septic shock or may have more non-specific findings such as fever, cough, nausea/vomiting, abdominal pain, and cutaneous lesions depending on the site of involvement. In children, the most common sites of IC are the lungs, liver, and spleen, but dissemination can occur to the other organs including the heart, eyes, or brain. Disseminated disease is an independent risk factor for death in children with IC [50].

The primary sites of IA are the lungs, skin, and sinuses [45]. The clinical presentation of fungal rhinosinusitis may include fever, rhinorrhea, nasal congestion, and facial pain; many cases, however, may not present with any symptoms and may be diagnosed based on imaging performed in a persistently febrile patient with profound and prolonged neutropenia. Cutaneous lesions can present as macules, papules, or nodular ulcerative lesions with or without surrounding erythema and tenderness.

Clinical presentation secondary to other molds, such as *Fusarium* or *Scedosporium*, is indistinguishable from IA. Mucormycoses deserve special mention since dissemination and death are higher due to IFD caused by these species when compared to IA [51].

Diagnosis

Early recognition and prompt treatment of IFD are crucial for optimal management. Diagnostic tests should include blood cultures (though often with low sensitivity), cultures of appropriate sterile sites (such as urine or CSF), and diagnostic biopsies of involved sites for culture and histopathology. Fungal biomarkers can be used as both a screening test during high-risk periods and adjunct diagnostic test in patients with suspected IFD, especially during the periods of prolonged fever and neutropenia. Galactomannan (GM) is a cell wall component released by *Aspergillus* species which can be detected in blood, bronchoalveolar lavage fluid, and cerebrospinal fluid. A cutoff value of a GM optical index of ≥0.5 in blood and a bronchoalveolar lavage fluid level of ≥1 is considered a positive test, though an optimum cutoff value is not well defined in children [52, 53]. Invasive fungal disease due to fungi other than *Aspergillus* species may have negative galactomannan tests. β-D-Glucan is a cell wall component found in many (but not all) species of fungi, and an elevated serum β-D-glucan assay can be caused by IC, IA, and other molds [53, 54]. The optimum cutoff value of β-D-glucan for a positive test is unknown in children, but ≥80 pg/ml is used in most studies [54]. Both GM and β-D-glucan assays have variable sensitivity and specificity among children and should be interpreted with caution. The sensitivity of GM has been reported to range from 65 to 82% in children with malignancy and IA [55, 56]; by contrast the β-D-glucan assay has high sensitivity for IFD (~90%) but suffers from poor specificity [57]. False-positive β-D-glucan can be due to systemic bacterial or viral coinfection, receipt of antibiotics (such as piperacillin-tazobactam or amoxicillin-clavulanate), hemodialysis, receipt of albumin or intravenous immunoglobulin, material containing glucan, oral mucositis, and other GI mucosal breakdowns [54]. Other PCR-based fungal diagnostic tests are under investigation but have low sensitivity and specificity.

GM and β-D-glucan monitoring twice weekly is suggested to evaluate treatment response in those with confirmed/probable disease and as a screening tool in patients at high risk for IFD [52, 53]. All PHO and HSCT patients with febrile neutropenia that persists beyond 4 days and/or those with suspected IFD should undergo computed tomography of the chest, abdomen, and pelvis and of other areas if indicated [53]. The most common findings on imaging suggestive of IFD are pulmonary nodules, especially those with a halo sign, air crescent sign, or cavitations. Hepatosplenic and renal nodules should also raise suspicion of IFD. Other studies to consider include an echocardiogram and dilated retinal examination, especially in patients with disseminated candidiasis. If symptoms of sinusitis or new lesions on the palate are present, a prompt nasal endoscopic examination and CT of sinuses are warranted.

Antifungal Prophylaxis

There are three main classes of antifungals used in patients with IFD: (1) polyenes, which include amphotericin B (AmB) and its lipid formulations (liposomal AmB is most commonly used in PHO and HSCT patients); (2) triazoles (fluconazole, itraconazole, voriconazole, and posaconazole); and (3) echinocandins (caspofungin, micafungin, anidulafungin). Antifungal prophylaxis should be considered in patients who are at high risk for IFD including HSCT recipients and those undergoing intensive remission-induction therapy or salvage-induction therapy [46, 53]. A high incidence of IFD has been reported in children with AML (newly diagnosed and relapsed) [58] and patients with relapsed ALL [46], and such patients may be considered candidates for prophylaxis. Among HSCT recipients, those with an unrelated donor or a partially matched donor are at higher risk of IFD [46].

Recent studies show that children with AML receiving antifungal prophylaxis have reduced rates of induction mortality and resource utilization compared to those who did not receive prophylaxis [59]. Posaconazole was found to be superior to fluconazole or itraconazole in reducing incidence of IFD in children [60]. Echinocandins have been shown to be as or more effective for IFD prophylaxis than triazoles, especially in HSCT recipients, with less adverse effects and can be an alternative option for prophylaxis [46].

The IDSA and the European Conference on Infections in Leukemia (ECIL-4) recommend using posaconazole, voriconazole, or micafungin during prolonged neutropenia to prevent IFD [20, 53]. Posaconazole is recommended for prophylaxis in patients with GVHD who are at high risk of IA [53]. Variable absorption of oral azoles in children should be taken into consideration when choosing oral antifungals.

Treatment

For patients with prolonged fever and neutropenia without an alternative explanation, consideration must be given to the possibility of an active fungal infection. Empiric antifungal therapy should be considered for neutropenic patients with persistent or recurrent fevers after 4–7 days of antibiotic therapy and whose overall duration of neutropenia is expected to be >7 days [20]. In low-risk patients, routine use of empiric antifungals is not recommended [20]. Liposomal amphotericin B or an echinocandin, both of which are fungicidal, are the first-line therapy for empiric antifungal treatment [20]. There is insufficient data to provide specific guidance for patients with concern for a new fungal infection who are already receiving mold-active (i.e., anti-*Aspergillus*) prophylaxis; however, some experts suggest switching to a different mold-active antifungal [18].

Surgical debridement of any fungal lesions or abscesses and prompt removal of CVC in the event of fungemia are crucial to reduce the progression of IFD.

Therapeutic drug monitoring (TDM) should be performed for patients receiving voriconazole, itraconazole, and posaconazole. There is extreme variability in triazole serum levels among pediatric patients owing to diversity in bioavailability in this population. For voriconazole TDM, a serum trough level between 1 and 5 mcg/dl has been considered safe and effective in preventing breakthrough IFD in children [53]. For posaconazole, a trough level of 0.7 mg/L–1 mg/L has been shown to be effective [53]. Due to increased toxicity associated with vinca alkaloids, high doses of cyclophosphamide, and anthracyclines, azoles should not be co-administered with these agents.

The antifungal agents most commonly used in children with PHO and HSCT and their indications are noted below (Table 16.4). Although combination antifungals are not well studied in children, they are used frequently in this population. Pediatric

Table 16.4 Antifungal agents used for treatment of invasive fungal diseases

Drug name	Indications	Organisms resistant or less active	Major adverse effects	Formulations available
L-AmB	First line: 1. IC but echinocandins preferred 2. Mucormycosis Second-line IA and other molds	*Aspergillus terreus, C. lusitaniae* but clinical significance is unknown	1. Nephrotoxicity 2. Electrolyte imbalance especially hypokalemia, hypomagnesemia, and hypocalcemia 3. Infusion reactions (chills, rigors, fevers)	IV
Fluconazole	Maintenance therapy for IC	*C. krusei* *C. glabrata*	Hepatic dysfunction Drug interactions due to CYP enzyme system	IV Oral (tablet, suspension)
Voriconazole	First line All molds except mucormycoses Second line IC	No activity against mucormycoses	Hepatic dysfunction Hallucinations Visual disturbances Drug interactions due to CYP enzyme system	IV and oral *TDM necessary
Posaconazole	Second-line agent for all molds Maintenance therapy for mucormycoses		Gastrointestinal symptoms (vomiting, nausea, diarrhea) Hepatic dysfunction Drug interactions due to CYP enzyme system	IV Oral (delayed release, suspension) *TDM necessary
Echinocandins: Micafungin Caspofungin Anidulafungin	First line: IC Second line: IA Other molds only as salvage therapy	*Cryptococcus* High MIC against *C. parapsilosis* *Trichosporon* spp.	Hepatic dysfunction	IV
Flucytosine	Only in CNS candidiasis in combination with L-AmB		Renal dysfunction Hepatic dysfunction Gastrointestinal symptoms	Oral capsules Suspension needs to be compounded *TDM necessary

IC invasive candidiasis, *IA* invasive aspergillosis, *IV* intravenous, **TDM* therapeutic drug monitoring, *L-AmB* liposomal amphotericin B data are variable regarding the benefit of combination antifungal therapy but overall report an increase in adverse events [45]; the risk of systemic toxicity must therefore be taken into account when considering the use of antifungal combinations. Combination therapy could be considered in patients with refractory disease or as salvage therapy. Granulocyte transfusions for profound or persistent neutropenia, adjunctive cytokines (e.g., granulocyte colony-stimulating factor [GCSF]), and reduction of immunosuppression and tapering of steroids are recommended as an adjunct to antifungal agents in the treatment of IFD [20].

In summary, children and adolescents with malignancy have additional risk factors for healthcare-associated infections. Meticulous attention to personal and oral hygiene, diet, environmental safety, and appropriate immunizations should be practiced in this high-risk population. The use of antimicrobial prophylaxis should be considered in periods of severe neutropenia to prevent bacterial and fungal infections as necessary. Prompt diagnosis and management strategies to prevent infectious complications are key to preventing morbidity and mortality in these immunocompromised hosts.

References

1. Raulji CM, et al. Daily bathing with chlorhexidine and its effects on nosocomial infection rates in pediatric oncology patients. Pediatr Hematol Oncol. 2015;32(5):315–21.
2. Thom KA, Kleinberg M, Roghmann MC. Infection prevention in the cancer center. Clin Infect Dis. 2013;57(4):579–85.
3. Padmini C, Bai KY. Oral and dental considerations in pediatric leukemic patient. ISRN Hematol. 2014;2014:895721.
4. American Academy of Pediatric Dentistry Clinical Affairs, C. and A. American Academy of Pediatric Dentistry Council on Clinical. Guideline on dental management of pediatric patients receiving chemotherapy, hematopoietic cell transplantation, and/or radiation. Pediatr Dent. 2005;27(7 Suppl):170–5.
5. Lake JG, et al. Pathogen distribution and antimicrobial resistance among pediatric healthcare-associated infections reported to the national healthcare safety network, 2011–2014. Infect Control Hosp Epidemiol. 2018;39(1):1–11.
6. Af Sandeberg M, et al. Antibiotic use during infectious episodes in the first 6 months of anti-cancer treatment-A Swedish cohort study of children aged 7–16 years. Pediatr Blood Cancer. 2017;64(7):e26397.
7. See I, et al. Mucosal barrier injury laboratory-confirmed bloodstream infection: results from a field test of a new National Healthcare Safety Network definition. Infect Control Hosp Epidemiol. 2013;34(8):769–76.
8. Torres D, et al. The Centers for Disease Control and Prevention definition of mucosal barrier injury-associated bloodstream infection improves accurate detection of preventable bacteremia rates at a pediatric cancer center in a low- to middle-income country. Am J Infect Control. 2016;44(4):432–7.
9. Marschall J, et al. Strategies to prevent central line-associated bloodstream infections in acute care hospitals: 2014 update. Infect Control Hosp Epidemiol. 2014;35(Suppl 2):S89–107.
10. O'Grady NP, et al. Guidelines for the prevention of intravascular catheter-related infections. Clin Infect Dis. 2011;52(9):e162–93.
11. Bundy DG, et al. Preventing CLABSIs among pediatric hematology/oncology inpatients: national collaborative results. Pediatrics. 2014;134(6):e1678–85.

12. Dandoy CE, et al. Rapid cycle development of a multifactorial intervention achieved sustained reductions in central line-associated bloodstream infections in haematology oncology units at a children's hospital: a time series analysis. BMJ Qual Saf. 2016;25(8):633–43.

13. Tomblyn M, et al. Guidelines for preventing infectious complications among hematopoietic cell transplantation recipients: a global perspective. Biol Blood Marrow Transplant. 2009;15(10):1143–238.

14. Gurry GA, et al. High rates of potentially infectious exposures between immunocompromised patients and their companion animals: an unmet need for education. Intern Med J. 2017;47(3):333–5.

15. Hemsworth S, Pizer B. Pet ownership in immunocompromised children--a review of the literature and survey of existing guidelines. Eur J Oncol Nurs. 2006;10(2):117–27.

16. Steele RW. Should immunocompromised patients have pets? Ochsner J. 2008;8(3):134–9.

17. Hammond SP, Baden LR. Antibiotic prophylaxis for patients with acute leukemia. Leuk Lymphoma. 2008;49(2):183–93.

18. Bucaneve G, et al. Levofloxacin to prevent bacterial infection in patients with cancer and neutropenia. N Engl J Med. 2005;353(10):977–87.

19. Cullen M, et al. Antibacterial prophylaxis after chemotherapy for solid tumors and lymphomas. N Engl J Med. 2005;353(10):988–98.

20. Freifeld AG, et al. Clinical practice guideline for the use of antimicrobial agents in neutropenic patients with cancer: 2010 update by the Infectious Diseases Society of America. Clin Infect Dis. 2011;52(4):427–31.

21. Yousef AA, et al. A pilot study of prophylactic ciprofloxacin during delayed intensification in children with acute lymphoblastic leukemia. Pediatr Blood Cancer. 2004;43(6):637–43.

22. Wolf J, et al. Levofloxacin prophylaxis during induction therapy for pediatric acute lymphoblastic leukemia. Clin Infect Dis. 2017;65(11):1790–8.

23. Felsenstein S, et al. Clinical and microbiologic outcomes of quinolone prophylaxis in children with acute myeloid leukemia. Pediatr Infect Dis J. 2015;34(4):e78–84.

24. Alexander S, Fisher RT, Gaur AH, et al. Effect of levofloxacin prophylaxis on bacteremia in children with acute leukemia or undergoing hematopoietic stem cell transplantation: a randomized clincial trial. JAMA. 2018;320:995–1004.

25. Shefer A, Strikas R, Bridges CB. Updated recommendations of the Advisory Committee on Immunization Practices for healthcare personnel vaccination: a necessary foundation for the essential work that remains to build successful programs. Infect Control Hosp Epidemiol. 2012;33(1):71–4.

26. American Academy of Pediatrics. Rotavirus infections. In: Kimberlin DW, et al., editors. 2018 redbook: report of the committee on infectious diseases. Grove Village: American Academy of Pediatrics; 2018. p. 700–4.

27. Sehulster L, et al. Guidelines for environmental infection control in health-care facilities. Recommendations of CDC and the Healthcare Infection Control Practices Advisory Committee (HICPAC). MMWR Recomm Rep. 2003;52(RR-10):1–42.

28. Klastersky J. Management of fever in neutropenic patients with different risks of complications. Clin Infect Dis. 2004;39(Suppl 1):S32–7.

29. Petty LA, et al. Repeated blood cultures in pediatric febrile neutropenia: would following the guidelines alter the outcome? Pediatr Blood Cancer. 2016;63(7):1244–9.

30. Hakim H, et al. Etiology and clinical course of febrile neutropenia in children with cancer. J Pediatr Hematol Oncol. 2009;31(9):623–9.

31. Ramphal R. Changes in the etiology of bacteremia in febrile neutropenic patients and the susceptibilities of the currently isolated pathogens. Clin Infect Dis. 2004;39(Suppl 1):S25–31.

32. Jones RN. Contemporary antimicrobial susceptibility patterns of bacterial pathogens commonly associated with febrile patients with neutropenia. Clin Infect Dis. 1999;29(3):495–502.

33. Irfan S, et al. Emergence of Carbapenem resistant Gram negative and vancomycin resistant Gram positive organisms in bacteremic isolates of febrile neutropenic patients: a descriptive study. BMC Infect Dis. 2008;8:80.

34. Zinner SH. Changing epidemiology of infections in patients with neutropenia and cancer: emphasis on gram-positive and resistant bacteria. Clin Infect Dis. 1999;29(3):490–4.
35. Montassier E, et al. Recent changes in bacteremia in patients with cancer: a systematic review of epidemiology and antibiotic resistance. Eur J Clin Microbiol Infect Dis. 2013;32(7):841–50.
36. Kumar P, et al. Management of febrile neutropenia in malignancy using the MASCC score and other factors: feasibility and safety in routine clinical practice. Indian J Cancer. 2014;51(4):491–5.
37. Lehrnbecher T, et al. Guideline for the management of fever and neutropenia in children with cancer and hematopoietic stem-cell transplantation recipients: 2017 update. J Clin Oncol. 2017;35(18):2082–94.
38. Hughes WT, et al. 2002 guidelines for the use of antimicrobial agents in neutropenic patients with cancer. Clin Infect Dis. 2002;34(6):730–51.
39. Taplitz RA, Kennedy EB, Flowers CR. Outpatient management of fever and neutropenia in adults treated for malignancy: American Society of Clinical Oncology and Infectious Diseases Society of America clinical practice guideline update summary. J Oncol Pract. 2018;14(4):250–5.
40. Klastersky J, et al. The Multinational Association for Supportive Care in Cancer risk index: a multinational scoring system for identifying low-risk febrile neutropenic cancer patients. J Clin Oncol. 2000;18(16):3038–51.
41. Freifeld AG, et al. Clinical practice guideline for the use of antimicrobial agents in neutropenic patients with cancer: 2010 update by the infectious diseases society of america. Clin Infect Dis. 2011;52(4):e56–93.
42. Castagnola E, et al. Invasive mycoses in children receiving hemopoietic SCT. Bone Marrow Transplant. 2008;41(Suppl 2):S107–11.
43. Wattier RL, et al. A prospective, international cohort study of invasive mold infections in children. J Pediatr Infect Dis Soc. 2015;4(4):313–22.
44. Corzo-Leon DE, et al. Epidemiology and outcomes of invasive fungal infections in allogeneic haematopoietic stem cell transplant recipients in the era of antifungal prophylaxis: a single-centre study with focus on emerging pathogens. Mycoses. 2015;58(6):325–36.
45. Georgiadou SP, et al. Invasive mold infections in pediatric cancer patients reflect heterogeneity in etiology, presentation, and outcome: a 10-year, single-institution, retrospective study. J Pediatr Infect Dis Soc. 2012;1(2):125–35.
46. Dvorak CC, et al. Antifungal prophylaxis in pediatric hematology/oncology: new choices & new data. Pediatr Blood Cancer. 2012;59(1):21–6.
47. Marty FM, Cosimi LA, Baden LR. Breakthrough zygomycosis after voriconazole treatment in recipients of hematopoietic stem-cell transplants. N Engl J Med. 2004;350(9):950–2.
48. Foster CE, et al. Trichosporonosis in pediatric patients with a hematologic disorder. J Pediatr Infect Dis Soc. 2017. https://doi.org/10.1093/jpids/pix031.
49. Steinbach WJ, et al. Results from a prospective, international, epidemiologic study of invasive candidiasis in children and neonates. Pediatr Infect Dis J. 2012;31(12):1252–7.
50. Zaoutis TE, et al. Risk factors for mortality in children with candidemia. Pediatr Infect Dis J. 2005;24(8):736–9.
51. Pana ZD, et al. Invasive mucormycosis in children: an epidemiologic study in European and non-European countries based on two registries. BMC Infect Dis. 2016;16(1):667.
52. Patterson TF, et al. Practice guidelines for the diagnosis and management of Aspergillosis: 2016 update by the Infectious Diseases Society of America. Clin Infect Dis. 2016;63(4):e1–e60.
53. Groll AH, et al. Fourth European Conference on Infections in Leukaemia (ECIL-4): guidelines for diagnosis, prevention, and treatment of invasive fungal diseases in paediatric patients with cancer or allogeneic haemopoietic stem-cell transplantation. Lancet Oncol. 2014;15(8):e327–40.
54. Pappas PG, et al. Clinical practice guideline for the management of Candidiasis: 2016 update by the Infectious Diseases Society of America. Clin Infect Dis. 2016;62(4):e1–50.
55. Dinand V, et al. Threshold of galactomannan antigenemia positivity for early diagnosis of invasive aspergillosis in neutropenic children. J Microbiol Immunol Infect. 2016;49(1):66–73.

56. Hayden R, et al. Galactomannan antigenemia in pediatric oncology patients with invasive aspergillosis. Pediatr Infect Dis J. 2008;27(9):815–9.
57. Koltze A, et al. Beta-D-glucan screening for detection of invasive fungal disease in children undergoing allogeneic hematopoietic stem cell transplantation. J Clin Microbiol. 2015;53(8):2605–10.
58. Science M, et al. Guideline for primary antifungal prophylaxis for pediatric patients with cancer or hematopoietic stem cell transplant recipients. Pediatr Blood Cancer. 2014;61(3):393–400.
59. Fisher BT, et al. Antifungal prophylaxis associated with decreased induction mortality rates and resources utilized in children with new-onset acute myeloid leukemia. Clin Infect Dis. 2014;58(4):502–8.
60. Doring M, et al. Antifungal prophylaxis with posaconazole vs. fluconazole or itraconazole in pediatric patients with neutropenia. Eur J Clin Microbiol Infect Dis. 2015;34(6):1189–200.

Nosocomial Infections in Pediatric Solid Organ Transplantation

17

Blanca E. Gonzalez and Johanna Goldfarb

Since the first kidney transplant was performed by Dr. Joseph Murray [1] in 1953, transplantation of solid organs has become standard of care for many conditions. This is largely related to improved organ procurement, development of standard surgical techniques, and advancements in the management of the immunosuppression required to maintain a transplanted organ. We have an improved understanding of the risks of immunosuppression and the need for the lowest possible doses to prevent infections which are so common after transplant. However, infections continue to account for significant morbidity [2, 3]. While many of the infections are opportunistic and related to the need for long-term immune suppression, a significant number are nosocomial and related to the surgery and/or the hospitalization after transplant and intermittently thereafter. Hospital stays are often prolonged in the immediate postoperative period and may follow a prolonged hospitalization prior to the transplant as an organ is symptomatically failing. Colonization with antibiotic-resistant hospital flora, therefore, is common, including multidrug-resistant organisms (MDROs). Interactions between these microorganisms and a patient with a dampened immune response can lead to host injury [4].

In order to understand fully the role of nosocomial infections in solid organ transplant recipients, we will first review the spectrum of infections and complications of this unique patient population over time.

B. E. Gonzalez (✉)
Cleveland Clinic Lerner College of Medicine of Case Western Reserve University, Cleveland Clinic Children's, Cleveland, OH, USA
e-mail: GONZALB3@ccf.org

J. Goldfarb
Cleveland Clinic Lerner College of Medicine of Case Western Reserve University, Cleveland, OH, USA

© Springer Nature Switzerland AG 2019
J. C. McNeil et al. (eds.), *Healthcare-Associated Infections in Children*,
https://doi.org/10.1007/978-3-319-98122-2_17

Timeline of Infections after Solid Organ Transplantation

In 1998, Rubin and Fishman noted that there is a timeline for the most frequent infections that occur after solid organ transplantation (Fig. 17.1) [2, 5]. This understanding of infection risk allows increased accuracy in evaluating patients who present with signs of infection after transplant and is crucial in planning and evaluating prevention strategies. This timeline will likely need reevaluation as newer immunosuppressive agents and approaches are developed and the period and type of maximal immune suppression evolve.

The goal of immunosuppression after transplantation is to prevent organ rejection by the host. The lowest possible doses of antirejection medications are used to minimize drug toxicity as well as reduce the risk of opportunistic infections [2, 6, 7]. Immunosuppression after transplantation can be categorized into three phases: induction, maintenance, and augmentation (at the time of rejection episodes) [3, 6, 7]. Induction occurs at or around the time of transplant and is aimed at preventing acute rejection by alloimmune T cell-mediated response. This strategy is also utilized to wean or avoid use of steroids, the first mainstay of transplant immune suppressive strategies, and to avoid use of renal toxic agents. Induction medications can be lymphocyte depleting (i.e., antithymocyte globulin (ATG) and anti-CD20 agents like alemtuzumab) or non-lymphocyte depleting (basiliximab). Some of the newer agents have long-lasting immune suppressive effects that can extend beyond 6 months and add additional risk for infection beyond the typical peri-transplant period [8].

During the maintenance period, the objective is to prevent rejection while optimizing graft function. Commonly used agents are calcineurin inhibitors (tacrolimus and cyclosporine), antimetabolite mycophenolate mofetil (MMF), mTOR inhibitors (sirolimus), and steroids (Table 17.1). Every attempt is made to limit the degree of immunosuppression while not losing the protective effect on the transplanted organ [3].

Episodes of rejection can occur at any point and are in general treated with increased immune suppression (i.e., augmentation), placing the patient at increased risk for opportunistic infections, regardless of time since transplant or the original course of immunosuppressive therapy.

Infections During the Posttransplant Period: 0–30 Days

Infections during the first month after transplant reflect multiple conditions including the state of the host at the time of transplant [2, 3, 5]. Many patients have been chronically ill and are extremely debilitated. It is not uncommon for patients to have been hospitalized in the weeks prior to the transplant and to have a history of multiple infections pretransplant. Most of the pretransplant infections are unrelated to immune suppression, though the debilitated state of chronic illness is a form of immune suppression and sometimes medications such as steroids are used pretransplant. Liver transplant candidates are frequently treated for repeated episodes of

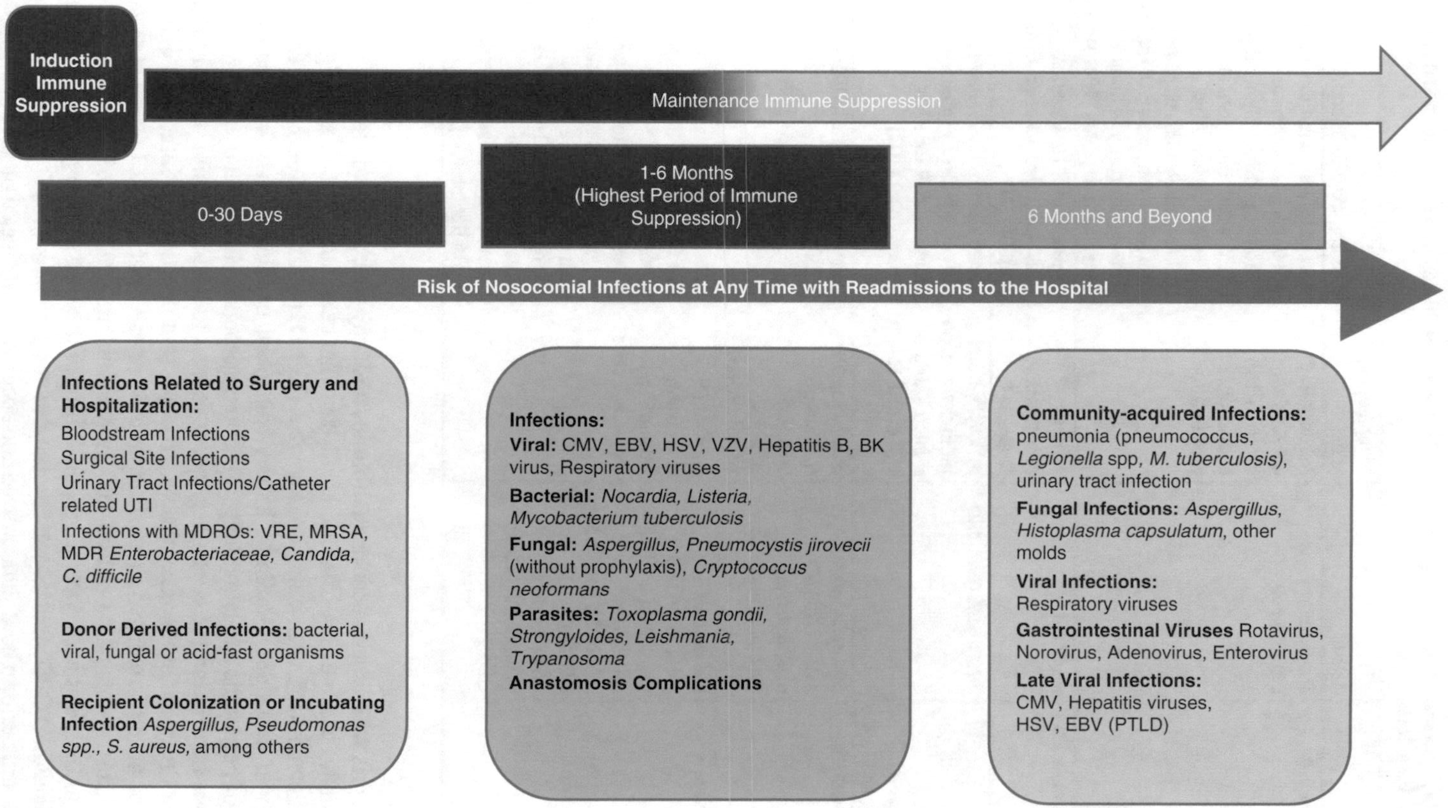

Induction Immune Suppression

Maintenance Immune Suppression

0-30 Days

1-6 Months (Highest Period of Immune Suppression)

6 Months and Beyond

Risk of Nosocomial Infections at Any Time with Readmissions to the Hospital

Infections Related to Surgery and Hospitalization:
Bloodstream Infections
Surgical Site Infections
Urinary Tract Infections/Catheter related UTI
Infections with MDROs: VRE, MRSA, MDR *Enterobacteriaceae*, *Candida*, *C. difficile*

Donor Derived Infections: bacterial, viral, fungal or acid-fast organisms

Recipient Colonization or Incubating Infection *Aspergillus*, *Pseudomonas spp.*, *S. aureus*, among others

Infections:
Viral: CMV, EBV, HSV, VZV, Hepatitis B, BK virus, Respiratory viruses
Bacterial: *Nocardia*, *Listeria*, *Mycobacterium tuberculosis*
Fungal: *Aspergillus*, *Pneumocystis jirovecii* (without prophylaxis), *Cryptococcus neoformans*
Parasites: *Toxoplasma gondii*, *Strongyloides*, *Leishmania*, *Trypanosoma*
Anastomosis Complications

Community-acquired Infections:
pneumonia (pneumococcus, *Legionella* spp, *M. tuberculosis*), urinary tract infection
Fungal Infections: *Aspergillus*, *Histoplasma capsulatum*, other molds
Viral Infections:
Respiratory viruses
Gastrointestinal Viruses Rotavirus, Norovirus, Adenovirus, Enterovirus
Late Viral Infections:
CMV, Hepatitis viruses, HSV, EBV (PTLD)

Fig. 17.1 Timeline of likely infections after organ transplantation. Adapted from Fishman [2]

Table 17.1 Common immunosuppressive agents used in solid organ transplantation and specific risks for infections

Type	Agent	Mechanism of action	Risk for specific infection
Calcineurin inhibitor	*Tacrolimus, cyclosporine*	*Inhibits IL-2 expression;* blocks T cell activation/ proliferation	Risk of infection not modified by choice of calcineurin inhibitor, possibly higher risk of CMV, worse outcomes in patients with hepatitis C. Tacrolimus when combined with MMF may be a risk for BK virus nephropathy in kidney transplant recipients [104, 105]
Corticosteroids	*Prednisone*	*Inhibits inflammatory responses*	Increased risk for Candida infections, herpes zoster, BSI, cellulitis [106]
mTOR (mammalian target of rapamycin) inhibitors	*Sirolimus/everolimus*	*mTOR inhibitor,* inhibits cytokine related T and B cell proliferation	Lower risk for CMV. Antifungal activity against *Cryptococcus*. Increased risk for PJP (everolimus) [107]
Antimetabolites	*Mycophenolate mofetil (MMF), azathioprine, cyclophosphamide*	*Blocks purine nucleotide synthesis,* inhibits transcription	Increased risk for CMV and VZV
Depleting agents	*Antithymocyte globulin (ATG)* polyclonal antibody *Basiliximab:* monoclonal antibody, CD25 *Alemtuzumab:* monoclonal antibody CD52	*Antibodies directed at lymphocytes.* Deplete T cells	*ATG:* Increased risk for CMV and BK virus [105] *Basiliximab:* CMV [105] *Alemtuzumab:* Higher risk for fungal infections when used to treat acute graft rejection. Higher risk for CMV and BK virus. Duration of immunosuppression is prolonged (up to 9 months) [105]

cholangitis with broad-spectrum antibiotics and may have received steroids to treat an immune cause of liver failure. Heart transplant candidates may be bridged for transplant with left ventricular assist devices (LVAD) putting them at risk for device-associated infections. Similarly, kidney transplant candidates may have had episodes of peritonitis and hemodialysis catheter-associated infections.

Graft-transmitted infections may occur related to acute bacterial or viral infections in the donor at the time of death, though some transmitted infections will be latent or have a prolonged incubation period and may not reactivate until after the immediate postoperative period [9]. Preventing transmission of infection from donor to recipient is in part the responsibility of the transplant organ procurement organizations (OPO) that coordinate the donation process [10]. They evaluate the donors and perform both standardized and specific testing based on epidemiological factors to detect active and latent infections. In coordination with transplant centers, careful selection of organs is made with the information provided by the OPO. Organs are accepted or rejected after weighing risks and benefits including the urgency of the need for a transplanted organ, infectious disease potential, and whether there is available prophylaxis or treatment for the possible transmitted infection [9, 10]. Asymptomatic infections in the donor as well as latent infections for which there is no routine screening may be transmitted silently to the recipients. Examples of such organ transmitted infections that convey high morbidity and mortality include parasitic infections such as chronic strongyloidiasis and more acute CNS viral infections such as West Nile and, very rarely, rabies [9, 11–13].

Just as after any surgery, transplant patients may suffer surgical complications including surgical site infections (the most frequent infections in the immediate postoperative period) and nosocomial infections. Wound-related infections are most common in liver transplant recipients followed by (in descending order) kidney, heart, and lung recipients [14]. If patients are colonized with MDRO going into transplantation, nosocomial infections with these pathogens can be especially challenging to treat. Lung transplant for cystic fibrosis is an especially difficult setting as patients have almost always acquired multiple potential pathogens that will remain in the host's bronchi and can cause infection at anastomoses [15–17]. Some of the risk factors associated with nosocomial infections include the often prolonged hospitalizations, intensive care unit admissions, and the use of indwelling catheters after transplantation. *Clostridium difficile* infection also often presents in this period [14].

Infections During Posttransplant Period: 1–6 Months

Opportunistic infections begin to predominate during the period of 1–6 months posttransplant [2, 3, 5]. This is a reflection of the sustained and high levels of immune suppression that often peak at 4–5 months. Reactivations of transplant-associated viruses including Epstein-Barr virus (EBV), cytomegalovirus (CMV), and herpes simplex virus (HSV) occur in this period and have become the target of prophylactic strategies, as these can be life-threatening after transplant. *Pneumocystis jirovecii* pneumonia (PJP) peaks in this period, a reflection of the extreme immune suppression. Infections with *Aspergillus* and other mold infections begin to occur, and preventative strategies must take these life-threatening and difficult to treat infections into account. Nosocomial infections are less frequent, unless continued hospitalization is required as is common after complex cases such as multi-organ transplants or those with failing organs or complicated medical issues that persist after transplant.

Infections During Posttransplant Period: 6 Months and Beyond

By the 6th month posttransplant, patients are usually at home and are starting to resume normal activities [2, 3, 5]; community-acquired infections become the major new threat. Therefore, counseling about safe living to avoid infection after transplant is pivotal and must be repeatedly taught during this period. Notably, opportunistic infections will continue to be a threat to patients in this time period.

Posttransplantation lymphoproliferative disorder (PTLD), the most serious complication of EBV in solid organ transplant recipients, is more common in the first year after transplant. EBV-naïve recipients receiving organs from a seropositive donor (situation which occurs frequently in the pediatric population) are at the highest risk for the development of PTLD, as well as patients who undergo heart or heart-lung transplant. Besides reduction of immunosuppression, many patients require therapy with chimeric anti-CD 20 antibodies or chemotherapy [18]. Side effects of these treatments in turn render patients more susceptible to infections.

Nosocomial Infections

As described above, it is during the immediate posttransplant period that the majority of nosocomial infections occur [2, 3, 14]. Central line-associated bloodstream infections (CLABSIs), ventilator-associated pneumonia (VAP), catheter-associated urinary tract infections (CAUTI), and surgical site infections (SSIs) occur in all hospitalized patients and are monitored by hospitals and reported as markers of quality of care to the National Healthcare Safety Network (NHSN) of the Centers for Disease Control and Prevention (CDC). Data are limited for transplant patients, however, as there are few studies that focus on nosocomial infections in transplant populations, especially in pediatrics [3, 14].

Bloodstream Infections (BSI)

Bloodstream infections (BSI) are the most serious and feared nosocomial infection. These are a significant cause of morbidity and mortality for the SOT recipient. BSI are most common early in the posttransplant period and commonly associated with the presence of venous catheters [14, 19–24].

A prospective surveillance study from Alberta, Canada, by Berenger et al., which included 2257 patients 15–79 years of age and 157 BSI [25], estimated the incidence of nosocomial BSI among SOT patients as 1.39 infections per 100 patient years at their institution. The highest risk was in multivisceral transplants followed by isolated intestinal and liver transplants. Forty-six percent occurred within the first month posttransplantation. CLABSI were most common in heart transplant recipients. UTI-related BSI was more common in kidney transplant recipients, and deep-seated organ space-related bacteremia was more prevalent after liver transplantation. Gram-positive organisms were the most common pathogens followed by gram-negative enterics and *Candida* species. While coagulase-negative staphylococcus (CONS) and *C. albicans* were associated with CLABSI, *E. coli* was associated with organ-specific infectious sources such as the urinary tract. In this study, CMV donor seropositivity was a risk factor for BSI after all SOT [25].

In pediatric small bowel and multivisceral transplantation, the rates of BSI are significant and can be close to 70%, with the majority occurring in the first 3 months post procedure in one series [20]. Catheters and intra-abdominal infections were the most common sources of the bacteremia and gram-positive organisms (CONS and *Enterococcus*) predominated. Overall, mortality was higher in those who experienced BSI due to *Candida* infections. Selective decontamination of the gut appeared in another study to have no impact on the number of CLABSIs or of bacterial infections after intestinal transplant, but it may shift the etiologic agents toward fungal infections over gram-negative enterics [26]. BSI are very common in children undergoing liver transplantation. In a pediatric study of 149 children undergoing living donor liver transplantation, BSI occurred in 21% of their patients in the first 30 days posttransplantation [23]. Gram-positive organisms were isolated in 58% of the BSI episodes followed by gram negatives in 21.5%. The most common organisms causing early BSI were CONS and *Klebsiella*. The majority of these infections were sourced to central venous lines and intra-abdominal infections [23]. In a comparable study, 25% of liver transplant recipients experienced BSI predominately due to central venous catheters followed by an intra-abdominal source [27]. UTI and pneumonia were much less common as sources of bacteremia in liver recipients. One of the risk factors identified as a predictor for BSI after liver transplant was degree of blood loss in the OR, which is likely a surrogate for a more technically complicated procedure. Notably, the 1-year mortality rate was higher in children who experienced a BSI in this study [27].

BSI are frequent after lung transplantation and may occur in up to 26% of pediatric lung recipients. The incidence is the highest in the first 30 days post lung transplantation and is associated with gram-positive organisms. In a study by Danziger et al., the rate of BSI in the first 30 days was 5.5/1000 catheter days and as high as 7.7/1000 catheter days in the first 7 days [19]. In descending frequency, gram-positive organisms (CONS followed by *Enterococcus* spp.), gram-negative bacilli (e.g., *Pseudomonas* spp.), and *Candida* spp. were the organisms identified. Furthermore, BSI in the first 30 days was a risk factor for death in the first year posttransplant. In another study looking specifically at BSI in the first 7 days posttransplantation in children with cystic fibrosis, *Staphylococcus aureus* was the most common isolate, and in 75% colonization was present pretransplantation. Higher ischemia time increased the risk of BSI, perhaps a reflection of the health of the donor tissue [28].

Similar to lungs, BSI in adult and pediatric heart transplant recipients range from 16% to 26% arising mainly in the early posttransplant period [14, 29]. The leading pediatric organisms causing BSI in this population are CONS, followed by *Enterobacter* spp. and *Pseudomonas* spp. Isolation of MDROs is common in pediatric heart transplant recipients [29].

BSI in pediatric kidney transplant recipients have not been well characterized. From adult data, BSI seldom occur in the immediate postoperative period. Rates oscillate between 3 and 5% in the first 30 days posttransplant and increase thereafter, at which time they are secondary to urinary tract infections (UTIs). Early BSI in this population are mainly caused by gram-negative organisms; however, *S. aureus* and CONS are common when the infections are sourced to catheters or intra-abdominal infections [14, 22].

Surgical Site Infections

Surgical site infections (SSIs) are a significant risk in children undergoing SOT. This is largely related to the surgical requirements and techniques utilized in pediatric transplantation. Organ size discrepancy is a frequent complication of pediatric transplant, as adult organs are often the only available organs and, hence, are frequently used in children. Placing an organ that is oversized for body space is associated with many complications including prolonged surgical times, inability to close the body space (requiring an open chest or abdomen during the immediate postoperative period), thrombosis and necrosis of the graft, and/or leakage at the anastomoses (related to pressure of the large organ in a small space) [3]. In liver transplant, the increased risk of wound infection after pediatric liver transplants is related to graft-to-recipient weight ratio >4 [30]. In pediatric heart transplantation, extreme weight mismatch is associated with the need for prolonged postoperative ventilation and ICU stay and ECMO support [31].

SSIs present with fever, accompanied by pain, induration, erythema, or drainage around the incision, usually within 30 days after transplant. However, because of immune suppression, fever may be absent and local signs delayed making the diagnosis more difficult. Limited data in children suggest that graft and patient survival is not adversely affected by these infections, unlike in adults where data are conflicting. However, in both pediatric and adult patients, SSIs result in prolonged hospitalizations and higher costs of care [14, 22, 32].

The high rate of SSI in pediatric liver transplantation, ranging from 25% to 33%, has been shown to correlate with prolonged surgical times, repeat surgeries, elevated WBC prior to surgery, female gender, HLA mismatches, and biliary anastomotic leaks [33, 34]. The most common pathogens include CONS followed by *Clostridium* spp., *Enterobacter*, and *S. aureus*. Given the wide spectrum of organisms involved, surgical prophylaxis is frequently targeted to cover common intraabdominal organisms although sometimes regimens are individualized to target pretransplant infecting organisms such as MDR gram negatives, methicillinresistant *S. aureus* (MRSA), and vancomycin-resistant *Enterococcus* (VRE) [35]. Regimens such as piperacillin/tazobactam with or without vancomycin are commonly used and recommended by the Infectious Disease Society of America (IDSA) surgical prophylaxis guidelines. In children without history of prior infections, however, ampicillin/sulbactam may be a reasonable alternative [35, 36].

Intestinal and multivisceral transplants in both adults and children are also associated with high rates of SSI; as many as 40% of patients will have a significant postoperative infection [37, 38]. Deep-seated infections and organ space infections with mixed bacterial flora *(Enterococcus, Staphylococcus, Streptococcus* spp.) are common. Delayed closure of the abdomen and use of meshes result in higher risk of infection [37]. No recommendations for surgical prophylaxis are available from the IDSA. Some experts recommend the combination of vancomycin, cefepime, and metronidazole or piperacillin/tazobactam plus an antifungal (i.e., fluconazole) for prophylaxis in these patients [35]. The duration of prophylaxis should be limited to less than 48 h. In a pediatric series by Florescu et al. of bacteremia after pediatric intestinal transplant, most infections occurred well after the prophylactic antibiotics were discontinued. This finding led to the shortening of the period of perioperative prophylaxis as it seemed to have no impact on the incidence of BSI [20].

While complete data on pediatric SSIs after heart and lung transplantation is lacking, it does appear that the rates of surgical site infections and mediastinitis are lower in children (3.8% in one study) undergoing heart transplant compared to adult data (incidence of SSI ranged from 8% to 15%) [14, 29]. In children, repeated sternotomies do not appear to place the patient at risk for complications, as in adult patients [19, 39, 40]. Risk factors identified in adult patients after heart transplant include repeat surgery, higher body mass, previous left ventricular assist devices (LVAD), and use of mTOR inhibitors. These risks have not been well established in pediatrics [14, 35]. Clinical presentations of infection include worsening pain out of proportion to findings and/or wound dehiscence. Gram-positive organisms predominate, but *Candida* are also significant pathogens [14, 22, 35, 41]. Prophylaxis is standard, and as with other cardiac surgery regimes, cefazolin is the antibiotic of choice [36]. Modifications can be made based on pretransplant surveillance, especially if a patient has had a preceding LVAD infection or is colonized by MRSA [35, 36].

Surgical site infections occur in approximately 5% after adult lung transplantation [14, 22, 35]. Empyema is the most frequent form (42%) followed by wound infections (29%), mediastinitis (16%), sternal osteomyelitis (6%), and pericarditis (6%) [42]. Most infections are related to gram-positive organisms (i.e., *S. aureus*), but gram negatives, including especially difficult to treat organisms, are common (e.g., *Pseudomonas* spp. and MDR *Acinetobacter, Klebsiella, E coli*). Fungi and *Mycobacteria* spp. have also been reported and can also be very resistant and challenging to treat. Since it is estimated that 35% of these SSIs are caused by colonizing organisms present prior to transplant, prophylaxis is complex, and most authorities suggest selecting agents with activity against colonizing pathogens of both donor and recipient [32, 42]. The recommendations by IDSA, however, still suggest the use of a first-generation cephalosporin for prophylaxis (a reminder of the importance of *S. aureus* in these infections).

Data for Rates of SSI after kidney transplant range from 4% to 26% in data from predominately adults. Deep-seated wound infections are slightly more common than superficial infections. Staphylococci and enterococci are the most common pathogens in this setting followed by gram-negative organisms; cefazolin is frequently recommended for prophylaxis [14, 35].

Pneumonia

A common complication in hospitalized adult patients requiring intensive care is pneumonia. This nosocomial infection is associated with high morbidity and prolonged hospital recovery with rehabilitation frequently required afterward. Although less common in children, when it does occur hospital-acquired pneumonia can be severe with prolonged recovery as in the adult. In a pediatric study evaluating the use of piperacillin/tazobactam for prophylaxis in pediatric transplant recipients, pneumonia was the most common postoperative infection developing in 6 of the 22 patients with bacterial infections [43].

Most hospital-acquired pneumonia occurs in the first month posttransplantation. This is most common after lung transplant and is estimated to occur in up to 60% of adult recipients [14, 22, 44, 45]. Pneumonia can occur after heart (20–35% of cases), liver (14–15%), and kidney (5–26%) transplant as well and is related to complex clinical courses with the need for prolonged intubation. This infection is associated with a reduced 1-year survival rate in adults [14]. The same risk factors that predispose other postoperative populations to VAP such as prolonged intubation, prior antibiotic exposure, and aspiration are risk factors for the transplant population with the added complication of a broader microbiological spectrum (related to chronic infections and greater antibiotic exposure [45]). Common pathogens to cause hospital-acquired pneumonia in the setting of SOT include *Pseudomonas, S. aureus, Acinetobacter,* and *E. coli* [44].

Lung transplant patients are at especially high risk for hospital-acquired pneumonia, likely related to chronic infections present prior to transplant and to the effects of immune suppression. Children with cystic fibrosis can have particularly virulent pathogens colonizing the bronchial tree and lungs [16, 19]. Pretransplant colonization with gram-negative bacilli has been identified as a risk factor for the development of pneumonia after lung and double lung transplant [14, 44, 46]. *Pseudomonas, S. aureus*, and *Aspergillus* are the most common organisms isolated. Targeted prophylaxis has decreased the incidence of these infections in lung transplant recipients [14, 44, 46].

A feared organism associated with nosocomial pneumonia in transplant recipients, and immunocompromised patients in general, is *Legionella* spp. including *Legionella pneumophila* and *Legionella micdadei* [47]. Water is the main reservoir of the organism, and *Legionella* is a rare cause of pneumonia in pediatric patients. Nonetheless outbreaks affecting immunocompromised children have been described. A report from Spain described five children in a kidney transplant unit who developed *Legionella* pneumonia [48]. Patients presented with fever and cough an average of 13 days after transplant. The shower and respiratory equipment were suspected to be the sources of infection prompting exhaustive measures to disinfect shower heads and the hospital water system.

It is very important to try to establish the etiological agent causing pneumonia in pediatric patients after SOT as it may have important treatment considerations. However, establishing microbiologic diagnosis may be difficult and often requires aggressive modalities such as bronchoalveolar lavage (BAL) or flexible bronchoscopy [49]. Notably, BAL in children has a higher diagnostic yield in the immunocompromised than in the general pediatric ICU population [50].

Urinary Tract Infections

Nosocomial urinary tract infections in pediatric hospitals have declined in incidence since the creation of infection control bundles and multicenter, national collaboratives aimed at preventing these infections. The Ohio Solutions for Patient Safety, a collaborative of over 100 children's hospitals, reported a reduction of CAUTI of greater than 60% since 2011 with a rate in 2016 of 1.005/1000 catheter days [51]. While there is no mention specifically of pediatric transplant patients in these reports, one presumes that this decline will also have a positive impact in the pediatric transplant population.

Urinary tract infections usually present with fever, dysuria, and suprapubic tenderness in older patients, but in younger children, the diagnosis may be more elusive, and a high index of suspicion must be maintained, especially in the immunocompromised host. Therefore, a urinalysis and urine culture should be part of the work-up of any hospitalized febrile child with a bladder catheter who has received an organ transplant and is in the intensive care unit.

Nosocomial UTIs occur in adult kidney transplant recipients with rates as high as 56%. Some of the risk factors identified include stent placements, bladder catheterization, female gender, and being a recipient of a deceased donor graft [14, 22]. The risk is reduced by removing catheters early and prophylaxis with trimethoprim/sulfamethoxazole. Organisms such as *E. coli, Klebsiella, Enterococcus*, and *Pseudomonas* species account for the majority of infections with a high prevalence of MDROs. In pediatric patients, UTIs are also common after transplant, but the exact incidence in hospitalized patients is unknown [52]. In a pediatric study of 110 patients who had undergone a kidney transplant, UTIs occurred in 36% of the patients at a mean of almost 12 months after transplant (range: 1 week to 8.9 years) [53]. The same pathogens are reported in pediatric kidney and adult kidney transplant recipients [54]. Pediatric liver transplant candidates also have a high incidence of urinary tract infections, especially younger children with biliary atresia; however posttransplant data are not available.

Urinary tract catheters are the largest risk factor for the development of UTI in the postoperative period. No data are available specifically for pediatric cardiac transplantation. However, in a study of 413 children admitted to an intensive care unit after cardiac surgery (unknown if transplant patients were included), the incidence of UTIs was 7% with all cases classified as CAUTI [55]. In the multivariate analysis, catheter days, presence of congenital abnormalities of kidney and urinary tract, and certain underlying syndromes such as Down and Noonan syndromes were associated with higher risk for the development of a UTI post cardiac surgery. The most common organisms isolated in this population were *Klebsiella, Candida* spp., and *E coli*.

Special Considerations and Situations

Multidrug-Resistant Organisms

The past decade has been marked by the emergence of multidrug-resistant (MDR) bacteria in hospital and community settings and by the limited availability of effective antimicrobial agents. Children are as affected as adult patients, but studies of newer drugs developed to treat these organisms in children lag behind those specifically for adults. A recent cohort study looking at the incidence and outcomes of MDR *Enterobacteriaceae* in 48 children's hospitals in the United States reported a rise in incidence from 0.2% in 2012 to 1.5% in 2015 [56]. A quarter of the infections were nosocomially acquired; older age and comorbidities increased the odds of acquiring these organisms. Consistent with adult data, these infections were associated with increase in length of hospital stay [56]. Importantly, in another pediatric study examining nosocomial infections in the PICU, history of SOT was a risk factor for the development of a nosocomial infection by an MDRO [57].

Transplant candidates and recipients are particularly vulnerable to acquiring these organisms. Frequent admission to the hospital and intensive care units for prolonged periods of time, placement of central venous and urinary catheters, surgical drains and devices, and history of treatment of repeated or chronic infections are all risk factors for colonization with MDRO. Specific risk factors for these infections identified in series of adult transplant recipients have been prior antibiotic exposure, length of stay in the hospital prior to transplant, previous transplant, and increasing age [58].

Commonly reported MDRO in the transplant populations include MRSA and VRE, extended spectrum beta-lactamase (ESBL)-producing *Enterobacteriaceae* and carbapenem-resistant *Enterobacteriaceae* (CRE*),* MDR *Pseudomonas,* and MDR *Acinetobacter* [59, 60]. In adult transplant recipients who develop BSI with *Klebsiella, Enterobacter,* and *Acinetobacter,* multidrug resistance is high with rates reaching up to 50% in certain centers [21, 24, 61].

These organisms are challenging to treat and are often associated with poor outcomes [62–64]. For example, VRE bacteremia was associated with high mortality in the first 30 days after liver transplant regardless of effective therapy. Pretransplant acquisition of carbapenem-resistant *Acinetobacter baumannii* was associated with posttransplant infections and poor outcomes in liver transplant recipients [65]. Data from single centers regarding infections with CRE in SOT recipients report alarming mortality rates that can reach 30% [63]. While more recent multicenter data have shown better outcomes, 20% of patient with a CRE infections still do not survive. Regardless, colonization with CRE should not automatically disqualify a patient as a transplant candidate [66] but should be taken as one factor in evaluating each patient for transplant.

What can be done to prevent these infections? Should patients be screened and decolonized prior to transplant? Pretransplant MRSA and VRE colonization in adults have become common, with rates as high as 8.5% and 12%, respectively, and both are associated with increased risk of infection [14, 22, 67]. A small retrospective study in intestinal transplant recipients who were actively screened reported that colonization pretransplant for MRSA and VRE was associated with increased risk of bacteremia compared to non-colonized patients [64]. A study from Italy screened patients with rectal swabs pre- and posttransplantation for the presence of carbapenem-resistant *Klebsiella pneumonia* and reported that while 18% of patients colonized pretransplant became infected, the risk was much higher (46.7%) when colonization occurred posttransplant [68]. There are very few pediatric studies examining colonization with MDRO and outcomes after transplantation. Paulsen et al. found that colonization with MRSA in children was as high as 11% at the time of the pretransplant evaluation. Two of the 28 patients who proceeded to transplantation were positive at the time of surgery, and 1 developed an MRSA infection despite receiving targeted prophylaxis [69]. Notably, the absolute risk of infection among those colonized with MDROs has been variable in the literature. In a study from Belgium of 100 children who were systematically screened pre- and posttransplant for MDROs (including *Enterobacteriaceae* and MRSA), no association with colonization with MDR strain and infection after transplant was found [70]. Data from pediatric lung transplant recipients with cystic fibrosis suggest that colonization with *B. cenocepacia* and *M. abscessus* is associated with poor posttransplant outcomes. The majority of centers will not perform lung transplants in children colonized with these difficult to treat organisms [71].

Decolonization may be reasonable for patients with MRSA colonization, though the best timing is unknown and the effect not likely to be sustained [72]. While screening for CRE and VRE has been used to cohort patients with these resistant organisms, screening is not recommended because of the lack of sufficient data to show any effect on outcomes [59, 61].

Clostridium difficile Infection (CDI)

Nosocomial *Clostridium difficile* infection (CDI) is a frequent problem in adult SOT patients [73]; however, data in children are scant. In adult transplant recipients, CDI is reported to occur most often after lung transplant (7–31%), followed by liver (3–19%), kidney (3.5–16%), heart (8–15%), and intestinal (9%) transplant [73]. In a single center pediatric study of 141 episodes of CDI, 9% occurred in patients who had undergone a solid organ transplant, and in a multivariate analysis, SOT was identified as a risk factor for CDI [74]. A study using a multi-institutional database estimated that the incidence in pediatric SOT was 3.5%, which was much higher than in the general population (0.6%) [75]. In addition, CDI in this population was associated with longer hospital stays and hospitalization costs. Another single center study estimated a high frequency of CDI in SOT recipients at approximately 10%, with a higher incidence in liver transplant recipients compared to kidney and heart transplant recipients. In this study, traditional risk factors such as recent hospitalizations or duration of antibiotic therapy were surprisingly not found to be risk factors for CDI, but the use of acid blocking agents was found to be protective [76].

In contrast to the hematopoietic stem cell transplant population where CDI infections may present with more subtle symptoms, children with CDI and SOT usually have the typical presenting features of diarrhea accompanied by abdominal pain and distention; more severe cases will develop leukocytosis and acute kidney injury [73, 76, 77]. One of the more problematic issues with CDI in the pediatric immunocompromised population is distinguishing colonization versus infection [78, 79]. Nucleic acid amplification tests (NAAT) have been adopted by most hospital laboratories to improve sensitivity. Importantly, this very sensitive but less specific assay may remain positive for a long time complicating the diagnosis [80, 81]. Updated IDSA guideline for the diagnosis and treatment of CDI recommends not testing for CDI unless there are at least three episodes of unexplained diarrhea in 24 h [82, 83]. Attempts to identify alternative causes of diarrhea are important, especially in children. In the study by Ciricillo et al., 16% of patients with a first episode of CDI also had a pathogen known to cause diarrhea such as norovirus, rotavirus, and adenovirus detected in stool in addition to *C. difficile*, casting doubt on the true etiology of the diarrhea [76]. It may be that CDI is overdiagnosed in some patients, especially those given the diagnosis of recurrent CDI; many cases of presumed CDI may actually only represent colonization with *C. difficile* [76]. It is important to keep in mind that in addition to viruses, medications utilized frequently in transplant can cause diarrhea (i.e., mycophenolate mofetil) [84, 85] and providers should consider this in the evaluation of transplant recipients with diarrhea.

Treatment of CDI in children should follow IDSA recommendations which have been recently updated [83, 86]. For multiple recurrences, fecal microbiota transplantation (FMT) has been done safely and successfully in a limited number of pediatric hematopoietic stem cell transplantation (HSCT) patients [87]. This procedure has also been performed in SOT patients. In a large series of immunocompromised patients (75 adults and 5 children), including 19 SOT patients, the success rate was 79% after first FMT with 15% requiring a subsequent FMT [88]. Recurrence of CDI after the initial FMT in SOT patients has been reported, including in a pediatric heart transplant recipient. It is unclear why some of these patients may fail initial treatment, but disruption of the GI tract by immunosuppression may play a role [89–91]. A multicenter study to determine the epidemiology of CDI in children after SOT is currently underway. A more thorough discussion of CDI is provided in Chap. 12.

Viral Nosocomial Infections

Viral infections constitute a major source of morbidity and mortality in the transplant recipient, especially in children. Outbreaks of respiratory and gastrointestinal viruses have been described among transplant recipients, including children [92, 93]. Transplant recipients may have more severe manifestations of disease and may shed viruses for prolonged periods of time, which has important implications for infection control and prevention [94, 95]. A pediatric study from Boston Children's Hospital evaluated the clinical features and outcomes of viral respiratory infections after HSCT and SOT for over a decade. In this study, 48% of the infections were nosocomial. RSV was the most common viral etiology followed by adenovirus, the latter being associated with worse outcomes [96]. In this study, the majority of infections occurred in lung/heart-lung and kidney transplant recipients. Influenza outbreaks have occurred in several transplant units involving mainly unvaccinated patients and hospital staff [93]. Such unfortunate events have helped to promote strict healthcare worker vaccination policies.

Gastrointestinal viruses such as adenovirus, rotavirus, and norovirus are also associated with prolonged disease duration and viral shedding. Norovirus diarrhea occurs perhaps more frequently than any other gastrointestinal virus among pediatric SOT recipients [97]. Ye et al. found that norovirus was the most common enteric virus isolated in their HSCT and SOT cohort of patients, and 25% of the cases were associated with healthcare transmission [97].

Prevention

Prevention of infections starts with the pretransplant evaluation (PTE), which should be approached as a risk assessment opportunity. The PTE is the time to evaluate for infections that can be treated before transplant or prevented by prophylaxis or vaccination. A thorough review of previous infections should include attention to bacterial cultures and to susceptibility patterns to help develop treatment and prevention strategies. Particular attention should be paid to the patient's history of medication allergies, especially antibiotics. If significant, referral for testing should be considered to verify allergies and pursue desensitization, especially in those colonized with resistant organisms who may need treatment with multiple classes of antibiotics. Inquiring about family history of infections for such organisms as MRSA may help identify those with risk of colonization so that decolonization, if indicated, can be planned. The vaccination status of not only the patient but also the entire family is important. Live virus vaccines are contraindicated in SOT candidates who are expected or may need to receive a transplant within 4 weeks; live virus vaccines, however, are not contraindicated for family members, and vaccines are crucial in preventing these viral infections in children. Yearly influenza virus vaccination should be mandatory for patients and their families.

Antibiotic prophylaxis is administered routinely during transplant with the main goal of preventing surgical site infections [35, 36]. IDSA surgical prophylaxis guidelines do not take into consideration unique situations, such as MDRO colonization [35, 36]. Anesi et al., in a very comprehensive review of SSIs in adult SOT patients, acknowledge that transplant centers may not follow the IDSA guidelines with regard to prophylaxis [35]. Adjusting prophylaxis based on local epidemiology therefore may be appropriate, underscoring the importance of sharing best practices among transplant centers. Whichever prophylaxis is utilized, antibiotics should be limited to short periods after transplant. An exception is after lung transplant where, in patients colonized with MDRO or difficult to treat bacteria, treatment may continue for 7–14 days posttransplant while anastomoses heal [35].

In addition, antibiotic administration within 60 min of incision (120 min for antibiotics that have prolonged infusion times such as vancomycin), weight-based dosing, and re-dosing during prolonged surgeries are practices that have reduced SSI in the general pediatric population and should be observed in the transplant recipient [98, 99].

Finally, strict adherence to infection prevention practices and a robust antimicrobial stewardship is imperative to prevent the emergence of resistant organisms and the nosocomial spread of infection in SOT patients [61]. The infection prevention practices that apply to all hospital populations should be followed and are discussed in detail in other chapters of this book. It is important to remember that even with ideal infection control practice, unexpected infections can occur and should be monitored with an eye toward patterns suggesting contamination of equipment or other fomites. Examples of such infections are an outbreak *of Rhizopus delemar* affecting immunocompromised patients at a children's hospital in Louisiana [100] and a worldwide outbreak of *Mycobacterium chimera* among patients who underwent cardiac surgery [101–103]. In the former, the infection was sourced to contaminated hospital linens and in the latter to contaminated heater-cooler devices. These events underscore that careful surveillance of these especially vulnerable patients for unusual infections is of utmost importance.

References

1. Harrison JH, Merrill JP, Murray JE. Renal homotransplantation in identical twins. Surg Forum. 1956;6:432–6.
2. Fishman JA. Infection in solid-organ transplant recipients. N Engl J Med. 2007;357(25):2601–14.
3. Green M, Michaels MG. Infections in pediatric solid organ transplant recipients. J Pediatric Infect Dis Soc. 2012;1(2):144–51.
4. Casadevall A, Pirofski LA. The damage-response framework of microbial pathogenesis. Nat Rev Microbiol. 2003;1(1):17–24.
5. Fishman JA, Rubin RH. Infection in organ-transplant recipients. N Engl J Med. 1998;338(24):1741–51.
6. Coelho T, Tredger M, Dhawan A. Current status of immunosuppressive agents for solid organ transplantation in children. Pediatr Transplant. 2012;16(2):106–22.
7. Malat G, Culkin C. The ABCs of immunosuppression: a primer for primary care physicians. Med Clin North Am. 2016;100(3):505–18.
8. Koo S, Marty FM, Baden LR. Infectious complications associated with immunomodulating biologic agents. Infect Dis Clin N Am. 2010;24(2):285–306.
9. Jr CS, Koval CE, van Duin D, de Morais AG, Gonzalez BE, Avery RK, et al. Selecting suitable solid organ transplant donors: reducing the risk of donor-transmitted infections. World J Transplant. 2014;4(2):43–56.
10. Giwa S, Lewis JK, Alvarez L, Langer R, Roth AE, Church GM, et al. The promise of organ and tissue preservation to transform medicine. Nat Biotechnol. 2017;35(6):530–42.
11. Basavaraju SV, Kuehnert MJ, Zaki SR, Sejvar JJ. Encephalitis caused by pathogens transmitted through organ transplants, United States, 2002-2013. Emerg Infect Dis. 2014;20(9):1443–51.
12. Le M, Ravin K, Hasan A, Clauss H, Muchant DG, Pasko JK, et al. Single donor-derived strongyloidiasis in three solid organ transplant recipients: case series and review of the literature. Am J Transplant. 2014;14(5):1199–206.
13. Mobley CM, Dhala A, Ghobrial RM. Strongyloides stercoralis in solid organ transplantation: early diagnosis gets the worm. Curr Opin Organ Transplant. 2017;22(4):336–44.
14. Dorschner P, McElroy LM, Ison MG. Nosocomial infections within the first month of solid organ transplantation. Transpl Infect Dis. 2014;16(2):171–87.
15. Faro A, Mallory GB, Visner GA, Elidemir O, Mogayzel PJ Jr, Danziger-Isakov L, et al. American Society of Transplantation executive summary on pediatric lung transplantation. Am J Transplant. 2007;7(2):285–92.
16. Sweet SC. Pediatric lung transplantation. Respir Care. 2017;62(6):776–98.
17. Yserbyt J, Dooms C, Vos R, Dupont LJ, Van Raemdonck DE, Verleden GM. Anastomotic airway complications after lung transplantation: risk factors, treatment modalities and outcome-a single-Center experience. Eur J Cardiothorac Surg. 2016;49(1):e1–8.
18. Green M, Michaels MG. Epstein-Barr virus infection and posttransplant lymphoproliferative disorder. Am J Transplant. 2013;13(Suppl 3):41–54; quiz.
19. Danziger-Isakov LA, Sweet S, Delamorena M, Huddleston CB, Mendeloff E, Debaun MR. Epidemiology of bloodstream infections in the first year after pediatric lung transplantation. Pediatr Infect Dis J. 2005;24(4):324–30.
20. Florescu DF, Qiu F, Langnas AN, Mercer DF, Chambers H, Hill LA, et al. Bloodstream infections during the first year after pediatric small bowel transplantation. Pediatr Infect Dis J. 2012;31(7):700–4.

21. Linares L, Garcia-Goez JF, Cervera C, Almela M, Sanclemente G, Cofan F, et al. Early bacteremia after solid organ transplantation. Transplant Proc. 2009;41(6):2262–4.
22. Moreno Camacho A, Ruiz CI. Nosocomial infection in patients receiving a solid organ transplant or haematopoietic stem cell transplant. Enferm Infecc Microbiol Clin. 2014;32(6):386–95.
23. Rhee KW, Oh SH, Kim KM, Kim DY, Lee YJ, Kim T, et al. Early bloodstream infection after pediatric living donor living transplantation. Transplant Proc. 2012;44(3):794–6.
24. Camargo LF, Marra AR, Pignatari AC, Sukiennik T, Behar PP, Medeiros EA, et al. Nosocomial bloodstream infections in a nationwide study: comparison between solid organ transplant patients and the general population. Transpl Infect Dis. 2015;17(2):308–13.
25. Berenger BM, Doucette K, Smith SW. Epidemiology and risk factors for nosocomial bloodstream infections in solid organ transplants over a 10-year period. Transpl Infect Dis. 2016;18(2):183–90.
26. Galloway D, Danziger-Isakov L, Goldschmidt M, Hemmelgarn T, Courter J, Nathan JD, et al. Incidence of bloodstream infections in small bowel transplant recipients receiving selective decontamination of the digestive tract: a single-center experience. Pediatr Transplant. 2015;19(7):722–9.
27. Shoji K, Funaki T, Kasahara M, Sakamoto S, Fukuda A, Vaida F, et al. Risk factors for bloodstream infection after living-donor liver transplantation in children. Pediatr Infect Dis J. 2015;34(10):1063–8.
28. Onyearugbulem C, Williams L, Zhu H, Gazzaneo MC, Das S, Lam F, et al. Determination of modifiable risk factors for infection in the early post lung transplant period for pediatric cystic fibrosis patients. J Heart Lung Transplant. 36(4):S276–S7.
29. Rostad CA, Wehrheim K, Kirklin JK, Naftel D, Pruitt E, Hoffman TM, et al. Bacterial infections after pediatric heart transplantation: epidemiology, risk factors and outcomes. J Heart Lung Transplant. 2017;36(9):996–1003.
30. Li JJ, Zu CH, Li SP, Gao W, Shen ZY, Cai JZ. Effect of graft size matching on pediatric living-donor liver transplantation at a single center. Clin Transplant. 2017;32
31. Kanani M, Hoskote A, Carter C, Burch M, Tsang V, Kostolny M. Increasing donor-recipient weight mismatch in pediatric orthotopic heart transplantation does not adversely affect outcome. Eur J Cardiothorac Surg. 2012;41(2):427–34.
32. Knackstedt ED, Danziger-Isakov L. Infections in pediatric solid-organ transplant recipients. Semin Pediatr Surg. 2017;26(4):199–205.
33. Hollenbeak CS, Alfrey EJ, Sheridan K, Burger TL, Dillon PW. Surgical site infections following pediatric liver transplantation: risks and costs. Transpl Infect Dis. 2003;5(2):72–8.
34. Yamamoto M, Takakura S, Iinuma Y, Hotta G, Matsumura Y, Matsushima A, et al. Changes in surgical site infections after living donor liver transplantation. PLoS One. 2015;10(8):e0136559.
35. Anesi JA, Blumberg EA, Abbo LM. Perioperative antibiotic prophylaxis to prevent surgical site infections in solid organ transplantation. Transplantation. 2017;102:21.
36. Bratzler DW, Dellinger EP, Olsen KM, Perl TM, Auwaerter PG, Bolon MK, et al. Clinical practice guidelines for antimicrobial prophylaxis in surgery. Am J Health Syst Pharm. 2013;70(3):195–283.
37. Surgical Site Infections After Intestinal and Multivisceral Transplantation [abstract]., Pub. L. No. suppl 3; 2015.
38. Silva JT, San-Juan R, Fernandez-Caamano B, Prieto-Bozano G, Fernandez-Ruiz M, Lumbreras C, et al. Infectious complications following small bowel transplantation. Am J Transplant. 2016;16(3):951–9.
39. Morales DL, Zafar F, Arrington KA, Gonzalez SM, McKenzie ED, Heinle JS, et al. Repeat sternotomy in congenital heart surgery: no longer a risk factor. Ann Thorac Surg. 2008;86(3):897–902. discussion 897-902.
40. Tortoriello TA, Friedman JD, McKenzie ED, Fraser CD, Feltes TF, Randall J, et al. Mediastinitis after pediatric cardiac surgery: a 15-year experience at a single institution. Ann Thorac Surg. 2003;76(5):1655–60.

41. Ramos A, Asensio A, Munez E, Torre-Cisneros J, Blanes M, Carratala J, et al. Incisional surgical infection in heart transplantation. Transpl Infect Dis. 2008;10(4):298–302.
42. Shields RK, Clancy CJ, Minces LR, Shigemura N, Kwak EJ, Silveira FP, et al. Epidemiology and outcomes of deep surgical site infections following lung transplantation. Am J Transplant. 2013;13(8):2137–45.
43. Wiesmayr S, Stelzmueller I, Mark W, Muehlmann G, Tabarelli W, Tabarelli D, et al. Experience with the use of piperacillin-tazobactam in pediatric non-renal solid organ transplantation. Pediatr Transplant. 2007;11(1):38–48.
44. Bonatti H, Pruett TL, Brandacher G, Hagspiel KD, Housseini AM, Sifri CD, et al. Pneumonia in solid organ recipients: spectrum of pathogens in 217 episodes. Transplant Proc. 2009;41(1):371–4.
45. Giannella M, Munoz P, Alarcon JM, Mularoni A, Grossi P, Bouza E, et al. Pneumonia in solid organ transplant recipients: a prospective multicenter study. Transpl Infect Dis. 2014;16(2):232–41.
46. Chan KM, Allen SA. Infectious pulmonary complications in lung transplant recipients. Semin Respir Infect. 2002;17(4):291–302.
47. Sivagnanam S, Podczervinski S, Butler-Wu SM, Hawkins V, Stednick Z, Helbert LA, et al. Legionnaires' disease in transplant recipients: a 15-year retrospective study in a tertiary referral center. Transpl Infect Dis. 2017;19(5)
48. Campins M, Ferrer A, Callis L, Pelaz C, Cortes PJ, Pinart N, et al. Nosocomial Legionnaire's disease in a children's hospital. Pediatr Infect Dis J. 2000;19(3):228–34.
49. Chan CC, Abi-Saleh WJ, Arroliga AC, Stillwell PC, Kirby TJ, Gordon SM, et al. Diagnostic yield and therapeutic impact of flexible bronchoscopy in lung transplant recipients. J Heart Lung Transplant. 1996;15(2):196–205.
50. Efrati O, Sadeh-Gornik U, Modan-Moses D, Barak A, Szeinberg A, Vardi A, et al. Flexible bronchoscopy and bronchoalveolar lavage in pediatric patients with lung disease. Pediatr Crit Care Med. 2009;10(1):80–4.
51. Lyren A, Brilli RJ, Zieker K, Marino M, Muething S, Sharek PJ. Children's Hospitals' solutions for patient safety collaborative impact on hospital-acquired harm. Pediatrics. 2017;140(3)
52. Parasuraman R, Julian K, Practice ASTIDCo. Urinary tract infections in solid organ transplantation. Am J Transplant. 2013;13(Suppl 4):327–36.
53. John U, Everding AS, Kuwertz-Broking E, Bulla M, Muller-Wiefel DE, Misselwitz J, et al. High prevalence of febrile urinary tract infections after paediatric renal transplantation. Nephrol Dial Transplant. 2006;21(11):3269–74.
54. Baskin E, Ozcay F, Sakalli H, Agras PI, Karakayali H, Canan O, et al. Frequency of urinary tract infection in pediatric liver transplantation candidates. Pediatr Transplant. 2007;11(4):402–7.
55. Kabbani MS, Ismail SR, Fatima A, Shafi R, Idris JA, Mehmood A, et al. Urinary tract infection in children after cardiac surgery: incidence, causes, risk factors and outcomes in a single-center study. J Infect Public Health. 2016;9(5):600–10.
56. Meropol SB, Haupt AA, Debanne SM. Incidence and outcomes of infections caused by multidrug-resistant Enterobacteriaceae in children, 2007-2015. J Pediatric Infect Dis Soc. 2017;7:36.
57. Foglia EE, Fraser VJ, Elward AM. Effect of nosocomial infections due to antibiotic-resistant organisms on length of stay and mortality in the pediatric intensive care unit. Infect Control Hosp Epidemiol. 2007;28(3):299–306.
58. Dumford DM 3rd, Skalweit M. Antibiotic-resistant infections and treatment challenges in the immunocompromised host. Infect Dis Clin N Am. 2016;30(2):465–89.
59. Cervera C, van Delden C, Gavalda J, Welte T, Akova M, Carratala J, et al. Multidrug-resistant bacteria in solid organ transplant recipients. Clin Microbiol Infect. 2014;20(Suppl 7):49–73.
60. Viehman JA, Clancy CJ, Clarke L, Shields RK, Silveira FP, Kwak EJ, et al. Surgical site infections after liver transplantation: emergence of multidrug-resistant Bacteria and implications for prophylaxis and treatment strategies. Transplantation. 2016;100(10):2107–14.

61. van Duin D, van Delden C, Practice ASTIDCo. Multidrug-resistant gram-negative bacteria infections in solid organ transplantation. Am J Transplant. 2013;4(13 Suppl):31–41.
62. Hand J, Patel G. Multidrug-resistant organisms in liver transplant: mitigating risk and managing infections. Liver Transpl. 2016;22(8):1143–53.
63. Pouch SM, Satlin MJ. Carbapenem-resistant Enterobacteriaceae in special populations: solid organ transplant recipients, stem cell transplant recipients, and patients with hematologic malignancies. Virulence. 2017;8(4):391–402.
64. Simkins J, Morris MI, Camargo JF, Vianna R, Beduschi T, Abbo LM. Clinical outcomes of intestinal transplant recipients colonized with multidrug-resistant organisms: a retrospective study. Transpl Int. 2017;30(9):924–31.
65. Freire MP, Pierrotti LC, Oshiro IC, Bonazzi PR, Oliveira LM, Machado AS, et al. Carbapenem-resistant Acinetobacter baumannii acquired before liver transplantation: impact on recipient outcomes. Liver Transpl. 2016;22(5):615–26.
66. Huprikar SCL, Pouch S, Pinheiro Freire M, Madan R, Kwak E, Satlin M, Hartman P, Pisney L, Henrique Mourão P, La Hoz R, Patel G. Prior infection or colonization with Carbapenem-resistant Enterobacteriaceae is not an absolute contraindication for solid organ transplantation. Am J Transplant. 2016;16(suppl 3):240.
67. Ziakas PD, Pliakos EE, Zervou FN, Knoll BM, Rice LB, Mylonakis E. MRSA and VRE colonization in solid organ transplantation: a meta-analysis of published studies. Am J Transplant. 2014;14(8):1887–94.
68. Giannella M, Bartoletti M, Morelli MC, Tedeschi S, Cristini F, Tumietto F, et al. Risk factors for infection with carbapenem-resistant Klebsiella pneumoniae after liver transplantation: the importance of pre- and posttransplant colonization. Am J Transplant. 2015;15(6):1708–15.
69. Paulsen GC, Danziger-Isakov L. Epidemiology and outcomes of pre-transplant methicillin resistant Staphylococcus Aureus screening in pediatric solid organ transplant candidates. 2015 American transplant congress abstracts. Am J Transplant. 2015;15(S3):1.
70. Dalex MS, Gautier C et al Impact of multidrug-resistant bacteria carriage in pediatric liver transplant recipients. Poster session #3: infectious diseases. Pediatr Transplant 2017;21:77–83
71. Benden C. Pediatric lung transplantation. J Thorac Dis. 2017;9(8):2675–83.
72. Garzoni C, Vergidis P, Practice ASTIDCo. Methicillin-resistant, vancomycin-intermediate and vancomycin-resistant Staphylococcus aureus infections in solid organ transplantation. Am J Transplant. 2013;13(Suppl 4):50–8.
73. Dubberke ER, Burdette SD, Practice ASTIDCo. Clostridium difficile infections in solid organ transplantation. Am J Transplant. 2013;13(Suppl 4):42–9.
74. Sandora TJ, Fung M, Flaherty K, Helsing L, Scanlon P, Potter-Bynoe G, et al. Epidemiology and risk factors for Clostridium difficile infection in children. Pediatr Infect Dis J. 2011;30(7):580–4.
75. Pant C, Deshpande A, Desai M, Jani BS, Sferra TJ, Gilroy R, et al. Outcomes of Clostridium difficile infection in pediatric solid organ transplant recipients. Transpl Infect Dis. 2016;18(1):31–6.
76. Ciricillo J, Haslam D, Blum S, Kim MO, Liu C, Paulsen G, et al. Frequency and risks associated with Clostridium difficile-associated diarrhea after pediatric solid organ transplantation: a single-center retrospective review. Transpl Infect Dis. 2016;18(5):706–13.
77. Alonso CD, Braun DA, Patel I, Akbari M, Oh DJ, Jun T, et al. A multicenter, retrospective, case-cohort study of the epidemiology and risk factors for Clostridium difficile infection among cord blood transplant recipients. Transpl Infect Dis. 2017;19(4)
78. Dominguez SR, Dolan SA, West K, Dantes RB, Epson E, Friedman D, et al. High colonization rate and prolonged shedding of Clostridium difficile in pediatric oncology patients. Clin Infect Dis. 2014;59(3):401–3.
79. Kim J. Editorial commentary: Clostridium difficile in pediatric oncology patients: more questions than answers. Clin Infect Dis. 2014;59(3):404–5.
80. Fang FC, Polage CR, Wilcox MH. Point-counterpoint: what is the optimal approach for detection of Clostridium difficile infection? J Clin Microbiol. 2017;55(3):670–80.

81. Polage CR, Gyorke CE, Kennedy MA, Leslie JL, Chin DL, Wang S, et al. Overdiagnosis of Clostridium difficile infection in the molecular test era. JAMA Intern Med. 2015;175(11):1792–801.
82. Nicholson MR, Osgood CL, Acra SA, Edwards KM. Clostridium difficile infection in the pediatric transplant patient. Pediatr Transplant. 2015;19(7):792–8.
83. McDonald LC, Gerding DN, Johnson S, Bakken JS, Carroll KC, Coffin SE, et al. Clinical practice guidelines for Clostridium difficile infection in adults and children: 2017 update by the Infectious Diseases Society of America (IDSA) and Society for Healthcare Epidemiology of America (SHEA). Clin Infect Dis. 2018;66(7):e1–e48.
84. Al-Absi AI, Cooke CR, Wall BM, Sylvestre P, Ismail MK, Mya M. Patterns of injury in mycophenolate mofetil-related colitis. Transplant Proc. 2010;42(9):3591–3.
85. Phatak UP, Seo-Mayer P, Jain D, Selbst M, Husain S, Pashankar DS. Mycophenolate mofetil-induced colitis in children. J Clin Gastroenterol. 2009;43(10):967–9.
86. Cohen SH, Gerding DN, Johnson S, Kelly CP, Loo VG, McDonald LC, et al. Clinical practice guidelines for Clostridium difficile infection in adults: 2010 update by the society for healthcare epidemiology of America (SHEA) and the infectious diseases society of America (IDSA). Infect Control Hosp Epidemiol. 2010;31(5):431–55.
87. Bluestone H, Kronman MP, Suskind DL. Fecal microbiota transplantation for recurrent Clostridium difficile infections in pediatric hematopoietic stem cell transplant recipients. J Pediatric Infect Dis Soc. 2017;7:e6.
88. Kelly CR, Ihunnah C, Fischer M, Khoruts A, Surawicz C, Afzali A, et al. Fecal microbiota transplant for treatment of Clostridium difficile infection in immunocompromised patients. Am J Gastroenterol. 2014;109(7):1065–71.
89. Alrabaa S, Jariwala R, Zeitler K, Montero J. Fecal microbiota transplantation outcomes in immunocompetent and immunocompromised patients: a single-center experience. Transpl Infect Dis. 2017;19(4)
90. Flannigan KL, Rajbar T, Moffat A, McKenzie LS, Dicke F, Rioux K, et al. Changes in composition of the gut bacterial microbiome after fecal microbiota transplantation for recurrent Clostridium difficile infection in a pediatric heart transplant patient. Front Cardiovasc Med. 2017;4:17.
91. Friedman-Moraco RJ, Mehta AK, Lyon GM, Kraft CS. Fecal microbiota transplantation for refractory Clostridium difficile colitis in solid organ transplant recipients. Am J Transplant. 2014;14(2):477–80.
92. Larcher C, Geltner C, Fischer H, Nachbaur D, Muller LC, Huemer HP. Human metapneumovirus infection in lung transplant recipients: clinical presentation and epidemiology. J Heart Lung Transplant. 2005;24(11):1891–901.
93. Malavaud S, Malavaud B, Sandres K, Durand D, Marty N, Icart J, et al. Nosocomial outbreak of influenza virus a (H3N2) infection in a solid organ transplant department. Transplantation. 2001;72(3):535–7.
94. Abbas S, Raybould JE, Sastry S, de la Cruz O. Respiratory viruses in transplant recipients: more than just a cold. Clinical syndromes and infection prevention principles. Int J Infect Dis. 2017;62:86–93.
95. Memoli MJ, Athota R, Reed S, Czajkowski L, Bristol T, Proudfoot K, et al. The natural history of influenza infection in the severely immunocompromised vs nonimmunocompromised hosts. Clin Infect Dis. 2014;58(2):214–24.
96. Lo MS, Lee GM, Gunawardane N, Burchett SK, Lachenauer CS, Lehmann LE. The impact of RSV, adenovirus, influenza, and parainfluenza infection in pediatric patients receiving stem cell transplant, solid organ transplant, or cancer chemotherapy. Pediatr Transplant. 2013;17(2):133–43.
97. Ye X, Van JN, Munoz FM, Revell PA, Kozinetz CA, Krance RA, et al. Noroviruses as a cause of diarrhea in immunocompromised pediatric hematopoietic stem cell and solid organ transplant recipients. Am J Transplant. 2015;15(7):1874–81.
98. Foster CB, Sabella C. Health care--associated infections in children. JAMA. 2011;305(14):1480–1.

99. Woodward C, Taylor R, Son M, Taeed R, Jacobs ML, Kane L, et al. Multicenter quality improvement project to prevent sternal wound infections in pediatric cardiac surgery patients. World J Pediatr Congenit Heart Surg. 2017;8(4):453–9.
100. Duffy J, Harris J, Gade L, Sehulster L, Newhouse E, O'Connell H, et al. Mucormycosis outbreak associated with hospital linens. Pediatr Infect Dis J. 2014;33(5):472–6.
101. Ninh A, Weiner M, Goldberg A. Healthcare-associated Mycobacterium chimaera infection subsequent to heater-cooler device exposure during cardiac surgery. J Cardiothorac Vasc Anesth. 2017;31(5):1831–5.
102. Perkins KM, Lawsin A, Hasan NA, Strong M, Halpin AL, Rodger RR, et al. Notes from the field: Mycobacterium chimaera contamination of heater-cooler devices used in cardiac surgery - United States. MMWR Morb Mortal Wkly Rep. 2016;65(40):1117–8.
103. van Ingen J, Kohl TA, Kranzer K, Hasse B, Keller PM, Katarzyna Szafranska A, et al. Global outbreak of severe Mycobacterium chimaera disease after cardiac surgery: a molecular epidemiological study. Lancet Infect Dis. 2017;17(10):1033–41.
104. Singh N. Infectious complications in organ transplant recipients with the use of calcineurin-inhibitor agent-based immunosuppressive regimens. Curr Opin Infect Dis. 2005;18(4):342–5.
105. Issa NC, Fishman JA. Infectious complications of antilymphocyte therapies in solid organ transplantation. Clin Infect Dis. 2009;48(6):772–86.
106. Rostaing L, Malvezzi P. Steroid-based therapy and risk of infectious complications. PLoS Med. 2016;13(5):e1002025.
107. Neff RT, Jindal RM, Yoo DY, Hurst FP, Agodoa LY, Abbott KC. Analysis of USRDS: incidence and risk factors for pneumocystis jiroveci pneumonia. Transplantation. 2009;88(1):135–41.

Infections in Pediatric Patients with End-Stage Renal Disease

18

Ayse Akcan-Arikan, Sarah J. Swartz,
and Poyyapakkam R. Srivaths

Introduction: Acquired Immune Dysfunction of ESRD

End-stage renal disease (ESRD) – defined as permanent loss of kidney function where either long-term dialysis or kidney transplantation is required to sustain life – is a multisystem disease, even when the primary cause is limited to isolated renal pathology. As kidneys have numerous functions outside of excretion of metabolic end products, many clinical conditions, such as anemia or metabolic bone disease, arise when normal renal function is lost. Dialytic therapies are only able to partially substitute for the toxin and fluid removal function, and only for limited periods of time during the day, as opposed to the continuous tight control provided by normally functioning kidneys. In fact, loss of residual renal function in patients on dialysis, even when it is a miniscule portion of normal function, leads to worsening metabolic control requiring increased dosages of supplemental and therapeutic medications, underscoring the important contribution of kidney function to overall health. A lesser-known aspect of ESRD is the adverse impact of abnormal renal function on host immunity. ESRD patients are prone to infections, have a high rate of malignancy – particularly skin cancer and non-Hodgkin lymphoma – and have poor response rates to routine vaccines dependent on T-cell-mediated antigens, highlighting ESRD as a state of acquired immune dysfunction [1].

Infection is one of the most important causes of mortality and morbidity in children with ESRD. There are currently about 9000 patients under the age of

A. Akcan-Arikan (✉)
Department of Pediatrics, Sections of Critical Care Medicine and Renal, Baylor College of Medicine, Houston, TX, USA
e-mail: aysea@bcm.edu

S. J. Swartz · P. R. Srivaths
Department of Pediatrics, Section of Renal, Baylor College of Medicine, Houston, TX, USA

© Springer Nature Switzerland AG 2019
J. C. McNeil et al. (eds.), *Healthcare-Associated Infections in Children*,
https://doi.org/10.1007/978-3-319-98122-2_18

21 years receiving renal replacement therapy, as per the US Renal Data System (USRDS) [2]. Although survival has somewhat improved over time, the mortality rate in pediatric ESRD remains much higher than the general population, with cardiovascular disease accounting for 40–50% of deaths and infections accounting for 20% [1]. Sepsis is common in patients on dialysis, and death from septicemia is 100–300-fold more likely in adults with ESRD compared to the general population [3, 4]. The increased predilection to sepsis persists throughout different decades, although somewhat decreases after the 6th to 7th decade [4]. Infection is widely reported as the second leading cause of death in dialysis patients [5]. Interestingly, over the last decade, some European centers have reported infections surpassing cardiovascular causes of mortality in pediatric chronic kidney disease patients [1, 6]. The reasons behind the impaired immunity of ESRD are multifactorial and include underlying disease and comorbidities; uremia; increased inflammatory and oxidative stress; malnutrition; changes in iron, calcium, and phosphorus metabolism; loss of the natural skin barrier; presence of indwelling catheters; increased exposure to healthcare-associated pathogens due to increased utilization of hospital resources (e.g., frequent hospitalization and routine outpatient and dialysis clinic visits); anemia; and vitamin D deficiency among others. Here we will consider some of the major pathways contributing to a higher risk of infection in this population in more detail.

Uremia

Alterations in the metabolic milieu due to the accumulation of toxins such as urea and other uremic toxins contribute to a state of functional immune deficiency in ESRD. More than 90 uremic toxins are retained in uremia and can be classified into three groups according to size as small, middle, and large; protein-bound toxins are also considered large as they are not easily removable by dialysis. The dialyzable middle molecular uremic toxins, such as granulocyte inhibitory protein I and II, interfere with neutrophil and lymphocyte function by inhibiting chemotaxis, adhesion, and oxidative killing capacity. In the era of biocompatible poly-flux membranes, these toxins are more readily removable but might still be retained, especially with suboptimal dialysis adequacy (which can be thought of as a measure of the effectiveness of dialysis). In addition, uremic retention solutes might alter apoptosis and necrosis of neutrophils [7]. For example, immunoglobulin light chains, middle molecules increased in uremia, inhibit apoptosis of neutrophils impacting an important regulatory step in the control of inflammation. Advanced glycation end products, also retained in ESRD, increase apoptosis of immune active cells; the same holds true for reactive oxygen species, oxidized lipoproteins, and uremic plasma in general. Moreover, uremia decreases the antigen-presenting capabilities of antigen-presenting cells (APCs) as well as leading to upregulation of Fas ligand, potentially contributing to enhanced apoptosis of immune effector cells [8, 9].

Immune Dysfunction

Both the innate and the acquired immune systems are impacted in ESRD [10]. Innate immunity is characterized by various pattern recognition receptors (PRR) – secreted, endocytic, and signaling – located on the surface of phagocytic cells that recognize pathogen-associated molecular patterns (PAMP) and trigger an immune response. Opsonins, such as mannose-binding lectin, are examples of secreted PRRs which bind to bacterial carbohydrates and initiate lectin complement activation. Endocytic PRRs are present on the surface of phagocytes, like macrophage scavenger protein receptor, and help clear bacteria from circulation. In ESRD, secreted PRRs are elevated and endocytic PRRs are increased. Signaling PRRs, like Toll-like receptors (TLRs), on the other hand, are downregulated. Signaling PRRs activate one of the key doorkeepers of inflammation, nuclear factor kappa B. TLRs also recognize PAMPs (such as endotoxin, RNA, and Tamm-Horsfall protein among others) and are thought to link innate and adaptive immunity. TLRs are major contributors to local defense against urinary tract infections; thus, UTIs may particularly impact ESRD patients due to impaired TLR signaling as well as decreased urine production and flow [11].

Dendritic cells are major contributors to local immunity in the kidney. They are the major APCs and participate in innate immunity via direct activation by PRRs and in adaptive immunity via antigen presentation. In addition, dendritic cells secrete cytokines to further modulate adaptive immunity. Importantly, dendritic cells have decreased endocytic capacity in ESRD patients [12]. Sera from dialysis patients can induce dendritic cell dysfunction in vitro by inhibiting maturation, leading to both decreased response to endotoxin stimulation and decreased capacity to secrete interferon gamma [13]. More frequent dialysis decreases the in vitro dysfunction that uremic plasma induces, suggesting that dialyzable soluble toxins are responsible for mediating dendritic cell dysfunction. Some of these deficiencies are reversed after kidney transplantation [14].

Despite increased subclasses with pro-inflammatory properties, monocytes from ESRD patients exhibit decreased endocytosis and impaired maturation, are hypoactive to endotoxin stimulation, and produce lower amounts of interleukin-1β and tumor necrosis factor (TNF)-α compared to those from healthy patients [15]. The same phenomena are seen when cultured monocytes are exposed to uremic plasma [16–18].

Neutrophil deficiency might also increase susceptibility to infections in the setting of ESRD [19]. The mechanism underlying this is not well understood but appears to be a functional deficiency, with normal cell counts but reduced intracellular killing ability. Historically, older hemodialyzers induced profound but transient neutropenia by sequestration of neutrophils in the lung due to complement activation caused by dialyzer blood contact. As current biocompatible dialyzers do not readily activate complement, this mechanism does not adequately explain the neutrophil dysfunction observed in ESRD patients. Uremic toxins may affect neutrophil function by interfering with chemotaxis. ESRD patients demonstrate inhibition of neutrophil glycolysis response to various stimuli (e.g., latex, Staph A, etc.) required to produce the ATP for NADPH oxidase. Enzymatic activity and release of myeloperoxidase (MPO), essential for adequate bacterial killing, are decreased in granulocytes from hemodialysis (HD) patients. This decreased bactericidal capacity of neutrophils might be partially restored by HD, supporting a mechanistic role of the accumulation of dialyzable toxins in neutrophil dysfunction [20]. Other hypothesized reasons for neutrophil dysfunction are iron overload, anemia, and increased cytosolic calcium levels [21]. Increased intracellular calcium inhibits mitochondrial oxygen consumption, decreasing ATP content and ultimately impairing energy-dependent phagocytosis [22].

Iron Overload/Iron Deficiency/Anemia

Anemia and perturbations in iron homeostasis, which are very common in the setting of ESRD, also likely play mechanistic roles in the susceptibility to infection in this population. Iron deficiency itself leads to immune dysfunction as iron is essential for immune processes such as lymphocyte mitogen responses, phagocytosis, respiratory burst, and MPO activity. Furthermore, excess iron has been demonstrated to be an infectious risk in animal studies. Iron-overloaded patients are believed to have abnormal neutrophil phagocytic function via unclear mechanisms perhaps related to the adverse impact of iron on superoxide production. Anemia adversely impacts tissue oxygenation and might have an adverse impact on the immune system. HD patients who were anemic had higher reported rates of infection-related hospitalizations in some studies [23, 24]. Neutrophil function has also been reported to correlate with hematocrit levels, and a marked increase in neutrophil glycolytic response is demonstrated after treatment with erythropoietin-stimulating agents [25].

Adaptive Immune System

Antigen-specific adaptive immune responses are also impacted in ESRD. Anergy to tuberculin test despite latent tuberculosis infection is well described in this population. Reduced responsiveness to vaccinations, specifically lower rates of response to vaccines containing T-cell-dependent antigens, and a more rapid decline of antibodies after vaccination are widely reported [26, 27]. Interestingly, innate and adaptive immunity are closely related through TLRs (a PRR). TLRs regulate the expression of costimulatory signal molecules (like CD80 or CD86) on APCs which are required to activate T cells in combination with the peptide-major histocompatibility antigen complex [10]. Thereby innate immunity is intimately connected to adaptive immunity via signaling PRRs, which are in turn downregulated in ESRD. Such complex interactions explain, at least in part, the impaired T-cell activation observed in ESRD. Helper T-cell (T_H) populations are also altered in ESRD with the T_H1/T_H2

ratio being increased. Additionally, APCs are overstimulated, and T-lymphocyte activation is impaired in the setting of ESRD [28]. Finally, humoral immunity may also be impaired in ESRD; despite normal quantitative immunoglobulin levels, decreased B-cell counts have been reported in these patients [18].

Acute and Chronic Inflammation

ESRD is characterized by a state of heightened inflammation and oxidative stress [29]. Several immune active proteins are excreted through the kidneys and are therefore retained in renal failure. Pro-inflammatory cytokine levels are increased in ESRD due to a combination of under-excretion, the presence of uremic toxins, oxidative stress, volume overload, and underlying diseases. Chronic inflammation due to sustained activation of CD14+ (endotoxin receptor) mononuclear cells in HD patients may explain impaired innate immunity; these chronically "primed monocytes" have decreased cytokine responses to endotoxin stimulation that are negatively correlated to C-reactive protein (CRP) levels [30, 31]. In pediatric HD patients, serum pro-inflammatory cytokine levels are elevated proportional to cumulative years on dialysis (often referred to as vintage) compared to healthy controls, suggesting a state of chronic inflammation [31]. The pro-inflammatory cytokines interleukin-1β and TNF-α are increased immediately after and remain elevated up to 24 h after an HD session, correlating positively with dialysis vintage and negatively with dialysis adequacy. Furthermore, inflammation and malnutrition are associated with pathologic calcifications; these in turn may be related to coronary calcification and increased cardiovascular mortality [32, 33]. In fact, the presence of HD catheters alone, even in the absence of infection, has been shown to alter CRP levels in children and induce "sterile inflammation;" interestingly, CRP levels decline after conversion of HD access from catheter to fistula [34]. Damage-associated molecular patterns, such as mitochondrial DNA and high-mobility group box-1 protein, are elevated in dialysis patients and associated with pro-inflammatory cytokine release [35]. Modern dialyzers are notably less inflammatory than older models; however, endotoxin leaks through back filtration from dialysate might contribute to increased inflammation in HD.

Malnutrition

Children with ESRD and moderate to severe growth failure are more likely to die and die of infectious causes [36, 37]. Growth failure might be an indicator of more severe disease, malnutrition, or due to an as yet unknown mechanism. Inflammation and malnutrition are closely linked in a bidirectional relationship. Infections are increased in adult ESRD patients with hypoalbuminemia, which might be a reflection of nutritional status.

Comorbidities

Underlying disease impacts immune response in ESRD. Nephrotic syndrome is common in children and not infrequently progresses to ESRD, particularly when due to focal segmental glomerular sclerosis. Hypoalbuminemia and edema characterize nephrotic syndrome and contribute to infection susceptibility, along with urinary loss of immunoglobulin, alternative complement factors, and other immune components [38]. In addition, immune modulation used to treat the underlying disorder causing renal disease, such as in systemic lupus erythematosus, also has adverse consequences on the host response to infections.

In summation, numerous factors contribute to susceptibility to infection in patients with ESRD. The contribution of HD and peritoneal dialysis (PD) catheters to infection susceptibility will be examined in detail in the corresponding sections.

Infections in Hemodialysis

Maintenance in-center HD remains the most common dialytic modality for ESRD patients and is common even among children. Infections are the leading cause of hospitalization in HD patients. An annual infection rate of 35% has been reported in adult HD patients, with most cases lacking a focal source (i.e., sepsis or bacteremia); however, access-related infections were responsible for 1/5 hospitalizations in this population [39]. One in three adult ESRD patients will have at least one infection-related hospitalization and, similarly, catheter-related infections increase the risk of hospitalization [40]. This number is even higher in pediatric HD patients, where the cumulative incidence of infection-related hospitalization is as high as 40% over 3 years [41].

HD catheter-related bloodstream infection (CRBSI) poses a great burden in the pediatric population since HD catheters are still the most common access for children receiving maintenance dialysis. Since venous access serves as a lifeline for dialysis patients, strategies to preserve the HD catheter while treating CRBSI are utilized more in this population compared to other populations with CRBSI (such as pediatric oncology patients).

Nearly 80% of new pediatric HD patients will start with a central venous catheter as their access for HD. Though the overall use of HD catheters decreases as the children get older, arteriovenous (AV) fistulas or grafts do not become the predominant vascular access for HD until young adulthood (18–21 years old) (Fig. 18.1). Since most of the infections observed in HD patients are thought to be secondary to dialysis catheter-related infections, one can clearly appreciate the disease burden posed by having an HD catheter in the pediatric population. This is underscored by Centers for Disease Control and Prevention (CDC) National Healthcare Safety Network (NHSN) study which revealed that among HD patients with a bloodstream infection, 63% had a central venous catheter in place [42].

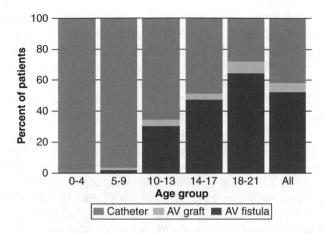

Fig. 18.1 Distribution of vascular access in incident pediatric dialysis patients. Age groups are divided by years of age. (Adapted from Ref. [2])

Epidemiology

Accurate information on the epidemiology of HD catheter-related bloodstream infections is hampered by a lack of a uniform definition used for reporting, particularly in children. Data has been reported either as infections per 1000 catheter days or infections per 100 patient-months with most reporting coming from single institutions. Rates of HD CRBSI reported vary from 0.5 to 8.6 infections/1000 catheter days [43–46]. A degree of the observed variability is likely attributable to diversity in definitions of CRBSI in these studies. Such discrepancies make understanding the scope and epidemiology of HD CRBSI challenging.

Staphylococcus aureus is the most common pathogen identified among HD CRBSI accounting for approximately 30% of cases; among these isolates 40–46% are methicillin-resistant [42, 47]. Numerous studies have illustrated an association between the need for dialysis and susceptibility to MRSA infection, and thus a high index of suspicion must exist for this organism [48, 49]. *S. epidermidis* and other coagulase-negative staphylococci are also common causes of these infections, accounting for just under 30% of cases [47]. Gram-negative organisms as a whole account for about 10–15% of infections. *Candida* species contribute to 2–3% of CRBSI in this population [42]. Antimicrobial susceptibilities usually follow local patterns, and it is important to be aware of local prevalence data for antibiotic resistance to guide empiric treatment.

Diagnosis

In 2009, the Infectious Diseases Society of America (IDSA) laid out strict criteria for diagnosing CRBSI [50]. This requires clinical symptoms such as fever, chills, and/or hypotension with no apparent source for infection and one of the following: (a) quantitative blood culture with colony count of microbes at least threefold greater from cultures obtained from the catheter when compared to peripheral culture; (b) differential time to positivity, growth of microbes from blood drawn from catheter hub at least 2 h before that drawn from a peripheral vein; and/or (c) growth of more than 15 colony-forming units (CFUs) from a 5 cm segment of catheter tip by roll plate culture or >10^2 CFUs by quantitative broth culture. This definition requires either a peripheral venous culture or the catheter tip to be obtained. However there are practical difficulties in following these criteria in patients receiving HD. Peripheral venous draws cannot always be accomplished in freestanding HD units, and drawing peripheral venous cultures has a potential of sclerosing the vein and thereby rendering the veins unusable as a future HD vascular access site. Also, many CRBSIs are treated by catheter salvage in this population, and therefore the catheter tip is not often available for culture. The most common practice in US outpatient HD units has been to draw two blood cultures from the catheter hub or to draw from both the catheter hub and the HD circuit [50, 51]. The IDSA guidelines do notably acknowledge that in cases when a peripheral blood culture cannot be obtained, samples may be obtained during HD from lines connected to the catheter [50].

Other common infections associated with HD catheters include exit site and tunnel infections. Exit site infections are defined as the presence of hyperemia, induration, or tenderness less than 2 cm from the HD catheter exit site. Extension of symptoms beyond 2 cm along the subcutaneous tract of the catheter tunnel defines a HD catheter tunnel infection [50].

Since 2014, the Centers for Medicare and Medicaid Services (CMS) has implemented mandatory reporting of HD catheter-related infections through the NHSN. The main events reported are (a) access-related bloodstream infections, a positive blood culture and the suspected source is a vascular access device; (b) local access site infection, an exit site infection without a positive blood culture; and (c) vascular access infection, a term encompassing either a local access infection or a bloodstream infection. Recent analysis of 2014 data including pediatric and adult dialysis units showed that the incidence of HD catheter infections was 2.16 per 100 patient-months. The risk of infection was far higher than that reported with AV fistulas and AV grafts, which were 0.26 and 0.39 infections per 100 patient-months, respectively [42].

Treatment

Treatment of these infections is complicated by the fact that HD catheters become colonized with skin microorganism within a short time after insertion. The microorganisms form biofilm, which provides protection to the organism and contributes to resistance to treatment. Treatment failure is often attributed to the difficulty of antibiotics to penetrate the biofilm.

Exit Site Infection

For patients with suspected exit site infection, cultures should ideally be obtained from the exit site before administration of antibiotics. Such infections may be successfully treated with oral antibiotics, with empiric choice geared toward treating gram-positive organisms while taking into account local resistance patterns [52]. Once the culture and susceptibilities are available, then antibiotics can be tailored to the specific organism. Generally treatment is provided for 7–14 days. For patients with poor response to therapy, consideration should be given to catheter removal and replacement at a separate site.

Tunnel Infection

Compared to exit site infections, tunnel infections are much more difficult to eradicate. They typically require treatment with intravenous antibiotics, after obtaining cultures of the exit site and the catheter. Tunnel infections generally require removal of the catheter and insertion of the new catheter at a separate site to achieve therapeutic success. Tunnel infections are often treated for up to 14 days depending on the organism and clinical course [53]; the IDSA guidelines recommend treating tunnel infections for 7–10 days following catheter removal assuming there are no signs of metastatic infection [50].

Catheter-Related Bloodstream Infection

For patients with known or suspected HD CRBSI, blood cultures should be obtained promptly and patients empirically managed with broad-spectrum antibiotics to cover gram-positive and gram-negative organisms (Fig. 18.2). Empiric antibiotics should generally include an agent active against methicillin-resistant *S. aureus* (MRSA); however, local susceptibility patterns and the individual patient's history of prior infections should ultimately guide antibiotic selection. An important consideration is to choose antibiotics with the least toxicity possible, which has prompted centers to consider third-generation cephalosporins for gram-negative coverage over aminoglycosides to reduce ototoxicity. Ease of administration is also a factor to consider as patients may be routinely seen three times a week to receive outpatient HD; thus, the use of medications which can be administered with dialysis may be convenient. When cultures are available and susceptibilities are known, antibiotics can be directly tailored to the specific organism. There are three general strategies to treat CRBSI in this population: (1) systemic antibiotics alone, (2) systemic antibiotics plus antibiotic lock for catheters, and (3) catheter removal/exchange. However, comparison between the three treatment strategies is challenging, as most evidence is derived from observational studies and there is limited data in children with ESRD.

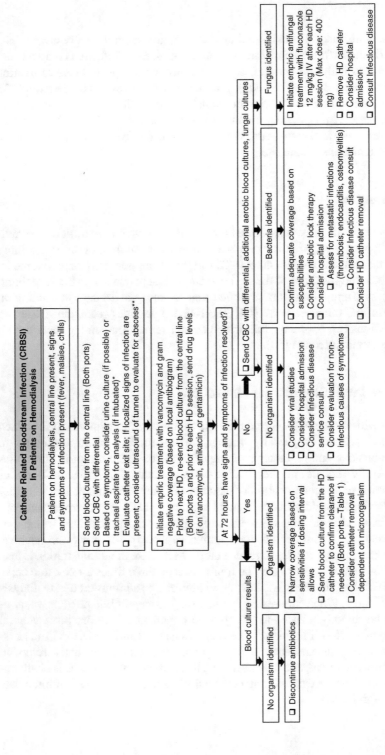

Fig. 18.2 Proposed algorithm for treatment of suspected catheter-related bloodstream infections in patients on hemodialysis. *If workup of symptoms reveals an alternative source of infection besides the venous catheter (such as the urine or respiratory tracts), treatment should be administered appropriate to these sources. **In the presence of a tunnel infection, the catheter should be removed promptly. (Reference: [50, 52, 53])

Systemic antibiotics alone can be utilized for patients with uncomplicated bloodstream infections if the organism is not exceptionally virulent or difficult to treat. CRBSIs that are unlikely to be successfully treated with systemic antibiotics alone (or are associated with risk of severe decompensation or dissemination) include those caused by *S. aureus*, *Pseudomonas* species, or fungi. Treatment is generally administered for 2 weeks, and as stated above, antibiotics may be administered to coincide with dialysis sessions. For methicillin-susceptible *S. aureus* (MSSA) infections, cefazolin can be given after dialysis three times a week and is preferred over vancomycin for the management of MSSA [50].

Antibiotic locks are useful adjuncts to systemic antibiotics in situations where line salvage is desired. Several observational studies have shown better treatment success in terms of line salvage than with systemic antibiotics alone [54, 55]. The largest study with antibiotic locks in pediatric ESRD patients was performed by Onder et al. They initially used antibiotic locks in HD catheter infections along with systemic antibiotics in cases with difficult to eradicate organisms and then ultimately in combination with systemic antibiotics for all HD catheter infections; a subset of patients also received prophylactic antibiotic locks. When compared to historical controls, antibiotic locks at the start of therapy decreased overall systemic antimicrobial exposure; the use of prophylactic locks, however, did not impact the rate of CRBSI in this population [56]. In cases of catheter retention, the IDSA recommends that repeat blood cultures be performed 1 week after the completion of therapy and the catheter removed if these new cultures become positive [50].

Catheter Removal and Exchange

In addition to antibiotics, catheter removal is warranted if there are persistent positive blood cultures or persistent clinical symptoms beyond 72 h after starting antibiotics. The infected catheter can be exchanged over a guidewire for a new catheter if no alternative sites are available [50]. If the patient has septic shock, fungal infection, infection due to a highly virulent or difficult to treat pathogen or tunnel infection, then the catheter should be removed promptly, and a new catheter should be inserted after 48 h. Alternatively, if the patient's symptoms rapidly resolve on antimicrobial therapy and there is no evidence of metastatic infection, the catheter may be exchanged for a new one over a guidewire [50].

Prevention

The best strategy to prevent catheter-related bloodstream infection is avoidance of venous catheters by using AV fistulas or AV grafts. However since catheter use cannot be completely eliminated, the CDC has recommended several core interventions to minimize the risk of infection (Table 18.1). An important consideration is the catheter insertion site. The subclavian catheter sites should be avoided due to risk of thrombosis. Femoral catheters are generally considered to have higher infection

Table 18.1 Hemodialysis catheter care bundle

Core intervention	Description
Surveillance	Monthly surveillance data using CDC NHSN definitions
Hand hygiene	Perform observations of hand hygiene as per hospital policy and share results with staff
Catheter care observations and staff education competency	1. Direct observations of access care 2. Perform competency evaluation for skills at hire and every 6–12 months 3. Continued training regarding infection prevention
Patient/caregiver education	Standardized education regarding access care, hand hygiene, recognizing signs of infections, home care for catheter
Vascular access assessment	Efforts to reduce catheters by addressing barriers for fistula placement
Skin antisepsis	Alcohol-based chlorhexidine preparations for dressing changes, using antibiotic ointment or measures such as chlorhexidine-impregnated discs
Catheter hub disinfection	Scrubbing the catheter hub with appropriate antiseptic before accessing every time

Modified from https://www.cdc.gov/dialysis/prevention-tools/core-interventions.html

risk, though this was not demonstrated in a large study of adults using HD catheters for acute kidney injury [57]; whether this finding is true for tunneled catheters is not known. Antimicrobial-coated tunneled catheters have not been shown to significantly reduce CRBSI and are not generally recommended at this time. Newer needleless connector systems like TEGO (Victus Inc., Miami, FL, USA) have been designed to decrease catheter hub manipulation. A retrospective analysis in an adult dialysis unit suggested there was approximately 10–12% reduction of CRBSI with the use of TEGO systems [58]. Prophylactic antibiotic lock therapy has been used to prevent CRBSI, but concerns regarding the emergence of antibiotic resistance have prevented CDC and other professional groups from advocating for its routine use for HD catheters. Other agents which could be used in lock prophylaxis such as taurine and ethanol have not been studied in a systematic fashion in the ESRD population. A randomized controlled trial in adult HD patients suggested that recombinant tissue plasminogen activator as a routine packing solution can decrease the rate of infections, and this is an area that is under investigation [59].

To summarize, CRBSI is a major cause of morbidity in pediatric HD patients. The age-old adage of prevention being better than cure is particularly true in this regard. Strategies to minimize catheter use and following core preventive measures play a central role in avoiding CRBSI in pediatric HD patients.

Peritoneal Dialysis Infections

Peritoneal dialysis (PD) is the preferred and most common form of chronic dialysis therapy in children with end-stage renal disease [60, 61]. Infectious complications including peritonitis and exit site or tunnel infections remain the most frequent and significant complications. They are associated with significant morbidity due to need for hospitalization, loss of school time, and potential need for PD catheter removal and/or change in chronic dialysis modality to HD. In addition, these infections are associated with increased mortality in the pediatric population [62, 63]. Peritonitis in the setting of PD results from bacteria reaching the peritoneum by either transluminal (touch contamination), periluminal (exit site or tunnel infection), enteric, hematogenous, and ascending routes.

Epidemiology

Peritonitis annualized rates vary in different parts of the world with 0.64 episodes per year of follow-up in North America [63]. Although many PD patients experience zero or only one episode of peritonitis, additional morbidity is observed in those with repeated episodes as this can result in peritoneal membrane dysfunction or scarring [64].

The majority of peritonitis episodes in children are caused by bacteria. Fungal peritonitis is responsible for less than 5% of all episodes [65, 66]. Gram-positive organisms have typically accounted for 40–50% of cases, gram-negative organisms for 20–30%, and culture-negative cases the remaining 20–30% of episodes of peritonitis [65, 67, 68]. As a single entity, *S. epidermidis* has been reported most commonly (11–22% of all cases) followed very closely by *S. aureus* (approximately 10–20%) [67, 68]. Fungal peritonitis is a relatively infrequent occurrence but often results in hospitalization and change in modality due to the need to remove the PD catheter for treatment. Data however suggests that preservation of the peritoneum is possible even in the setting of fungal peritonitis with prompt treatment [69].

Two or more episodes of peritonitis can be characterized as relapsing, recurrent, or repeated episodes depending on the timing of their occurrence [70]. An episode occurring within 4 weeks of completion of antibiotics for a prior infection with the same organism or sterile episode is defined as relapsing peritonitis. An episode that occurs within 4 weeks of completion of antibiotics for a prior infection but with a different organism is defined as recurrent peritonitis. An episode that occurs greater than 4 weeks from completion of therapy for a prior episode is defined as repeat peritonitis. Relapsing episodes of peritonitis are not counted as an additional episode when calculating peritonitis rates for epidemiology purposes.

Diagnosis

A diagnosis of peritonitis should be considered in any patient with abdominal pain and/or cloudy PD effluent. Other symptoms can include fever, chills, anorexia, and vomiting; severe infections can present as septic shock. Diagnosis is based on an effluent white blood cell count greater than 100/mm^3 with at least 50% neutrophils on an uncentrifuged specimen. A standardized diagnostic evaluation includes collecting 50–100 mL sample from either first cloudy effluent bag or manual drain which is then centrifuged at $3000 \times g$ for 15 min with decantation of the supernatant, resuspension, and culture of the sediment. For children on automated PD without a daytime dwell or no effluent present at the time of evaluation, the peritoneal effluent should be obtained from a dwell after a minimum of 1–2 h [70]. Notably, cloudy PD effluent can also occur with chemical peritonitis, eosinophilic peritonitis, hemoperitoneum, necrotizing pancreatitis, chylous effluent, malignancy, or if the fluid is obtained from a dry abdomen, and these must be considered in the differential diagnosis.

Treatment

The optimal treatment of peritonitis involves instillation of intraperitoneal antibiotics to allow for direct delivery of high drug concentrations to the site of infection. Antibiotics are also readily absorbed across the peritoneal membrane leading to therapeutic blood levels. Once systemic levels are obtained, the body acts as a reservoir for continuous diffusion back into the peritoneal cavity [71]. Intraperitoneal antibiotics are typically delivered initially at a loading dose followed by a maintenance dose to achieve desired therapeutic levels. Recommendations for dosing of intraperitoneal antibiotics are available in the "Consensus Guidelines for the Prevention and Treatment of Catheter-Related Infections and Peritonitis in Pediatric Patients Receiving Peritoneal Dialysis" published in 2012 by the International Society for Peritoneal Dialysis (ISPD 2012 guidelines) [70]. Intraperitoneal antibiotics should be initiated as soon as possible once the diagnosis of peritonitis is made, with most studies suggesting that intraperitoneal administration is superior to intravenous antibiotics [72]. For the rare patients with septic shock secondary to PD-associated peritonitis, consideration should be given to empiric systemic (i.e., intravenous) antimicrobial therapy as well. Selection of empiric antibiotics should include coverage for both gram-positive and gram-negative organisms. ISPD 2012 guidelines recommend monotherapy with intraperitoneal cefepime pending culture results, although center-specific antibiograms need to be considered. Cefepime provides broad-spectrum coverage for both gram-positive and gram-negative organisms. Intraperitoneal vancomycin should be included in empiric therapy in patients with known MRSA colonization, prior MRSA infection, or where there is high community prevalence of MRSA (>10% of S. aureus resistant to methicillin/oxacillin). Thus, depending on local epidemiology, empiric combination therapy may be reasonable. Infection with MRSA is associated with more severe peritonitis, lower cure rates, and higher morbidity with need for PD catheter removal [73]. Once an organism is identified, intraperitoneal therapy should be modified to narrow coverage based on susceptibilities. If a *Pseudomonas* species is identified, ISPD 2012 guidelines recommend adding a second agent with a different mechanism of action (such as a fluoroquinolone or aminoglycoside). If a culture remains negative after 72 h and clinical signs and symptoms have improved, combined empiric therapy for both gram-positive and gram-negative organisms should be continued for treatment of culture-negative peritonitis. Length of therapy has been largely guided by expert opinion based on organism with a typical treatment duration of 2–3 weeks (Table 18.2).

Table 18.2   Treatment duration for peritoneal dialysis-associated peritonitis

Length of therapy	Organism
2 weeks	Gram-positive bacteria (excluding *Staphylococcus aureus*)
	Gram-negative bacteria (excluding *Pseudomonas* species or *Stenotrophomonas* species)
	Culture-negative peritonitis
3 weeks	*S. aureus* (MSSA or MRSA)
	Pseudomonas spp. or *Stenotrophomonas* spp.
	Drug-resistant gram-negative bacteria
	Polymicrobial infection
	Anaerobes

MSSA indicates methicillin-susceptible *S. aureus*; MRSA indicates methicillin-resistant *S. aureus*
Adapted from Ref. [70]

Conservative management with antibiotic therapy is not always successful, and a nidus of infection can persist despite adequate and appropriate therapy. Many bacteria and all fungi can form biofilm or colonize the PD catheter, preventing eradication of the infection. In such situations, symptoms of abdominal pain may be persistent, or a patient may develop relapsing peritonitis. Typically peritonitis symptoms improve within 72 h and resolve within 5 days of appropriate therapy; if persistent symptoms or refractory peritonitis develop, infection is unlikely to respond to medical therapy alone. PD catheter removal is indicated in such situations to prevent morbidity and mortality from uncontrolled peritonitis and to protect the peritoneal membrane from scarring to allow for future use [70]. ISPD 2012 guidelines [70] outline indications for PD catheter removal including the presence of refractory peritonitis, relapsing peritonitis, peritonitis with concomitant exit site or tunnel infection, fungal peritonitis, peritonitis in the setting of intra-abdominal pathology, and repeatedly relapsing or refractory exit site or tunnel infection. For patients with severe sepsis related to PD-associated peritonitis, early removal of the catheter should be considered. In the setting of fungal peritonitis, following catheter removal antifungal therapy should be continued for at least two weeks after complete resolution of clinical symptoms of infection [70].

Exit Site and Tunnel Infections

Exit site and tunnel infections are important risk factors for peritonitis. Exit site infection is defined by the presence of purulent drainage with or without erythema, swelling, or tenderness at the PD catheter-skin interface although erythema without drainage can be an early indication of infection. Diagnosis, however, can be subjective, leading to the recommendation to standardize the assessment of the exit site. A scoring system was developed by Schaefer et al. to help monitor the PD catheter exit site and tunnel on a regular basis (Table 18.3) [74]. The scoring system takes into account the presence of swelling, crust, erythema, pain on pressure, and secretion in the assessment; the site is assumed to be infected in the setting of a cumulative score

Table 18.3 Peritoneal dialysis catheter exit site scoring

Finding	0 points	1 point	2 points
Swelling	No	<0.5 cm (at exit site only)	Includes tunnel (part or in entirety)
Crust	No	<0.5 cm	>0.5 cm
Redness	No	<0.5 cm	>0.5 cm
Pain	No	Slight	Severe
Secretion	No	Serous	Purulent

Adapted from Ref. [70, 74]

of ≥4 irrespective of culture results or ≥2 with a positive culture [70, 74]. Infections are most often secondary to *S. aureus* or *Pseudomonas* species [75–77]. ISPD 2012 guidelines recommend treatment typically with an oral antibiotic for a minimum of 2 weeks and for at least 7 days after resolution of infection and a minimum of 3 weeks if infection is caused by *S. aureus* or *Pseudomonas* species or an antibiotic-resistant pathogen. For infections due to MRSA, both intraperitoneal and intravenous vancomycin is generally recommended [70]. Catheter removal is recommended in the setting of exit/tunnel infections with concomitant peritonitis or in those who are severely ill.

Prevention

Preoperative care, catheter insertion practices, postoperative catheter care, chronic exit site and catheter care, management of exit site and tunnel infections, and technique of the dialysis procedure have been identified as primary drivers important in the prevention of peritonitis [78]. For example, a better annualized peritonitis rate and longer time until first episode of peritonitis has been associated with placement of a double-cuff Tenckhoff catheter with a swan-neck tunnel configuration and downward exit site [64]. The ISPD 2012 guidelines additionally outline practice recommendations for the prevention of PD-associated infections [70]. Recommended prevention measures include the administration of antibiotics with PD catheter insertion, delaying initiation of dialysis for at least 2 weeks to allow healing, and application of daily topical antibiotic (mupirocin and gentamicin) to the sealed exit site in conjunction with sodium hypochlorite solution. These practices have been shown to reduce the incidence of exit site infections and peritonitis [79–82]. In addition, the ISPD 2012 guidelines recommend the use of prophylactic antibiotics and antifungals for invasive interventional procedures such as gastrostomy tube placement and other gastrointestinal, dental, and genitourinary procedures and touch contamination events, which are associated with an increased risk for peritonitis. Through a multicenter collaborative effort, "Standardizing Care to Improve Outcomes in Pediatric ESRD (SCOPE)," best practice standardized care bundles have been developed which encompass PD catheter insertion practices, patient and caregiver training, and follow-up care; these efforts have successfully decreased peritonitis rates among children on chronic PD in participating centers [83]. As compliance increased with the follow-up bundle in the first 3 years of the collaborative, the mean monthly peritonitis rates decreased significantly, from 0.63 to 0.42 episodes per patient-year [67]. Finally, routine exit site care with cleansing, application of topical antibiotic, and immobilization are key in infection prevention [84–87].

In summary, peritoneal dialysis-related infections remain the most significant complication of peritoneal dialysis in children. Peritonitis is the primary reason for change in modality and/or technique failure due to problems with ultrafiltration, development of abdominal adhesions, and persistent infection or secondary fungal infection. PD-related infections are associated with hospitalizations and increased healthcare costs. Recognition and timely initiation of antibiotics are central to the preservation of the peritoneum. Adherence to best practices as outlined by ISPD 2012 guidelines and incorporation of quality improvement practices have the potential to reduce infection rates and improve outcomes for children on peritoneal dialysis.

Conclusion

Pediatric ESRD patients are a vulnerable population at risk for healthcare-associated infections due to increased susceptibility to infections brought about by their underlying pathophysiology along with unique considerations in regard to required dialysis access. The consistent practice of preventive measures is essential in decreasing further resource utilization, morbidity, and mortality associated with infectious complications in these children.

References

1. Groothoff JW. Long-term outcomes of children with end-stage renal disease. Pediatr Nephrol. 2005;20:849–53.
2. United States Renal Data System. 2016 USRDS annual data report: epidemiology of kidney disease in the United States. Bethesda, MD: National Institutes of Health, National Institute of Diabetes and Digestive and Kidney Diseases; 2016.
3. Powe NR, Jaar B, Furth SL, Hermann J, Briggs W. Septicemia in dialysis patients: incidence, risk factors, and prognosis. Kidney Int. 1999;55:1081–90.
4. Sarnak MJ, Jaber BL. Mortality caused by sepsis in patients with end-stage renal disease compared with the general population. Kidney Int. 2000;58:1758–64.
5. Dalrymple LS, Go AS. Epidemiology of acute infections among patients with chronic kidney disease. Clin J Am Soc Nephrol. 2008;3:1487–93.
6. Groothoff JW, Offringa M, Grootenhuis M, Jager KJ. Long-term consequences of renal insufficiency in children: lessons learned from the Dutch LERIC study. Nephrol Dial Transplant 2017. https://doi.org/10.1093/ndt/gfx190
7. Glorieux G, Vanholder R, Lameire N. Uraemic retention and apoptosis: what is the balance for the inflammatory status in uraemia? Eur J Clin Investig. 2003;33:631–4.
8. Jaber BL, Cendoroglo M, Balakrishnan VS, Perianayagam MC, King AJ, Pereira BJ. Apoptosis of leukocytes: basic concepts and implications in uremia. Kidney Int Suppl. 2001;78:S197–205.
9. Hauser AB, Stinghen AE, Kato S, et al. Characteristics and causes of immune dysfunction related to uremia and dialysis. Perit Dial Int. 2008;28(Suppl 3):S183–7.

10. Kato S, Chmielewski M, Honda H, et al. Aspects of immune dysfunction in end-stage renal disease. Clin J Am Soc Nephrol. 2008;3:1526–33.
11. Lofaro D, Vogelzang JL, van Stralen KJ, Jager KJ, Groothoff JW. Infection-related hospitalizations over 30 years of follow-up in patients starting renal replacement therapy at pediatric age. Pediatr Nephrol. 2016;31:315–23.
12. Choi HM, Woo YS, Kim MG, Jo SK, Cho WY, Kim HK. Altered monocyte-derived dendritic cell function in patients on hemodialysis: a culprit for underlying impaired immune responses. Clin Exp Nephrol. 2011;15:546–53.
13. Lim WH, Kireta S, Russ GR, Coates PT. Uremia impairs blood dendritic cell function in hemodialysis patients. Kidney Int. 2007;71:1122–31.
14. Lim WH, Kireta S, Thomson AW, Russ GR, Coates PT. Renal transplantation reverses functional deficiencies in circulating dendritic cell subsets in chronic renal failure patients. Transplantation. 2006;81:160–8.
15. Ando M, Shibuya A, Yasuda M, et al. Impairment of innate cellular response to in vitro stimuli in patients on continuous ambulatory peritoneal dialysis. Nephrol Dial Transplant. 2005;20:2497–503.
16. Lim WH, Kireta S, Leedham E, Russ GR, Coates PT. Uremia impairs monocyte and monocyte-derived dendritic cell function in hemodialysis patients. Kidney Int. 2007;72:1138–48.
17. Verkade MA, van Druningen CJ, Vaessen LM, Hesselink DA, Weimar W, Betjes MG. Functional impairment of monocyte-derived dendritic cells in patients with severe chronic kidney disease. Nephrol Dial Transplant. 2007;22:128–38.
18. Verkade MA, van Druningen CJ, Op de Hoek CT, Weimar W, Betjes MG. Decreased antigen-specific T-cell proliferation by moDC among hepatitis B vaccine non-responders on haemodialysis. Clin Exp Med. 2007;7:65–71.
19. Chonchol M. Neutrophil dysfunction and infection risk in end-stage renal disease. Semin Dial. 2006;19:291–6.
20. Anding K, Gross P, Rost JM, Allgaier D, Jacobs E. The influence of uraemia and haemodialysis on neutrophil phagocytosis and antimicrobial killing. Nephrol Dial Transplant. 2003;18:2067–73.
21. Alexiewicz JM, Smogorzewski M, Fadda GZ, Massry SG. Impaired phagocytosis in dialysis patients: studies on mechanisms. Am J Nephrol. 1991;11:102–11.
22. Srivaths PR, Silverstein DM, Leung J, Krishnamurthy R, Goldstein SL. Malnutrition-inflammation-coronary calcification in pediatric patients receiving chronic hemodialysis. Hemodial Int. 2010;14:263–9.
23. Ishida JH, Johansen KL. Iron and infection in hemodialysis patients. Semin Dial. 2014;27:26–36.
24. Ishida JH, Marafino BJ, McCulloch CE, et al. Receipt of intravenous iron and clinical outcomes among hemodialysis patients hospitalized for infection. Clin J Am Soc Nephrol. 2015;10:1799–805.
25. Veys N, Vanholder R, Ringoir S. Correction of deficient phagocytosis during erythropoietin treatment in maintenance hemodialysis patients. Am J Kidney Dis. 1992;19:358–63.
26. Litjens NH, Huisman M, van den Dorpel M, Betjes MG. Impaired immune responses and antigen-specific memory CD4+ T cells in hemodialysis patients. J Am Soc Nephrol. 2008;19:1483–90.
27. Kruger S, Seyfarth M, Sack K, Kreft B. Defective immune response to tetanus toxoid in hemodialysis patients and its association with diphtheria vaccination. Vaccine. 1999;17:1145–50.
28. Kim JU, Kim M, Kim S, et al. Dendritic cell dysfunction in patients with end-stage renal disease. Immune Netw. 2017;17:152–62.
29. Seibert E, Zohles K, Ulrich C, et al. Association between autonomic nervous dysfunction and cellular inflammation in end-stage renal disease. BMC Cardiovasc Disord. 2016;16:210.
30. Kim HW, Woo YS, Yang HN, et al. Primed monocytes: putative culprits of chronic low-grade inflammation and impaired innate immune responses in patients on hemodialysis. Clin Exp Nephrol. 2011;15:258–63.
31. Goldstein SL, Currier H, Watters L, Hempe JM, Sheth RD, Silverstein D. Acute and chronic inflammation in pediatric patients receiving hemodialysis. J Pediatr. 2003;143:653–7.

32. Wang AY, Woo J, Wang M, et al. Association of inflammation and malnutrition with cardiac valve calcification in continuous ambulatory peritoneal dialysis patients. J Am Soc Nephrol. 2001;12:1927–36.
33. Hilderman M, Qureshi AR, Al-Abed Y, et al. Cholinergic anti-inflammatory pathway activity in dialysis patients: a role for neuroimmunomodulation? Clin Kidney J. 2015;8:599–605.
34. Goldstein SL, Ikizler TA, Zappitelli M, Silverstein DM, Ayus JC. Non-infected hemodialysis catheters are associated with increased inflammation compared to arteriovenous fistulas. Kidney Int. 2009;76:1063–9.
35. Cao H, Ye H, Sun Z, et al. Circulatory mitochondrial DNA is a pro-inflammatory agent in maintenance hemodialysis patients. PLoS One. 2014;9:e113179.
36. DeRusso PA, Ye W, Shepherd R, et al. Growth failure and outcomes in infants with biliary atresia: a report from the Biliary Atresia Research Consortium. Hepatology. 2007;46:1632–8.
37. Furth SL, Hwang W, Yang C, Neu AM, Fivush BA, Powe NR. Growth failure, risk of hospitalization and death for children with end-stage renal disease. Pediatr Nephrol. 2002;17:450–5.
38. McIntyre P, Craig JC. Prevention of serious bacterial infection in children with nephrotic syndrome. J Paediatr Child Health. 1998;34:314–7.
39. Allon M, Depner TA, Radeva M, et al. Impact of dialysis dose and membrane on infection-related hospitalization and death: results of the HEMO Study. J Am Soc Nephrol. 2003;14:1863–70.
40. Dalrymple LS, Mu Y, Nguyen DV, et al. Risk Factors for Infection-Related Hospitalization in In-Center Hemodialysis. Clin J Am Soc Nephrol. 2015;10:2170–80.
41. Chavers BM, Solid CA, Gilbertson DT, Collins AJ. Infection-related hospitalization rates in pediatric versus adult patients with end-stage renal disease in the United States. J Am Soc Nephrol. 2007;18:952–9.
42. Nguyen DB, Shugart A, Lines C, et al. National Healthcare Safety Network (NHSN) dialysis event surveillance report for 2014. Clin J Am Soc Nephrol. 2017;12:1139–46.
43. Ramage IJ, Bailie A, Tyerman KS, McColl JH, Pollard SG, Fitzpatrick MM. Vascular access survival in children and young adults receiving long-term hemodialysis. Am J Kidney Dis. 2005;45:708–14.
44. Paglialonga F, Esposito S, Edefonti A, Principi N. Catheter-related infections in children treated with hemodialysis. Pediatr Nephrol. 2004;19:1324–33.
45. Onder AM, Chandar J, Coakley S, Abitbol C, Montane B, Zilleruelo G. Predictors and outcome of catheter-related bacteremia in children on chronic hemodialysis. Pediatr Nephrol. 2006;21:1452–8.
46. Ma A, Shroff R, Hothi D, et al. A comparison of arteriovenous fistulas and central venous lines for long-term chronic haemodialysis. Pediatr Nephrol. 2013;28:321–6.
47. Patel PR, Shugart A, Mbaeyi C, et al. Dialysis event surveillance report: national healthcare safety network data summary, January 2007 through April 2011. Am J Infect Control. 2016;44:944–7.
48. Laupland KB, Ross T, Gregson DB. Staphylococcus aureus bloodstream infections: risk factors, outcomes, and the influence of methicillin resistance in Calgary, Canada, 2000-2006. J Infect Dis. 2008;198:336–43.
49. Nguyen DB, Lessa FC, Belflower R, et al. Invasive methicillin-resistant Staphylococcus aureus infections among patients on chronic dialysis in the United States, 2005-2011. Clin Infect Dis. 2013;57:1393–400.
50. Mermel LA, Allon M, Bouza E, et al. Clinical practice guidelines for the diagnosis and management of intravascular catheter-related infection: 2009 update by the Infectious Diseases Society of America. Clin Infect Dis. 2009;49:1–45.
51. Quittnat Pelletier F, Joarder M, Poutanen SM, Lok CE. Evaluating approaches for the diagnosis of hemodialysis catheter-related bloodstream infections. Clin J Am Soc Nephrol. 2016;11:847–54.
52. Vascular Access Work G. Clinical practice guidelines for vascular access. Am J Kidney Dis. 2006;48(Suppl 1):S248–73.
53. Miller LM, Clark E, Dipchand C, et al. Hemodialysis tunneled catheter-related infections. Can J Kidney Health Dis. 2016;3:2054358116669129.

54. Allon M. Prophylaxis against dialysis catheter-related bacteremia with a novel antimicrobial lock solution. Clin Infect Dis. 2003;36:1539–44.
55. Dogra GK, Herson H, Hutchison B, et al. Prevention of tunneled hemodialysis catheter-related infections using catheter-restricted filling with gentamicin and citrate: a randomized controlled study. J Am Soc Nephrol. 2002;13:2133–9.
56. Onder AM, Billings AA, Chandar J, et al. Antibiotic lock solutions allow less systemic antibiotic exposure and less catheter malfunction without adversely affecting antimicrobial resistance patterns. Hemodial Int. 2013;17:75–85.
57. Marik PE, Flemmer M, Harrison W. The risk of catheter-related bloodstream infection with femoral venous catheters as compared to subclavian and internal jugular venous catheters: a systematic review of the literature and meta-analysis. Crit Care Med. 2012;40:2479–85.
58. Brunelli SM, Njord L, Hunt AE, Sibbel SP. Use of the Tego needlefree connector is associated with reduced incidence of catheter-related bloodstream infections in hemodialysis patients. Int J Nephrol Renovasc Dis. 2014;7:131–9.
59. Hemmelgarn BR, Moist LM, Lok CE, et al. Prevention of dialysis catheter malfunction with recombinant tissue plasminogen activator. N Engl J Med. 2011;364:303–12.
60. Zaritsky J, Warady BA. Peritoneal dialysis in infants and young children. Semin Nephrol. 2011;31:213–24.
61. Alexander S, Warady B. The demographics of dialysis in children. In: Warady B, Schaefer F, Fine R, Alexander S, editors. Pediatric dialysis: Kluwer Academic Publishers:Springer; 2004.
62. United States Renal Data System. 2015 USRDS annual data report: epidemiology of kidney disease in the United States. Bethesda, MD: National Institutes of Health, National Institute of Diabetes and Digestive and Kidney Diseases; 2015.
63. North American Pediatric Renal Trials and Collaborative Studies. 2011 Annual Dialysis Report; 2011.
64. North American Pediatric Renal Trials and Collaborative Studies. 2008 Annual Dialysis Report; 2008.
65. Vas S, Oreopoulos DG. Infections in patients undergoing peritoneal dialysis. Infect Dis Clin N Am. 2001;15:743–74.
66. Warady BA, Feneberg R, Verrina E, et al. Peritonitis in children who receive long-term peritoneal dialysis: a prospective evaluation of therapeutic guidelines. J Am Soc Nephrol. 2007;18:2172–9.
67. Sethna CB, Bryant K, Munshi R, et al. Risk factors for and outcomes of catheter-associated peritonitis in children: The SCOPE collaborative. Clin J Am Soc Nephrol. 2016;11:1590–6.
68. Schaefer F, Feneberg R, Aksu N, et al. Worldwide variation of dialysis-associated peritonitis in children. Kidney Int. 2007;72:1374–9.
69. Warady BA, Bashir M, Donaldson LA. Fungal peritonitis in children receiving peritoneal dialysis: a report of the NAPRTCS. Kidney Int. 2000;58:384–9.
70. Warady BA, Bakkaloglu S, Newland J, et al. Consensus guidelines for the prevention and treatment of catheter-related infections and peritonitis in pediatric patients receiving peritoneal dialysis: 2012 update. Perit Dial Int. 2012;32(Suppl 2):S32–86.
71. Manley HJ, Bailie GR. Treatment of peritonitis in APD: pharmacokinetic principles. Semin Dial. 2002;15:418–21.
72. Ballinger AE, Palmer SC, Wiggins KJ, et al. Treatment for peritoneal dialysis-associated peritonitis. Cochrane Database Syst Rev. 2014:CD005284.
73. Huang SS, Platt R. Risk of methicillin-resistant Staphylococcus aureus infection after previous infection or colonization. Clin Infect Dis. 2003;36:281–5.
74. Schaefer F, Klaus G, Muller-Wiefel DE, Mehls O. Intermittent versus continuous intraperitoneal glycopeptide/ceftazidime treatment in children with peritoneal dialysis-associated peritonitis. The Mid-European Pediatric Peritoneal Dialysis Study Group (MEPPS). J Am Soc Nephrol. 1999;10:136–45.
75. Piraino B. Peritonitis as a complication of peritoneal dialysis. J Am Soc Nephrol. 1998;9:1956–64.

76. Piraino B. Infectious complications of peritoneal dialysis. Perit Dial Int. 1997;17(Suppl 3):S15–8.
77. Piraino B. Management of catheter-related infections. Am J Kidney Dis. 1996;27:754–8.
78. Redpath Mahon A, Neu AM. A contemporary approach to the prevention of peritoneal dialysis-related peritonitis in children: the role of improvement science. Pediatr Nephrol. 2017;32:1331–41.
79. Strippoli GF, Tong A, Johnson D, Schena FP, Craig JC. Antimicrobial agents for preventing peritonitis in peritoneal dialysis patients. Cochrane Database Syst Rev. 2004:CD004679.
80. Sardegna KM, Beck AM, Strife CF. Evaluation of perioperative antibiotics at the time of dialysis catheter placement. Pediatr Nephrol. 1998;12:149–52.
81. Auron A, Simon S, Andrews W, et al. Prevention of peritonitis in children receiving peritoneal dialysis. Pediatr Nephrol. 2007;22:578–85.
82. Chua AN, Goldstein SL, Bell D, Brewer ED. Topical mupirocin/sodium hypochlorite reduces peritonitis and exit-site infection rates in children. Clin J Am Soc Nephrol. 2009;4:1939–43.
83. Neu AM, Miller MR, Stuart J, et al. Design of the standardizing care to improve outcomes in pediatric end stage renal disease collaborative. Pediatr Nephrol. 2014;29:1477–84.
84. Jones LL, Tweedy L, Warady BA. The impact of exit-site care and catheter design on the incidence of catheter-related infections. Adv Perit Dial. 1995;11:302–5.
85. van Esch S, Krediet RT, Struijk DG. 32 years' experience of peritoneal dialysis-related peritonitis in a university hospital. Perit Dial Int. 2014;34:162–70.
86. Uttley L, Vardhan A, Mahajan S, Smart B, Hutchison A, Gokal R. Decrease in infections with the introduction of mupirocin cream at the peritoneal dialysis catheter exit site. J Nephrol. 2004;17:242–5.
87. Bernardini J, Bender F, Florio T, et al. Randomized, double-blind trial of antibiotic exit site cream for prevention of exit site infection in peritoneal dialysis patients. J Am Soc Nephrol. 2005;16:539–45.

Index

© Springer Nature Switzerland AG 2019
J. C. McNeil et al. (eds.), *Healthcare-Associated Infections in Children*,
https://doi.org/10.1007/978-3-319-98122-2

Printed in the United States
By Bookmasters